NO MAGIC BULLET

NO MAGIC BULLET

A Social History of Venereal Disease
in the United States Since 1880

Expanded Edition

ALLAN M. BRANDT

New York   Oxford
OXFORD UNIVERSITY PRESS
1987

OXFORD UNIVERSITY PRESS

Oxford   New York   Toronto
Delhi   Bombay   Calcutta   Madras   Karachi
Kuala Lumpur   Singapore   Hong Kong   Tokyo
Nairobi   Dar es Salaam   Cape Town
Melbourne   Auckland

and associated companies in
Beirut   Berlin   Ibadan   Nicosia

Library of Congress Cataloging in Publication Data

Brandt, Allan M.
No magic bullet.

Bibliography: p.
Includes index.
1. Venereal diseases—United States—History.
I. Title.
RC201.47.B73   1985   362.1'9695'100973   84-18991
ISBN 0-19-503469-4
ISBN 0-19-504237-9 (pbk.)

Illustration credits: 1, 2–9, 19 — the American Social Hygiene Association Papers, Social Welfare History Archives Center, University of Minnesota; 10, 12,
14–18, 20–21 — the National Archives, Washington, D.C.; 11 — Thomas
Parran, "The Next Great Plague To Go," *Survey Graphic* 25 (July 1936); 13 —
Library of Congress Federal Theatre Project Collection at George Mason University Libraries, Fairfax, Virginia; Appendix — the *STD Fact Sheet*, U.S. Department of Health and Human Services, Division of Sexually Transmitted Diseases, Center for Prevention Services, Centers for Disease Control, Atlanta,
Georgia, 1981. All illustrations reproduced by permission.

8 10 9

To my parents

Preface to the Expanded Edition

When *No Magic Bullet* was first published in early 1985, the extent and consequences of the AIDS epidemic were far from clear. This remains true. But in the time since then a great deal has become clear. One thing is certain: the epidemic is a public health threat of great magnitude. AIDS is a disease which will be with us for some time; there will be no simple answers to the complex social and medical problems it poses. Contemporary events are dangerous ground for any historian, but the history of sexually transmitted diseases speaks clearly to the current health crisis and may serve to inform how we come to understand AIDS. This new edition thus has an added chapter which analyzes the meaning and impact of the early years of the AIDS epidemic and puts it in historical perspective.

AIDS, a terrifying and tragic epidemic, reminds us of the power of biological forces in determining the quality and meaning of human existence. These biological forces, however, are shaped and transformed by social and cultural forces. By examining attitudes and responses to the disease, we may be able to understand better the process by which disease is defined. And ultimately, this understanding may facilitate rational interventions that will slow and ultimately stop the course of this epidemic.

Cambridge, Massachusetts   A.M.B.
August 1986

Preface

Thorns on the rose. The dark side of love. The risk of passion. Venereal diseases typically have been portrayed in such ways as these in the last hundred years. Sexually transmitted diseases are, indeed, a potential hazard of sexual intimacy, a persistent, troublesome, sometimes tragic irony of our time. This book is devoted to tracing the historical record of this distinctive set of infectious diseases from the late nineteenth century to the current epidemics of herpes and Acquired Immune Deficiency Syndrome (AIDS). It is my hope that an understanding of the past may help to inform our assessment of these contemporary health problems. We need to understand these diseases as social phenomena as much as we need to know more about them from a scientific standpoint. Only when we recognize that diseases have a history—that they are more than discrete biological entities—and that their causes are complex and varied, will we be able to address them effectively and humanely.

I have incurred more than the typical number of debts over the years that I have worked on this book. Without the unfailing kindness of my family, friends, and colleagues this study would never have appeared. Financial support from Columbia University, the Mrs. Giles Whiting Foundation, the Rockefeller Archives Center, and Harvard University greatly eased the material burdens of this project.

Although for many years venereal diseases have been subject to secrecy and taboo, there is nevertheless a wealth of historical materials. I have been fortunate to work in a number of libraries and archives that preserved the substantive materials for this book. The Social Welfare History Archives Center of the University of Minnesota provided invaluable assistance. David Klaassen's historical and archival skills make this archive one of the finest to work in. Randy Wallach and William Wallach also provided generous assistance and guidance through these materials. The staffs of the Library of Congress, the National Archives, the Centers for Disease Control, the Rockefeller Archives Center, the

New York Academy of Medicine, the National Library of Medicine, the Francis A. Countway Library of the Harvard Medical School, and especially the Columbia University Libraries all provided advice and counsel that made my work easier.

My friends have listened to me rant and rave about venereal disease for many years. In particular my colleagues at the Project on Values and Ethics in Health Care at the College of Physicians and Surgeons, Columbia University, helped me to refine and rethink my understanding about the role of values in medical practice. Kim Hopper, Stephanie Kiceluk, Beth Langan, and Michael Meyer were especially helpful. The spirit of critical inquiry which the Project engendered was a testament to the vision of the late Bernard Schoenberg. The topic for this study was arrived at in conversations with Herman Ausubel. With his death, I lost an acute and thoughtful critic, but even more, a kind and generous friend.

William McLaughlin read and generously commented on the earliest drafts of this manuscript. My daily conversations with him helped to move this study from disparate ideas to actual prose. Alan Gardner and Jay Schechter taught me how to think critically about society and politics. They represent for me all the finest attributes of scholarship, intellect, and friendship.

Many individuals reviewed drafts and sections of this book when it was in various states of disrepair. Henry Aranow, Harry Brandt, Joan Jacobs Brumberg, Peter Buck, Diane Cats, Harold Cook, Leon Eisenberg, Rashi Fein, Diana Long Hall, Steven Marcus, Harry Marks, Sonya Michel, Regina Morantz, David Rothman, Barbara Sicherman, Walter Metzger, Carla Millhauser, Ellen Smith, and Stephen Whitfield all provided critiques which have considerably improved the manuscript. The administrative and secretarial skills of Pamela Webb-Mitchell also are greatly appreciated. Sheldon Meyer and Pamela Nicely of Oxford University Press provided excellent editorial advice.

Barbara Gutmann Rosenkrantz has been an unusually supportive friend and thoughtful colleague. Conversations with her contributed to the development of this book, and her comprehensive knowledge of American medicine and public health has deeply influenced me.

Without the ongoing support and friendship of Mary Dearborn this book would have remained work-in-progress. Her incisive intelligence, not to mention her excellent editorial skills, have improved my work immeasurably. I will always be grateful to her.

William Leuchtenburg has been an outstanding teacher, with all that this implies: critical, thoughtful, responsive, and kind. He has set a model for me of patience, sensitivity, and scholarship that I can only hope to emulate in my own career.

Whatever shortcomings and errors remain are, of course, my own damn fault.

Cambridge, Massachusetts   A.M.B.
May 1984

Contents

NO MAGIC BULLET

INTRODUCTION

Sex, Disease, and Medicine

The most remarkable change in patterns of health during the last century has been the largely successful conquest of infectious disease. Less than one hundred years ago diphtheria, tuberculosis, pneumonia, typhoid, and dysentery constituted this nation's greatest health threats; epidemics could devastate a city or town with tragic speed. In 1918 an outbreak of Spanish influenza claimed more victims than did combat in World War I.[1] Today these diseases are largely under control if not virtually unknown. Although there is considerable debate about the reasons for the decline of these infections—some credit medical advances while others have stressed a rising standard of living, better nutrition, and natural changes in the host-parasite relationship—there is no doubt that we have much less to fear from infectious disease than we did even a generation ago.[2]

Yet, strikingly, venereal diseases are inadequately controlled, if controlled at all. Given the power of the contemporary media, it seems impossible to be unaware of the current problem. Herpes, a viral infection that is often transmitted sexually, is according to most reports epidemic, affecting perhaps as many as 20 million Americans. With no effective treatments available, it threatens to become endemic. Even more ominous is the new disease known as Acquired Immune Deficiency Syndrome (AIDS). Found primarily among homosexual males, in most cases this disease poses a lethal threat. Again, there is no known effective treatment. Yet even syphilis and gonorrhea, diseases for which cures have been developed, remain in dramatically high proportions. Gonorrhea constitutes the most prevalent bacterial infection on earth, with over one hundred million cases occurring annually; more than two million of which occur in the United States.[3] Why, if we have been successful in fighting infectious disease in this century, have we been unable to deal effectively with venereal disease?

To answer this question, we must examine venereal disease not only as a biological entity, but as a disease that has engaged certain attitudes and values; beliefs about its causes and consequences that in turn affect responses to the problem. A society's response to those who are ill, its employment of medical discoveries and resources, is closely related to its most basic assumptions and

3

beliefs.[4] I have attempted, therefore, to trace shifting attitudes and perceptions concerning venereal disease among both laypeople and physicians during the last century. In addition, I have sought to evaluate the impact of these beliefs and values upon medical practice, public health and military programs, and social behavior in general.

Although no single agency regulates sexuality—social reformers, families, and public institutions, as well as popular culture, all exert influence in this area— in the twentieth century, Americans increasingly turned to physicians for advice, counsel, and treatment for sexual diseases and problems. Physicians throughout the last hundred years have presented divergent views concerning the meaning of venereal diseases and approaches to their control. Recent studies have rightly cautioned against seeing the medical profession as a monolithic entity.[5] Yet despite disagreement and internal debate among doctors, the debate over venereal disease increasingly took place within professional circles, rather than between professionals and laypeople. Contention among physicians did not call into question their essential authority in sexual matters.

But the response to venereal disease was not always limited to private exchanges in the doctor's office; in the twentieth century there have been major public interventions that provide the central focus for this study. As the costs of venereal disease became clear, both public health and military officials sought to address the problem of these infections, transforming a previously secreted medical issue into a social dilemma. Their public pronouncements and policies—from municipal ordinances requiring doctors to report cases to authorities to military orders calling for compulsory chastity—reflected prevailing views of the problem at various historical moments. To what extent were the responses of physicians, public health officials, and the military to venereal disease determined by social values, sexual concerns, and scientific advances? Because of my concern with the relationship of scientific and medical advances to social attitudes and professional practice regarding venereal disease, this study begins in the last decades of the nineteenth century, when researchers made the first dramatic breakthroughs concerning the specific causative agents of the venereal diseases.

The social history of venereal disease reveals major trends in the development of modern medicine. Perhaps more than any other single theme, twentieth-century medicine has been characterized by the search for "magic bullets"—specific treatments to root out and destroy infecting microorganisms. This biomedical model has come to define the role and nature of the medical enterprise. In this paradigm, individuals become infected with a parasite that causes dysfunction of some sort; disease is defined as a deviation from a biological norm.[6] Social conditions, environmental phenomena, and other variables are generally discounted as causes of disease. The physician dispenses "magic bullets" that restore the patient to health. This book suggests that this paradigm is too restrictive; to find the solution to problems of disease we must look beyond the model of the magic bullet.

Although I have been concerned with professional and institutional issues, I have attempted to link these activities to social definitions of venereal diseases.

This focus on disease as it is socially defined forces a reorientation in historical approach, a different set of priorities; the frame of reference is expanded beyond the narrower field of clinical medicine. This study, therefore, directs attention to various "social constructions" of venereal disease—the particular symbols which American society came to associate with these diseases and their victims. By assessing the symbols and images which diseases attract we can come to understand the complex phenomena of illness. The symbols reflect social values—patterns of judgment about what is good or bad that guide perceptions and practice. They tell us how a disease is regarded, how we believe it is caused, who its victims are, and what they are like. Some diseases are viewed as the result of a sinister environment beyond our control; others are blamed on the individual victim and his or her personality and behavior.[7] Examining these constructions can help us to recover the values at the core of medicine, and to make decisions about their meaning for the medical task. Our ability to recognize and interpret these symbols substantially affects medical practice and public health.

Fundamental to the notion that disease is socially constructed is the premise that it is profoundly shaped by both biological and cultural variables. Attitudes and values concerning disease affect the perception of its pattern of transmission, its epidemiological nature. Only if we understand the way disease is influenced by social and cultural forces—issues of class, race, ethnicity, and gender—can we effectively address its biological dimension. A "social construction" reveals tacit values, it becomes a symbol for ordering and explaining aspects of the human experience. In this light, medicine is not just affected by social, economic, and political variables—it is embedded in them.

Since the late nineteenth century, venereal disease has been used as a symbol for a society characterized by a corrupt sexuality. Venereal disease has typically been used as a symbol of pollution and contamination, and cited as a sign of deep-seated sexual disorder, a literalization of what was perceived to be a decaying social order.[8] Venereal disease makes clear the persistent association of disease with dirt and uncleanliness as well, revealing pervasive cultural attitudes and values. We have known since the late nineteenth century that venereal diseases are caused by microorganisms, and yet the persistent association of dirt and disease is remarkable. The very term which the venereal disease control movement took for itself in the twentieth century—social hygiene—makes explicit this association.

Within the social constructions of venereal disease in the last century a number of important values have been expressed; themes that reflect longstanding historical traditions regarding sexual behavior.[9] In particular, venereal disease came to be seen as an affliction of those who willfully violated the moral code, a punishment for sexual irresponsibility. These infections were employed to argue for a more restricted sexuality. So long as these social *uses* of the diseases have dominated medical and public approaches, therapeutic approaches to the problem have necessarily remained secondary. Because of the nature of these diseases, individuals often have suffered a double jeopardy: the physiological consequences of the disease itself, as well as the deep psychological stigma.

Venereal disease provided evidence for those seeking to demonstrate—for a variety of reasons—that attempts to regulate sexuality had failed, that the idealized unified social values of American society were threatened. In this respect, many discussions of venereal disease became a rhetorical vehicle for demanding reform of American sexual mores. Much of the writing about venereal disease was, therefore, prescriptive. But venereal disease also is indicative of actual sexual behavior and practice, and programs and policies for its treatment often forced physicians to confront the disquieting distance between ideals and behavior.

This book, then, poses two related questions about venereal disease in American society. First, what does venereal disease reveal about sexual attitudes and practices, as well as larger social values? And second, how have attitudes and beliefs concerning sexuality affected medical and public health practices for the control of these infections? I want to demonstrate that the symbols that we use not only affect the way we come to think about a problem, but also dramatically affect the material reality; practice and policy are fundamentally influenced by the symbols we attach to a particular disease. I have sought to investigate the impact of values on health care, as well as the impact of medicine on social values and behavior.

Since the late nineteenth century, the venereal diseases have raised a number of deeper social conflicts which continue to generate controversy in American society. First, the tension between morality and secular rationalism: moral approaches have frequently clashed with scientific instrumentalism in the debates concerning venereal disease. Second, venereal disease fundamentally broached the modern dilemma of individual versus social responsibility. The problem of venereal disease made these conflicts explicit; addressing venereal disease forced a consideration of the notion that in modern society the sacrosanct, private world of sexuality might indeed have social implications of enormous moment, inviting the interest and control of public institutions. In this respect, the social history of venereal disease has significant implications not just for health policy, but for the polity as well.

If the three elements of this study—sex, disease, and medicine—could be considered seriatim, the problem of venereal disease would be far easier to assess. Venereal disease, however, by its very nature has historically been defined by the interrelation of these three issues. The basic contention of this work is that venereal disease has engaged a number of social fears about class, race, ethnicity, and in particular, sexuality and the family. Venereal disease—in its social constructions—has been used during the last century to express these anxieties. In turn, the social and cultural uses of venereal disease as a means of controlling sexuality have greatly complicated attempts to deal effectively with the diseases from a therapeutic standpoint. Venereal disease became a rallying point for concerns about sexual mores and a more generally perceived social disorder. In its transformation from a biological entity to a social symbol, venereal disease has defied control.

I

"Damaged Goods":
Progressive Medicine and Social Hygiene

1

Progressive reformers and social critics identified a myriad of ills surrounding the dramatic alterations in American life during the late nineteenth and early twentieth century. Few problems evoked more fear than the perceived "crisis of the family." During the Victorian years the middle-class family had become, preeminently, an institution devoted to child-rearing and the maintenance of the home. No longer fulfilling the basic economic functions of earlier periods, the home had become a private place, given over to motherhood, childhood, and domesticity.[1] Acute observers at the turn of the century saw trends within the family itself that threatened this ideal. Medical doctors in particular came to share these concerns when it became accepted that venereal disease constituted a special danger to the family.

The growing tendency toward later marriages and smaller families and the precipitous rise in the number of divorces foretold the demise of the middle-class family, the bulwark of American society, in the minds of Progressive social critics. The depressed economic conditions of the late nineteenth century led members of the middle class to postpone marriage in order to support their families in their accustomed manner. Family size was often limited to maintain this standard of living; by 1900 the average American family had only 3.56 children, down from 6.14 in 1840.[2] In addition, the heightened emotional demands placed upon the family caused more marriages to end in the courts. In the years between 1870 and 1920 the divorce rate increased by a factor of fifteen.[3] Moreover, a growing number of women, particularly the best educated, passed up domestic life altogether to pursue careers.

Critics charged that the American family, in a flight of selfishness, was failing in its primary responsibility, the "reproduction of the race." When social scientists reported that couples of Anglo-Saxon descent were falling behind their immigrant counterparts in producing children, Theodore Roosevelt raised the pitch of concern by proclaiming that the great white middle class was committing "race suicide," borrowing the phrase from the noted sociologist E.A. Ross. Roosevelt argued that men and women were "shirking" their most important duty to the state. "Shame to those who choose to lead their lives in a round of cheap self-indulgence and vapid excitement," declared the former president in 1911. Although Roosevelt suggested that both men and women must bear the responsibility for this trend, he agreed with most observers, especially physicians, who blamed women for this "unnatural" inclination to suppress the maternal instinct.[4]

American physicians, dedicated to the ideal of a domestic, affective family, assessed these trends with considerable anxiety. Indeed, in the new urban-industrial, secularized world many physicians viewed the "health" of the family as a primary professional domain. "No apology will be required," noted an editorial in *American Medicine* in 1911, "for presenting certain phases of the question [of marriage] as topics for medical discussion, and it will be freely conceded that the modern physician should be as concerned with these as with anything else that has any bearing whatsoever on the mental and moral as well as the physical welfare of human beings."[5] The new trend for women to seek careers, the editorial suggested, reduced the numbers of suitable brides, concluding that "marriage should be encouraged, never discouraged."

Within the profession, the specter of venereal diseases—and new knowledge about the impact of these diseases on the family—fueled anxieties regarding the future of domestic life. Venereal diseases provided a palpable sign of degeneration, as well as a symbol of a more general cultural crisis. Recent scientific advances concerning the pathology and treatment of venereal diseases granted physicians new stature and increased authority in the assessment of a variety of related problems from the changing role of the family and marriage to sex roles and morality.

Physicians devoted to the venereal problem became an influential force in Progressive reform. "Progressive physicians" were generally those doctors who committed themselves to the larger political and social currents of reform during the first two decades of the twentieth century. Progressivism was no single movement, but rather a diverse configuration of principles, ideas, and practices for social reformation.[6] Although these ideas attracted professionals from a number of fields, the input of the medical profession has yet to be fully explored; reformers tended to emphasize how social problems affected their particular domains, and doctors were no exception. These Progressive physicians helped to pull together two of the most significant threads of the complex Progressive ideology: the desire for a rigorously defined moral order and a growing reliance on technical expertise. Indeed, Progressive physicians were quick to suggest the relationship of social pathology to medicine. In their evaluations of health and disease, these doctors reflected larger concerns about the major transformations in American life in the postbellum years. Many of these concerns—the growth of the cities, the increase in immigration, as well as the changing nature of the family—could be seen in their assessment of venereal disease, as well as other medical problems such as tuberculosis and mental illness. Venereal diseases offered physicians an opportunity to develop a comprehensive approach to health and disease, for here was a massive problem that clearly demanded the broadest possible view of the doctor's task from an educational, social, and clinical perspective. In fact, venereal disease, as a social construct, provided a means of organizing and explaining many of the social dilemmas which Progressivism sought to address.

2

For physicians who treated venereal diseases, claims of the family's decline rang true. A generation of scientific progress had clarified the devastating impact of syphilis and gonorrhea within the family unit. Though most physicians had long accepted the social stigma attached to these maladies, considering them just rewards for moral turpitude, the knowledge that profligate men "visited" these sins upon their wives and children led to a dramatic reversal in professional attitudes. The "discovery" of venereal *insontium*—infections of the innocent— in the last decades of the nineteenth century generated a movement to prevent these diseases and to demand adherence to a strict sexual code.[7] There followed a virtual redefinition of venereal disease from the classic "carnal scourge" to "family poison," a redefinition that would illuminate the relationship of science, morals, and disease in the new century.

The physician's new approach proceeded from a growing body of evidence detailing the pathology of venereal diseases. From the sixteenth century until well into the nineteenth century, most doctors assumed gonorrhea and syphilis were manifestations of the same disease. Only in 1837 did the eminent French venereologist Phillipe Ricord establish the specificity of the two diseases through a series of experimental inoculations from syphilitic chancres.[8] Ricord was also among the first physicians to differentiate primary, secondary, and tertiary syphilis, the three stages of infection. By the late nineteenth century the systemic dangers of syphilis had been identified in a series of pathbreaking studies. Because syphilitic infections appear to resolve after the initial inflammatory reaction, chronic ailments resulting from the disease had long been thought to be distinct clinical entities. Rudolph Virchow, one of the leading figures in the development of modern germ theory, established that the infection could be transferred through the blood to the internal organs, and that syphilis was in fact a systemic condition.[9]

Subsequent research demonstrated syphilis to be the cause of a variety of serious illnesses. By 1876, cardiovascular syphilis had been clearly documented in the medical literature. If spread to the spinal cord, the infection could cause muscular incoordination and partial paralysis (tabes, locomotor ataxia, paresis), or eventually complete paralysis. Ultimately affecting the brain, syphilis also led to insanity in some cases.[10] By the early twentieth century, doctors reported that mental institutions were filled with patients whose illnesses could be traced to syphilitic infections. "The elimination of these diseases," remarked one physician, "would render one-third, possibly one-half, of our institutions for defectives unnecessary."[11]

These discoveries of the nefarious spread of syphilis to the internal organs, made clear that the disease was much more dangerous than many doctors had previously assumed. The late indications of syphilis, often seemingly unrelated to the initial symptoms, prompted William Osler, then the most distinguished clinician in the United States, to tell his students at the Johns Hopkins Medical School, "Know syphilis in all its manifestations and relations, and all other things clinical will be added unto you." "In one direction our knowledge was widened greatly," he noted in 1909. "It added terror to an already terrible disorder."[12] Because of misunderstandings of the pathology of the disease, as well as a desire to avoid the moral opprobrium attached to venereal infection, physicians often ascribed deaths due to syphilis to other causes. "A convenient and somewhat elastic medical nomenclature lends itself to this policy of concealment," explained one doctor. "A vast number of morbid conditions which should be charged to venereal infection are entered under some non-compromising name which does not indicate its real value." As Osler remarked, "Men do not die of the diseases that afflict them," at least in the reports of many physicians.[13]

Long after the ravages of syphilis had become clear, physicians continued to consider gonorrhea a relatively minor, nonspecific, inflammatory disorder. Doctors practicing in the mid-nineteenth century frequently suggested that excessive sexual intercourse was a primary cause of infection and, with interesting logic, often recommended marriage as a cure for the afflicted. Indeed, many doctors believed that gonorrhea need not always originate from another infection. The asymptomatic nature of the disease in women even led to the idea that virtually all women carried gonorrhea without damage and could transmit it to their partners. "One denied the right of a woman *not* to have gonorrhea; she possessed it permanently, immanently," wrote a French physician. "She was contagious without having been contagioned. The woman was considered dangerous *ipso facto*.[14] Victorian notions of motherhood and domesticity in the United States, however, would not long accommodate such suggestions.

By the end of the nineteenth century substantial progress had been made toward a fuller understanding of gonorrhea. In 1879 Albert Neisser, a German dermatologist, made a fundamental contribution not just to venereal research, but to the germ theory of disease when he identified the gonococcus as the organism responsible for infection. The bacteria that Neisser viewed under the microscope—small, bead-like growths—were among the first to be identified with a specific disease. In subsequent studies of the pathology of gonorrhea, it was soon demonstrated that the bacteria could cause arthritis, as well as a variety of systemic ailments including meningitis, pericarditis (inflammation of the tissue surrounding the heart), and peritonitis (inflammation of the tissues lining the walls of the abdominal and pelvic cavities).[15] Gonorrhea, previously considered a "trivial disease" no worse than a common cold, now joined syphilis as a serious venereal malady.

Even though it had been known for centuries that these diseases could be communicated through sexual contact, only in the mid-nineteenth century did physicians come to center attention on the devastating impact of syphilis and gonorrhea within the family. Two of Ricord's students, Paul Diday and Alfred Fournier, examined the pathologic effects of syphilis upon pregnancy and newborn children. Diday described the deformities of infants born of syphilitic parents; the mother, he suggested, usually infected the fetus, after receiving the disease from her husband.[16] Fournier, perhaps the greatest clinical syphilographer of the nineteenth century, wrote extensively about the repercussions of syphilis in marriage, describing a condition of "congenital syphilis" in which children, born healthy, suffered serious effects of the disease years later.[17]

In 1872 an American physician, Emil Noeggerath, demonstrated the disastrous results of gonorrheal infections in women. Noeggerath discovered the so-called "latency period" of gonorrhea, in which an asymptomatic man actually still harbors the infection, and can communicate it in sexual relations. Latent gonorrhea in men, according to Noeggerath, explained "why so many healthy, blooming young girls begin to suffer and fail as soon as they enter the bonds of marriage." He also attributed high rates of sterility to gonorrhea, estimating that "about ninety per cent of sterile women are married to husbands who have suffered from gonorrhea either previous to, or during marriage."[18] Given the fact that gonorrhea remains today a leading cause of sterility, it is likely that in the late nineteenth century, before the introduction of any effective treatment, it was among the most significant causes.

Noeggerath's work was exceptional in that Europeans dominated most research concerning the transmission and pathology of venereal disease during the late nineteenth century. American physicians, however, avidly followed the results of these studies. Indeed, during these years, when American medical education was substantially inferior to European, many Americans traveled overseas to augment their training and participate first-hand in scientific research.[19] A young American dermatologist, Prince Albert Morrow, spent a year in Europe after completing his medical training at New York University Hospital in 1873. Morrow contacted some of the leading figures in venereal research, including Alfred Fournier, whose *Syphilis and Marriage* Morrow translated into English in 1880.[20]

Fournier posed questions raised by the new knowledge of the pathologic impact of syphilis. When could a syphilitic man marry without endangering wife and offspring? Was the physician's responsibility to the patient or society? Vividly outlining the potential dangers of introducing infection into the family, Fournier argued that professionals must take action to prevent the spread of syphilis. These themes had particular resonance for American physicians, who were already concerned about the future of the family. In Morrow's preface to the American edition of *Syphilis and Marriage,* he explained:

> There is scarcely a subject in the entire domain of medicine of greater practical importance to the profession and to the public, not only on account of the nature of the pathological questions presented, but also on account of the family and society interests involved, and which it is the physician's manifest duty to protect.[21]

Although substantial progress was made during the nineteenth century toward an understanding of the etiology and pathology of the venereal diseases, physicians, despite their increasing apprehension, could offer little therapeutic hope for those afflicted. Most physicians treated syphilis with mercury, either orally, in vapor baths, or topically. They based the use of mercury on the ancient theory of humors and health. Mercury caused salivation, which, it was believed, removed the humors causing the ailment. Hot vapor baths worked in a similar fashion by causing profuse perspiration.[22] Modern observers have suggested that high doses of heavy metal therapy probably neared lethal rates, with many symptoms attributed to syphilis likely the result of mercury intoxication. Patients with gonorrhea probably fared little better from the efforts of physicians. Most doctors employed oral medications which, they argued, when excreted through the urethra would have an antiseptic effect. Some injected chemicals directly into the urethra, but usually this had no beneficial impact, and may actually have been harmful. Until the advent of the sulfa drugs in the late 1930s, Ricord's dictum held true: "A gonorrhea begins and God alone knows when it will end."[23]

Treatments at this time indicated the nature of prescientific therapeutics as well as professional attitudes toward sexually transmitted diseases. For a therapy to be considered effective by both doctor and patient it had to elicit some outward, empirical effect.[24] In this regard, most venereal treatments certainly fulfilled and exceeded expectations. Massive doses of mercury and iodides of potasium often led to serious complications: loss of teeth, tongue fissures, and hemorrhaging of the bowel. The initial chancre, however, naturally disappeared in the course of the disease, and doctor and patient usually credited the treatment. These therapies, however, also entailed considerable pain, demonstrating the punitive position of the profession regarding diseases communicated in "immoral congress." One New York physician suggested at mid-century a "Hot Water Retrojection" therapy in which he injected quarts of water heated to 180 degrees Fahrenheit until "sometime after the point of toleration had been reached." Another well-known physician, Frederick Hollick, prescribed a measure, no less heroic, for the treatment of a complication of gonorrhea known as chordee, a curvature of the penis which caused pain upon erection. Hollick recommended that the organ be placed "with the curve upward on a table and struck a violent blow with a book . . . and so flattening it."[25] By the end of the nineteenth century, better informed physicians had abandoned such efforts, leaving patients to suffer only from the disease, not the "cure." Indeed, as doctors sought to discourage premarital and extramarital sex, cure of the venereal sufferer became a questionable goal, and many argued with increasing frequency that the diseases were treatable but incurable.

The state of venereal therapeutics in the late nineteenth century explains, in part, the high estimates of the incidence of infection. In 1901 the New York County Medical Society appointed Prince Morrow to chair a Committee of Seven to assess the problem of venereal disease in New York City. After an investigation of local practitioners, the Committee presented absolutely staggering rates of infection in their report. Quoting statistics from a variety of sources, Morrow contended that as many as 80 of every 100 men in New York City had been infected at one time or another with gonorrhea. He considered it to be the most prevalent of all diseases in the adult male population. According to his report, from 5 to 18 percent of all men harbored syphilitic infections.[26] Because few hospitals or health departments collected venereal statistics, seeking to spare patients and families from the social stigma attributed to them, doctors frequently cited the figures collected by the military as the most reliable. The admission rate for venereal disease in the Army in 1909 neared 200 per 1000 men, and over one-third of all days lost from duty resulted from these infections. Morrow pointed out that these statistics, because they counted only new infections, did not reflect total venereal morbidity, which probably reached much higher rates due to the chronic nature of syphilis and gonorrhea. Indeed, he argued that venereal infections were more prevalent—and dangerous—than all other infectious diseases combined. "It is a conservative estimate," he later declared, "that fully one-eighth of all human suffering comes from this source."[27]

Critics within the profession challenged these figures, charging that fanatics and moralists inflated venereal statistics to generate publicity and fuel the public's fears. "Here we might see the hopeless amateur," wrote Dr. John S. Fulton, "beginning without a knowledge of whole numbers, proceeding without a sense of fractions, achieving a childish confusion of ratios, factoring and developing out of those miraculous numbers which seem to be the chief sustenance of a crusading zeal." Richard Cabot, the renowned Boston physician, concluded in his study of venereal incidence that Morrow's figures were "wild guesses published for campaign purposes."[28]

The perception of a venereal epidemic, however, prevailed in the medical literature. Morrow, responding to Cabot's critique, noted caustically that, if his figures on venereal morbidity in Boston were correct, "the citizens of Boston and vicinity . . . are vastly more virtuous than the citizens of New York and Baltimore." Even Cabot had reported that 35.5 percent of his sample at the Massachusetts General Hospital had admitted having had gonorrhea. Morrow discounted personal testimony as certain to produce a low count. "It is never safe to array a man's honesty against his sense of shame," he explained. "The venereal specialist perhaps more than any other is impressed with the adage, 'the world is given to lying.' " Many physicians continued to endorse the assessment of the Committee of Seven that "morbidity of venereal disease exceeds that of all other diseases combined."[29]

The debate about the rates of venereal disease reveals the uncertain nature of diagnostics during this period. In the years just prior to the introduction of stained smear microscopy to detect gonococcus and complement fixation tests for syphilis, venereal diagnostics were based on a number of highly subjective criteria. Given the widespread concern about venereal disease and its impact on the family, it seems likely that many symptoms, particularly involving the genitals, probably led to the diagnosis of venereal infection. The suggestion, knowledge, or inference of immoral behavior by a patient also may have led to a tendency to identify non-specific infections as venereal. In any event, the poor state of therapeutics accounts for rates of venereal infection that far exceed contemporary estimates; because there was no effective treatment, there was more disease. Even today, venereal disease is underreported and rates of infection are only projected on the basis of collected data. As William Osler noted in 1917, "Syphilis . . . remains the despair of the statistician."[30] Nevertheless, in this era before the advent of effective therapeutics, the venereal diseases clearly constituted a health problem of enormous dimensions.

3

New knowledge concerning the pathology of venereal disease, coupled with the reports of its epidemic proportions, galvanized the American medical profession to take action. Already uneasy about the future of the family, Progressive physicians suggested that the impact of "innocent infections" gave the crisis greater immediacy. Their suggestions evoked an inevitably repeated scenario, in which a married man, or one about to be married, would visit a prostitute and acquire a venereal infection. Ignorant of the nature of his new affliction, he would infect his wife; soon pregnant, she would pass the disease to the newborn. American doctors examined the sequelae of venereal disease spread in this fashion with growing alarm.

Prince Morrow became the leading figure in publicizing the problem among his medical colleagues. Born in Mt. Vernon, Kentucky, in 1846, the son of a prominent planter and politician, he had graduated from Princeton College (Kentucky) in 1863. After returning from Europe in 1874 he began practicing dermatology and syphilology in New York City. In 1882 he was appointed clinical lecturer at New York University, and two years later he became clinical professor of genito-urinary diseases. After completing the report of the Committee of Seven, Morrow returned to Europe to attend the Second International Conference on Venereal Disease in Brussels, at which the continent's leading experts discussed the venereal problem in all its ramifications.[31] Morrow returned to the United States committed to founding an American group to educate the profession and the public to the dangers of the venereal peril. First, however, he set out to write a full exposition of the disastrous implications of introducing venereal disease into marriage.

Published in 1904, Morrow's *Social Diseases and Marriage* attracted a wide medical audience to the problems of venereal disease in American society. Morrow chronicled the potential danger to women, children, and "the race," a danger he called the "morbid irradiations into family and social life."[32] Progressive physicians like Morrow came to view venereal disease as a threat to the very foundations of the Victorian, child-centered family; the susceptibility of innocent women and children seemed not only criminal, but treasonous.

Morrow outlined the impact of syphilis upon children in considerable detail in *Social Diseases and Marriage*. Physicians at this time conceived of any ailment passed to the newborn as "hereditary," even though not necessarily the result of genetic defect.[33] As Morrow observed: "No other disease is so susceptible of hereditary transmission, and so fatal to the offspring." Those children who survived infections at birth, he suggested, faced lives of suffering. Syphilis, Morrow argued, because of its effects on offspring, "is an actual cause of the degeneration of the race." Fournier had demonstrated the predisposition of these children to meningitis, severe mental retardation, and hydrocephalus, in addition to any number of serious constitutional disorders. "The souls of infants born only to die or suffer, cry out against the infamy of uncured syphilis," announced one well-known venereal specialist.[34]

The tragic results of gonorrheal infections in children evoked a powerful reaction within the profession. The discovery that the gonococcus could cause blindness in the newborn was, perhaps, the most frequently cited repercussion of venereal *insontium*. "The public should know," Morrow declared, "that opthalmia neonatorum [blindness at birth] is the fateful expression of ignorance and criminal carelessness, the working of that relentless law of Nature which visits the sins of the fathers upon the children."[35] In 1884 Karl S. F. Credé, a German obstetrician, had found that the infection that caused blindness occurred as the infant passed through the birth canal. Credé demonstrated that neonatal gonorrheal blindness could be prevented by introducing a drop of 2 percent silver nitrate solution into the child's eyes immediately after birth.[36] Almost thirty years later, however, large numbers of children still lost their eyesight from these infections because this prophylactic measure had not been universally adopted. According to the most commonly cited figures, 25 percent of all the blind in the United States had suffered from opthalmia neonatorum.[37]

The impact of gonorrhea on women appeared even more ominous to Progressive physicians. Morrow, anxious to dispel the notion that gonorrhea was a minor disease in women, argued that it was more dangerous to them than syphilis. "In the female the local and general effects of gonorrhea are apt to be much more serious and permanent, owing to the character and extent of the structures involved," he explained. Following the work of Noeggerath, Morrow discussed the grave constitutional complications of gonorrhea. Though previously assumed to be limited to the urinary tract, the infection, recent research had demonstrated, could be spread to the cervix, uterus, fallopian tubes and ultimately through the blood stream, endangering the lives of its victims. In particular, Morrow directed attention to the effects of gonorrhea on the woman's reproductive function, estimating that 50 percent of all women infected eventually would become sterile. Gonorrheal infections, he argued, "extinguish her conceptional capacity, and condemn her to a lifelong invalidism or the sacrifice of her reproductive organs to save her life.[38] A similar concern led E. L. Keyes, one of the most prominent venereologists in the United States, to attribute 60 to 80 percent of pelvic inflammations in women that required hysterectomy or removal of the ovaries to gonorrhea.[39]

The serious repercussions of untreated venereal disease for the individual woman created grave concern for womanhood itself within the medical profession. In 1906 the American Medical Association responded by sponsoring a "Symposium on the Duty of the Profession to Womanhood." Dr. Albert H. Burr of Chicago explained, "However unfortunate the effects may be on the male offender, the pathologic relations of gonorrhea to the pelvic organs of the helpless wives is a stupendous calamity. If this one disease could be eliminated from wedded life, gynecology as a specialty would shrink to small proportions." Viewing gonorrhea as the primary cause of sterility, members of the profession sought to defend motherhood from its effects. "The flower of our land, our young women, the mothers of our future citizenship," noted Dr. Abraham Wolbarst, "are being mutilated and unsexed by surgical life-saving measures because of these diseases." Burr concluded that venereal disease posed a greater threat to the family than did the much-detested practices of birth control and abortion: "The ban placed by venereal disease on fetal life outrivals the criminal interference with the products of conception as a cause of race suicide."[40]

For Morrow, the impact of venereal diseases upon a woman's ability to conceive called into question the very notion of "race suicide." He criticized the term because it implied that the low birth rate resulted from voluntary dispositions to limit family size. "There is ample reason for believing," he noted, "that in a large proportion of cases the low birth rate is not a result of choice but of incapacity." Morrow described cases of "one-child sterility" in which a woman, infected by her husband, had an uneventful, chronic, latent infection which, through the birth of the first child, was spread throughout the uterus, becoming virulent. The first born thus became the last born. Small families thus stemmed not from a selfish desire for a higher standard of living, as many social critics had suggested, but rather from the father's philandering. Morrow recorded a series of case histories riddled with tragedy:

> It is common to hear women who constantly suffer from uterine torture employ such words as these: "When I was a young girl I was quite well. It is only since my marriage that I have become ill!" And every day this confidence, this plaintive refrain saddens the gynecologist. It is continual and inexorable. From the discolored and suffering faces we may guess a whole past of debility, and the *origin is always* marriage.[41]

On the basis of the 1890 census, Morrow estimated that one in every seven marriages would prove sterile due to venereal infections. By suggesting that infertility was typically involuntary, Morrow denied the reality that many American women had begun to limit family size by choice.[42] Morrow's view demonstrated the widespread medical concern about the declining size of the white, middle-class family and provided a means for members of the profession to join the debate about the future of domesticity.

In these discussions of the impact of venereal disease upon the family, physicians endorsed a traditional Victorian view of the nature and role of women. Though their defense of women and the concomitant attack on immoral men could be mistaken for an incipient feminism—indeed, the public campaigns attracted a number of feminists—in reality, these doctors accepted a common image of women as innocent, weak, and helpless. The belief that gonorrhea wreaked special havoc in women substantiated the popular view of the biologically determined shortcomings of the female species.[43] Widespread notions of woman as innocent victim were repeatedly conveyed in the medical literature on venereal disease. "While she may not appreciate its pathological significance," wrote Morrow, "she suffers most keenly from the knowledge that her husband has soiled her with an impure disease." Most importantly, venereal disease often made it impossible for a women to fulfill what Progressive physicians saw to be her primary domestic responsibility, motherhood; "In missing maternity," Morrow explained, "she has missed her highest destiny in being created woman."[44] These views make clear the way in which disease functioned metaphorically to define gender roles. Venereal disease had specifically different meaning for the infected man or woman, meanings that revealed powerful assumptions about the nature of the family and sexuality. These infections served as yet another means of defining the separate spheres of gender identity. When physicians came to the defense of women, it was to a sentimental, domestic, objectified ideal, one that bore little resemblance to the emerging "new woman." Women suffered both the consequent dangers of venereal infection as well as the constraints of medical beliefs concerning gender.

4

As venereal disease became a focus for Progressive fears concerning the future of the family in the first years of the twentieth century, physicians increasingly considered it their responsibility to protect the institution of marriage from the introduction of disease. This new duty, however, generated a crisis in contemporary medical ethics. In the past, doctors had assisted the male patient in concealing their ailments; indeed, some hid the nature of the disease from the patient himself. Action of this sort, however, based on the premise of the confidentiality of the physician-patient exchange, held the risk of promoting infection of the innocent woman and her children. As Prince Morrow observed, "The medical profession has not appreciated its share of the responsibility for these tragic results."[45] Was it the doctor's obligation to see that a spouse be treated or a prospective bride warned of potential contamination? Physicians on both sides of the Atlantic debated this question with some vehemence.

Traditionally, all transactions between doctor and patient had been deemed strictly confidential. In no instance had the so-called "medical secret" prevailed so completely as in cases of venereal infection. In the era before scientific therapeutics, the confidence of the doctor-patient relationship had provided the fundamental basis for professional authority; medical care was predicated on this intimacy.[46] The questioning of the primacy of the medical secret marked a subtle yet significant shift in the role of the physician from protecting the patient from social conventions to demanding his or her allegiance to these mores.

During the course of the nineteenth century, the principles of confidentiality had been widely codified. More than one-half of the states forbade testimony from physicians in legal proceedings without the patient's consent.[47] Many doctors suggested that revealing a patient's venereal infection violated this principle— not to mention the tenets of Hippocrates. Indeed, many doctors argued, to label a patient a venereal carrier inflicted irreparable harm, given the stigma that accompanied these diseases. Some physicians expressed concern that if the nature of a man's infection were fully explained to his spouse, many marriages would be terminated. Dr. John Fordyce, a genito-urinary specialist at the College of Physicians and Surgeons in New York, claimed: "If the etiological element of many of the diseases which arise after marriage . . . were known to the wife, what domestic calamities would follow!" Other physicians suggested that a weakened dedication to confidentiality would encourage venereal patients to turn to quacks—already a common practice—or to conceal their infections.[48]

Progressive physicians, however, increasingly pointed to the tragic results in cases in which the carrier refused to reveal his infection to his spouse. Dr. John Stokes of the Mayo Clinic characterized the medical secret as a "blind policy of protecting the guilty at the expense of the innocent." Prince Morrow emphasized the doctor's obligation to prevent further infections. "Does not his silence and inaction," he asked, "make [the physician] an accomplice, a *particeps criminis?*" A prominent New York attorney, William A. Purrington, argued that a physician acted within the law if protecting an innocent from possible infection: "A physician who knows that an infected patient is about to carry his contagion to a pure person, and perhaps to persons unborn, is justified both in law and morals, in preventing the proposed wrong by disclosing his knowledge if no other way is open."[49]

On the issue of the medical secret, American doctors achieved no consensus. Morrow, for example, despite his inherent sympathy for the innocent woman, argued that the secret "was in the interest of the social order." Some physicians suggested the possibility of "forging" a history of extra-genital infection and then informing the wife, "to take the keen edge off the situation."[50] E.L. Keyes cautioned that in some cases preventing a diseased man from marrying could be worse than allowing him the risk of infecting his new wife. "To prohibit matrimony in a given case may wreck a man's life even more completely than syphilis could blast his wife's." Charlotte Perkins Gilman, the well-known feminist writer and theorist, dissected the problem of the medical secret in her novel, *The Crux*, published in 1911. When Dr. Bellair, a woman physician, tries to convince Dr. Hale, a male colleague, to reveal a patient's infection to his fiancée, he responds, "You know how I feel about this. It is a matter of honor—professional honor. You women don't seem to know what the word means. I've told that good-for-nothing young wreck that he has no right to marry for years yet if ever. That is all I can do. I will not betray the confidence of a patient." An exasperated Dr. Bellair replies, "Not if he had smallpox, or scarlet fever, or the bubonic plague? Suppose a patient of yours had the leprosy, and wanted to marry your sister; would you betray his confidence?"[51] She marches off to tell the unfortunate woman to break off her engagement. As Gilman made clear, the medical secret was closely tied to the ideology of male supremacy and loyalty in Victorian America. Clearly, many physicians acted to uphold a double standard at the same time that they decried its impact on the family.

The unmasking of the medical secret often did bring marriages to an end. Just as physicians ascribed falling birth rates to venereal infections, so, too, did many attribute a large percentage of the growing number of divorces to these diseases. Doctors noted that the venereal diseases often served as *les maladies revelatrices*, providing proof of infidelity. Commenting on the consequences, Morrow explained:

> No other commentary upon the intolerable situations created by the introduction of these diseases into the family is needed than the fact that so many women, loyal to the highest ideals of marriage, devoted to home and family, are driven to the divorce courts as a refuge. No one can condemn a self-respecting woman for separating from a man who has dishonored her with a shameful disease.

As Dr. Robert N. Willson of Philadelphia observed, "Many a divorce comes as a godsend to an already infected wife who can no longer cherish the transmitter of an eternal woe."[52] The image of woman as victim inspired the reform of divorce laws during the late nineteenth century; by the first years of the twentieth century, courts increasingly recognized the introduction of venereal disease into marriage as proper grounds for disunion. Women often disguised, however, these grounds in their petition; "cruelty" or "non-support" frequently concealed the true cause. Morrow called this a "shame that cannot be named for a shame," because of the humiliation it would cause the woman. "Divorce increasing?" asked Dr. William Lee Howard, a popular medical commentator. "Of course; cannot you all see why? Divorce increases in direct ratio to the increase in venereal diseases. We cannot stop the effect until we stop the cause."[53]

5

Fears about the impact of venereal diseases on the future of the family led physicians to ally with the nascent eugenics movement in the first decades of the twentieth century. The initial impetus behind eugenics was the differential in birth rates between native-born Americans and newly arriving immigrants.[54] Morrow, noting that "degenerates" were multiplying at faster rates than the "respectable" middle class, attributed this problem to the high incidence of sterility caused by venereal disease, thereby making a connection between "respectability" and disease that would seem to contradict the very premises of the eugenics movement. "The function of eugenics is to produce a race healthy, well-formed and vigorous by keeping the springs of heredity pure and undefiled, and improving the inborn qualities of the offspring," wrote Morrow. "The effect of venereal diseases is to produce a race of inferior beings, by poisoning the sources of life, and sapping the vitality and health of the offspring." Though venereal diseases were not transmitted through the "germ plasm," or genes, in a strictly hereditarian sense, Morrow argued that they were the proper domain of eugenic interest because of their influence on the future of "the race." "The syphilitic, the consumptive and the epileptic, the alcoholic—each produces his kind," he explained. He considered venereal disease "directly antagonistic to the eugenic ideal."[55]

Physicians now frequently asserted that their expertise should be consulted prior to any hasty marriages. Morrow cautioned against unions based solely on emotion and romance. "Young women should know," he wrote, "that marriage is not all romance and sentiment, that dissipated men make unsafe husbands and unsound fathers, and that the halo of romantic interest thrown around the man with a profligate past by fiction writers is a symbol of shame, a signal of danger for his wife and chilren."[56] Recognizing this threat to the family, several states enacted "eugenic marriage laws" that required that a prospective groom be examined by a physician and receive a certification of health before obtaining a marriage licence. In 1899 Michigan became the first state to make venereal disease a bar to matrimony, directing that all men swear to their health before taking marriage vows. By 1913 a total of seven states had laws designed

to eliminate venereal contagion in the family. Although some of these enactments required men to undergo medical examinations, none of these states
required that prospective brides be examined, on the premise that such a procedure would be an affront to a respectable woman.[57]

Because diagnostic procedures were imperfect and many practitioners un-
trained, physicians were forced to admit that these laws were less than fully
effective. As Edward L. Keyes explained, "In the present state of medical
knowledge, a few weeks of preparation and a willingness to perjure himself,
may enable the patient with infectious syphilis to defy the most conscientious
examination."[58] Supporters of these statutes argued that they nevertheless served
an important educational purpose. In fact, the existence of these so-called
"eugenic marriage laws" indicate that medical authority had been invoked *prior*
to the development of effective diagnostics and therapeutics. Indeed, most states
did not require serologic and microscopic tests even after they came into practice, continuing to rely on the personal credibility of the doctor, rather than
laboratory diagnosis. The growing stature of the medical profession was clearly
a function of shifting cultural precepts as well as scientific advance.[59]

Though some physicians centered attention on the eugenic implications of
venereal disease in marriage, others emphasized the dangers posed by venereal
disease among the influx of immigrants entering the United States in the last
years of the nineteenth century and early twentieth century. From 1897 to 1907
more than 650,000 Europeans per year crossed the Atlantic.[60] The fear expressed by nativists that these "degenerate racial stocks" from Southern and Eastern
Europe would pollute the Anglo-Saxon gene pool or soon outnumber the respectable middle class attracted a considerable audience. The Immigration Act
of 1891 excluded "persons suffering from a loathsome or dangerous contagious
disease," which the Public Health Service interpreted to include venereal infections. Because of the great expense, however, only those immigrants who
showed external signs of infection—open chancres, ataxia, dementia—received
full examinations for syphilis and gonorrhea. Though the actual number of immigrants found to be infected remained low, critics suggested that this was the
result of inadequate exams. In 1907 the United States Immigration Commission noted that "it seems probable that a considerable number of persons afflicted with venereal disease are admitted to this country, and that such diseases
have been spread in many communities as a result of immigration." Lax diagnostic procedures came under increasing attack. As one observer remarked upon
learning that all aliens did not receive mandatory venereal tests: "Why, that is
just as if a man were to pay for a strong gate for his wheat field and not put a
fence all the way around!"[61]

Some physicians, influenced by nativist views, singled out immigrant populations as particularly prone to venereal infection. A widely circulated theory
held that some immigrants, following a common folk remedy of intercourse
with a virgin, raped their own children as a means of attempting to rid themselves of infection. "It has been brought to my notice many times that among
certain classes, especially ignorant Italians, Chinese, and Negroes, it is an accepted belief that, if a man infected with an obstinate venereal disease have

intercourse with a virgin the latter will develop the disease and he will be cured," explained Dr. W. Travis Gibb, examining physician for the New York Society for the Prevention of Cruelty to Children. Other doctors suggested that poor conditions in American cities contributed to immorality and the spread of venereal diseases. "Much of the vice we see around us," noted Dr. Howard Kelly of Johns Hopkins, "is bred in the pestilential hot house atmosphere of dark, dirty, ill-ventilated homes, which induces abnormal cravings in ill-conditioned bodies."[62] Fear of sexually transmitted diseases became closely tied to growing anxieties about the city and urban masses. As Dr. L. Duncan Bulkey reported:

> Syphilis is everywhere seen to be a disease more especially belonging to communities, and flourishing most luxuriantly wherever there is crowding or massing together of individuals. . . . Syphilis is, therefore, most abundantly met with in cities, and its frequency is commonly seen to diminish in a pretty direct ratio to the suburban or rural character of the people.[63]

Venereal infections among immigrants might well have been considered of little concern to the native-born middle class if not for two reasons. First, many observers suggested that the foreign-born furnished the bulk of prostitutes in American cities, and physicians believed prostitutes to be the primary locus of infection.[64] And second, doctors now asserted that venereal diseases could be transmitted without sexual contact in any number of ways.

The most innocent behavior could lead to venereal infection, according to many physicians. Metal drinking cups attached to public water fountains, eating utensils, towels and bedding, all were noted as possible points of transmission of both syphilis and gonorrhea. "The methods by which non-venereal syphilis may be acquired are innumerable," explained Bulkey in his definitive study of syphilis *sine coitu*, "and relate to every conceivable circumstance surrounding life."[65] Bulkey catalogued records of extra-genital infections caused by whistles, pens, pencils, toilets, medical procedures, tattoos, and toothbrushes, to name only a few. Physicians most often noted epidemics of vulvo-vaginitis among young girls—a gonorrheal infection—which they usually traced to the school lavatory.

Innocent acquisition of a venereal disease did nothing to relieve the personal anguish of the venereal victim. In an anonymous short story in a popular monthly magazine one woman poignantly described the agony and stress that accompanied an innocently transmitted infection. After manifesting the standard symptoms of early syphilis, the woman visited a physician:

> At first it was unbelievable. I knew of the disease only through newspaper advertisements [for patent medicines]. I had understood that it was the result of sin and that it originated and was contracted only in the underworld of the city. I felt sure that my friend was mistaken in diagnosis. When he exclaimed, "Another tragedy of the public drinking cup!" I eagerly met his remark with the assurance that I did not use public drinking cups, that I had used my own cup for years. He led me to review my summer. After recalling a number of times when my thirst had forced me to go to the public fountain, I came at last to realize that what he had told me was true.

She lived in fear of transmitting the catastrophe to another innocent:

> Every day I expected to be accused of unspeakable things and turned adrift. . . .
> Even though I was not discovered I had perhaps a more direful possibility to face.
> Daily, hourly, momentarily, I was haunted by the dread of passing on the disease
> to another. . . . Every act of my life was carefully weighed under the influence of
> that feverish fear. . . . I was strained, tense—afraid, afraid. Night and day, day
> and night I bore my burden of fear.

Venereal disease remained a stigma; the possibility of innocent infections only
implied a larger susceptible population. The woman concluded by arguing for
the total social isolation of the infected, all the more ironic for her own tor-
ment: "If each state would pass and enforce stringent laws causing persons so
diseased to be isolated, just as lepers are, there would be more hope in repressing the evil."[66] Despite the contributions of germ theory to the understanding
of venereal disease, it continued to be an essentially morally-defined malady.

Since it is now known that syphilis and gonorrhea are almost never communicated in non-sexual ways, it seems that the frequent diagnosis of extra-
genital infections around the turn of the century reveals certain professional and
public value-laden assumptions about sexuality and disease. In some cases,
physicians pointed to these infections as a means of attempting to reduce the
stigma of venereal disease, both for patients and doctors. Until the "discovery"
of these innocent infections, some members of the profession had refused to
treat venereal diseases, and those who did held little professional stature. Members of the American Urological Association, founded in 1902, complained of
being considered only "clap doctors."[67] The belief in non-sexual transmission
served to make treatment more respectable. For members of the middle class,
these infections provided a safety-valve; patients could acquire a venereal disease within the boundaries of Victorian morality. Many physicians who became infected, for example, suggested that they had received the contagion in
the course of treating their patients—a possibility that today would be considered highly unlikely.[68]

The substantial professional interest and popular anxiety that extra-genital infections generated also reflected concern about the changes in American society
during the late nineteenth century, particularly the heterogeneity and unhy-
gienic nature of the burgeoning cities. Innocent infections promoted apprehen-
sions of the city, the working class, and the new immigrant populations, ultimately encouraging racism and nativism. Progressive unease about hygiene,
contagion, and cleanliness were evoked in the belief that in the brief contacts
of everyday life—at the grocery, in the park, at the barber shop—these infections, originally obtained in "immoral" circumstances, could be passed to na-
tive, middle-class "moral" Americans. Fear of contamination justified a distaste
for social contact with the urban masses. As one commentator suggested: "It is
not well to use such articles (wash-basins and towels) in public places, as for
instance, in shops or railway stations where they are free to all." If venereal
disease could be spread so easily, no one was safe from contagion. As Dr. Howard Kelly, one of the nation's most distinguished gynecologists, noted in richly
metaphorical language:

The personal services of the poor must daily invade our doors and penetrate every nook in our houses; if we care for them in no wise beyond their mere service, woe betide us. Think of these countless currents flowing daily in our cities from the houses of the poorest into those of the richest, and forming a sort of civic circulatory system expressive of the life of the body politic, a circulation which continually tends to equalize the distribution of morality and disease.[69]

L. Duncan Bulkey cited these infections as a motivation for public anti-venereal campaigns in the urban ghettos:

Venereal diseases, with their manifold and direful results so frequently reaching to and working havoc among those who are innocent, will never be checked until in some way even the lowest levels of society are influenced toward their prevention.

Until disease and immorality were controlled within the working class, these physicians argued, the entire society would be imperiled. "The tide [of venereal disease] has been raising [sic] continually," concluded Kelly, "owing to incessant impouring of a large foreign population with lower ideals."[70] Venereal disease had become, preeminently, a disease of the "other," be it the other race, the other class, the other ethnic group.

6

Though the medical profession discussed the impact of venereal disease on American society with increasing vigor in the first years of the twentieth century, the public had remained largely ignorant on the subject. The tenets of Victorian respectability precluded open debate on these diseases, heavily cloaked in what physicians now called "the conspiracy of silence." Some doctors admitted that they had actually contributed to this state of affairs by hiding diagnoses of syphilis and gonorrhea from their patients and upholding the "medical secret." Dr. Robert N. Willson described the nature of the conventions that surrounded sexually transmitted diseases:

Medical men are walking with eyes wide open along the edge of a slough of despair so treacherous and so pitiless that the wonder can only be that they have failed to warn the world away. Not a signboard! Not a caution spoken above a whisper! All mystery and seclusion. . . . As a result of this studied propriety, a world more full of venereal infection than of any other pestilence.

Prince Morrow concluded succinctly: "Social sentiment holds that it is a greater violation of the properties of life publicly to mention venereal disease than privately to contract it."[71]

The press remained reticent on the subject of sexual diseases, refusing to print accounts of their effects. The only references to venereal ailments that ever punctuated their pages were euphemisms like "rare blood disease." These same magazines and newspapers accepted, however, advertisements for venereal nostrums and quacks. Morrow accused such periodicals of an unabashed hypocrisy. "Many newspapers which do not hesitate to speak freely of prostitution," he wrote, "which lay bare disgusting details of private intrigues in language which conveys a distinct conception of an immoral act, yet shrink from mentioning the pathologic consequence of that act as something unprintable." When Edward Bok, editor of the *Ladies' Home Journal*, broke convention and published a series of articles on venereal disease in 1906, he lost some 75,000 subscribers.[72] Although several Progressive social welfare journals such as *Survey* and *Charities and Commons* followed the *Journal's* suit with accounts of the venereal menace, newspapers refused to join the anti-venereal campaign. In 1912 the silence received official endorsement when the U.S. Post Office confiscated copies of Margaret Sanger's pamphlet, *What Every Girl Should Know*, because it considered the references to syphilis and gonorrhea "obscene" under the Comstock Law. "The mention of . . . these diseases is interdicted by the best forms of good society," lamented Morrow.[73]

Members of the medical profession called for an end to the veil of secrecy concerning venereal disease. They blamed ignorance and prudishness for the high incidence of syphilis and gonorrhea and their drastic impact on the family. "We are dealing with the solution of a problem," wrote Dr. Egbert Grandin, "where ignorance is *not* bliss but is misfortune, and where, therefore, it is folly not to be wise." The recent public health campaign for the eradication of tuberculosis provided an often-cited model for bringing venereal disease to public attention. As the long-term effects of syphilis and gonorrhea had become better known to physicians, the "conspiracy of silence" appeared increasingly intolerable. "I cry aloud against this state of affairs, for it is criminal, utterly criminal," wrote Dr. D.E. Standard of Missouri.[74]

Physicians increasingly sought publicity for the venereal problem, insisting that public enlightenment would have an immediate ameliorative impact on the incidence of venereal diseases. "No evil ever flourished long in the world's history after the limelight of knowledge had uncovered it," declared Grandin, "and I am convinced that neither gonorrhea nor syphilis can thrive in any community where force of public opinion is exerted against them." A heightened public consciousness, doctors argued with undaunted optimism, would alleviate the venereal problem. "Venereal disease must be made a subject of gossip," commented Dr. William A. Evans, "a gossip which must be instructive and elevating."[75]

In this spirit Prince Morrow founded the American Society for Sanitary and Moral Prophylaxis in early 1905 to "prevent the spread of diseases which have their origin in the social evil." Morrow envisioned the organization as a center for the diffusion of information about venereal disease. The grandiose title, however, belied an inauspicious beginning; only twenty-five physicians attended the meeting of the Society at the New York Academy of Medicine. This group, discouraged by the number of empty chairs, adjourned to a smaller room. Though the organization drew its first members primarily from the ranks of the medical profession, it soon attracted a number of prominent social reformers. Morrow encouraged lay membership, explaining, "To correct these evil conditions there should be a union of all the social forces which work for good in the community." Venereal disease, he contended, could not be considered solely within the physician's domain. "The evil is composite in its causes," Morrow argued, "and to be successfully combatted the cooperative efforts of different social groups is required." Like many Progressive voluntary organizations, the ASSMP attracted a coalition of support from those involved in the settlement movement, charity groups, moral reformers, and the church, in addition to physicians. Morrow, who became the first president of the ASSMP, sought to make it "the medium of communication between the medical profession and the public."[76] Membership in the Association doubled between 1906 and 1910, from 344 to almost 700, with women comprising 30 percent. Soon other cities including Philadelphia, Baltimore, Detroit, and Milwaukee established similar groups, and together they formed the American Federation for Sex Hygiene in 1910 under Morrow's leadership. The ASSMP remained, however, the most active and powerful affiliate.[77]

True to Progressive precepts, the ASSMP viewed education and publicity as a radical force, a virtual panacea. "An aroused public conscience would no longer tolerate such social infamies," declared Morrow. Citing the recently exposed scandals of the trusts, the insurance companies, and the proprietary medicines, he attempted to place the campaign against venereal disease in the mainstream of contemporary reform. Morrow advocated that the ASSMP become the vehicle for piercing the "conspiracy of silence":

> Now the role of muck-raker is considered neither dignified nor desirable, the work of delving in the filth of human weakness and depravity is unsavory, even repulsive; it can be undertaken only from a sense of duty, but the muck is there and needs to be raked. . . . The public should know that the introduction of venereal infection into marriage constitutes its chief social danger and at the same time makes up the saddest chapter in the martyrdom of women.[78]

Although the Association directed attention to the related issues of prostitution and public health, it initially concentrated on publicity and education to stay the tide of venereal disease. These physicians and reformers argued that, once enlightened about the causes and impact of venereal disease, citizens would realize their moral duty to remain chaste and healthy. Morrow believed that "sexual errors are due largely to this enforced ignorance." Robert N. Willson, the leader of the social hygiene movement in Philadelphia, called for the "sane, quiet, complete sex-education of the American people," as the only means of eliminating venereal disease.[79]

Although the ASSMP contended that parents should teach their children about sex, members frequently asserted that most parents were incapable of this task. Their failure to fulfill the responsibility of sex education left their children to the dubious wisdom of the streets. "If [curiosity] is not satisfied from pure sources," Prince Morrow explained, "it will be fed from impure and tainted sources." Willson endorsed this view, noting, "The guttersnipe is far more apt in gaining the ear of your boy than his pastor; his lesson sinks deeper and is more lasting!"[80] Reformers, therefore, increasingly demanded professional sex education in the school. In its first year the ASSMP established a Committee on Education which sponsored a full program including lectures and conferences, as well as pamphlets for parents and children. Morrow argued that sexual enlightenment was similar to other "former parental duties . . . [now] relegated to the educator." The ASSMP lobbied for sex instruction in the classroom, sexually segregated, with teachers of the same sex. By 1919 the U.S. Public Health Service had endorsed sex education in the schools, commenting, "As in many other instances, the school must take up the burden neglected by others."[81]

Late-Victorian notions of sexual morality infused all educational efforts. In particular, physicans considered the male sexual drive with foreboding. Among Progressives concerned with order and control, few instincts created so much apprehension. As Dr. Frederic H. Gerrish explained to the Massachusetts Medical Society, "If one is justified in ascribing motives to Nature, it may be fairly said that, in her anxiety to provide for the preservation of the race, she has oversexed mankind." Instruction for men thus centered on their duty to repress impulse, as well as their responsibility to women and "the race." Sex, many physicians had come to argue, should be limited exclusively to marriage and then, only for procreation; otherwise, it was merely a self-indulgent act. Rose Woodallen Chapmen detailed this view of male sexuality for her readers in the *Ladies' Home Journal*: "You will readily understand that power fraught with such tremendous consequences was not instituted for the gratification of the lower nature, but for procreation."[82] Eliminate sex outside marriage, physicians suggested, and a host of social maladies—from venereal disease to prostitution—would disappear.

Continence, therefore, became the hallmark of all sexual prescription. Members of the medical profession sought to dismiss the frequently cited view that men required sex to maintain their physical and psychic health. During the nineteenth century some commentators on sexual matters had advised that failure to "exercise" the sexual organs could lead to atrophy and weakness, eventual impotence, and physical decline.[83] Morrow and most late-Victorian physicians came to reject this view outright. Morrow pointed to instances of celibate laybrothers who, after leaving the convent and marrying, were "exceptionally prolific."[84] Indeed, most doctors now emphasized the necessity of not expending too much semen. According to these physicians, the testes secreted "cells" from the semen into the blood-stream that caused the development of masculine features, and reaching the brain, provided for intelligence, inventiveness, and imagination. Though they no longer suggested that masturbation could lead to debilitating physical illness, as some earlier experts had argued, they nevertheless warned that the practice did lead to loss of "self-respect, willpower, and mental force." Morrow concluded that "perfect inhibition is the sign of perfect health."[85]

In addition to violating values of discipline, restraint, and deferred gratification, the double standard contributed to the high incidence of venereal disease and innocent infections. "The double standard of sexual living is subversive of every standard of right and justice," claimed Dr. Winfield Scott Hall in his widely circulated primer, *Instead of Wild Oats*.[86] According to an overwhelming consensus of physicians, both partners should reach the marriage bed as virgins. Morrow, for instance, called for an end to the traditions of bachelor life, especially the raucous parties preceding marriage. All too often, he argued, these festivities would lead to a fateful liaison in the waning hours of bachelorhood, whose impact could be traced in a series of subsequent familial tragedies.

Physicians and educators urged that demands for sexual restraint be placed in the context of eugenics, and that restraint be considered a responsibility to the future of the race. Frank D. Watson of the New York School of Philanthropy reminded his students of the "sacredness of the germ-plasm": It was the man's "obligation and privilege," he contended, "to pass on that germ-plasm uncontaminated and unimpaired." The noted psychologist G. Stanley Hall remarked, "Man is prone to mortgage posterity by consuming, in his own self-gratification, energies that belong to the future."[87] In sum, Victorian physicians and psychologists had developed a highly-defined physiological argument for the need for sexual control.

Instructors did not, however, always base their appeal for sexual restraint on such high-minded premises. They often invoked the dread of infection as a powerful control on immorality and disease. In devising an educational approach, Morrow believed it valuable to describe the impact of venereal diseases in considerable detail. "I have always felt that the doctrine of consequences should be fully expounded as the fear of infection will sometimes restrain men from an evil life when educational or moral considerations fail," he explained. "As a matter of fact all hygienic precepts are based upon the consequences which result from the infraction of Nature's laws." Morrow considered fear—"fear of microbes"—the "protective genius of the human body." Only a well-developed awe of infection, suggested Dr. Abraham Wolbarst, could control the sexual drive in men. "The sexual instinct is imperative and will only listen to fear," he noted. "Ninety-nine out of one hundred persons could be frightened into being good by the fear of evil consequences." If educators established the proper attitude, physicians believed, men would think twice before pursuing the temptations of the double standard. "There should be taught such disgust and dread of these conditions," declared Dr. Margaret Cleaves, "that naught would induce the seeking of a polluted source for the sake of gratifying a controllable desire."[88] Seen by doctors as an authoritative ally in venereal disease control, the specter of unseemly infection would be raised throughout the twentieth century.

Given the emphasis on the "loathsome" aspects of venereal infection, some physicians expressed concern that sex education could have the undesired effect of causing "impure" thought. Max J. Exner, a well-known expert on sex education, cautioned that undue attention to the "sordid aspects of the sex question" would undoubtedly have a deleterious impact on impressionable adolescents. Exner suggested that in many colleges "sex thoughts and sex imaginations are allowed to dominate the stage." Sex educators hoped that instruction would curb "morbid curiosities," and erase sexuality from consciousness. Maurice Bigelow, who taught sexual hygiene at Columbia University Teachers College, considered day-dreaming about sex to be more dangerous than actual masturbation because it could be practiced constantly.[89] Dr. B.S. Talmey called this "mental masturbation." For certain individuals, Dr. Ferdinand C. Valentine contended, any education in sexual matters could be dangerous:

Each venereologist has met psychopaths to whom each curve in nature or art suggests female breasts, nates, or genitalia. For such not even the slightest education

would be advisable. Indeed, it would be harmful, because every step thereof would
to them contain lubricious suggestions.

Even so strong an advocate of sex education as Dr. Woods Hutchinson cautioned that much of the material produced by the sex hygiene campaign smacked
of "rank sensationalism, hysterical overstatement, sloppy sentimentality and
eroticism disguised as maudlin pseudopiety."[90]

Educators proposed that instruction in sex should be integrated into existing
courses so as not to attract undue interest. A frequent suggestion was the inclusion of sex hygiene in courses on biology and zoology. Doctors recommended
teaching about reproduction of plants in elementary education, eventually moving
on to animals. "The normal processes of reproduction in plants and lower animals should be taught," wrote Morrow, "unfolding the beauties and mysteries
of the great law of reproduction which runs through out all animate nature."
The essential goal was to impart new knowledge while maintaining an illusion
of non-communication. "Sex knowledge . . . can often be conveyed without
the slightest consciousness on their part that what they are receiving is sex instruction," explained Maurice Bigelow.[91]

The educational campaign confronted Victorian notions of "pure" womanhood. The "conspiracy of silence" had reigned supreme regarding women, and
many doctors felt women should be spared the "degrading" experience of receiving sexual knowledge. According to many reports, women often entered
marriage with no knowledge about sex. In the early years of the twentieth century, some doctors continued to suggest that sex education might disrupt marriages, because women might come to understand the cause of many of their
gynecological ailments.[92] Physicians of the Progressive years, however, now
questioned the wisdom of the *femina tabula rasa* in sexual matters. "For centuries, we, as physicians, have been covering up the fact that [the wife's] trouble lay at the door of her newly wedded husband, who, though demanding
chastity and purity of womanhood at her hands, brought to her the filthy gonorrheal virus," wrote Dr. D.E. Standard.[93] Education for women threatened a
significant break with the Victorian tradition which had placed a premium on
modesty and innocence among mothers.

Although physicians, reformers, and feminists called for the sexual enlightenment of women, educational precepts differed considerably from those
devised for men. Just as education for men followed the Victorian assumption
that men were sexually aggressive, instruction for women focused on the notion
of the passionless, dutiful woman. Because many doctors presumed that most
women were sexually anesthetic, they placed little emphasis on the need to instill control in the prescriptive literature directed to women. "There are but few
Messalinas, hopeless sexual perverts," noted Dr. Frederic H. Gerrish. "The vast
majority have no very pronounced sexual feelings; and a majority are altogether
deficient in this respect."[94] Indeed, this apparent lack of interest in sex among
women was typically cited as an aspect of their moral superiority.

Women, physicians urged, should be taught to demand a higher moral standard from men. Though sexual education for men centered on repression of

the sex drive, for women it concentrated primarily upon warnings about men. "Shall the mother advise her girls of their high privilege in life, or shall they learn first of these things in gossip, or as sometimes occurs, from an infected or infectious husband?" asked Dr. Robert N. Willson. "The woman, at least, must be given the opportunity of knowledge, and the right to intelligently choose between the diseased and the clean." Prince Morrow argued that only with informed motherhood could the crisis of the family be resolved: "These crimes against the family will continue until women know, as they have a perfect right to know, the facts which so vitally concern their own health and the health and lives of their children." Feminists joined the physicians in the sex hygiene movement, insisting upon their right to defend themselves against the hazards of the double standard of morality. As Charlotte Perkins Gilman told a meeting of the American Society for Sanitary and Moral Prophylaxis: "With motherhood we should have maturity and that knowledge which is power and protection."[95]

Doctors expressed the greatest concern about women of the working class, who they believed could more easily be led astray. In 1908 the Massachusetts Association of Boards of Health published a circular for young women, warning them of the possible consequences of premarital sex. "Among the most serious dangers which threaten young women, especially those of the wage-earning class," noted the pamphlet, "is the danger of sexual relations outside of marriage to which they are led by such harmless pleasures as dancing." Moreover, conditions in factories and slums often made prostitution seem an attractive alternative, according to many social workers. Doctors suggested that admonitions about illicit disease and unwanted pregnancy would prove valuable to women tempted to try the life of the streets. "The inducements in the way of dress, jewelry and amusements which are used to overcome the scruples instinctive to every woman would have far less weight if the consequences of indulgence were clearly understood," explained Dr. Margaret Cleaves.[96]

Although sex education during the Progressive years remained for the most part on a highly superficial and euphemistic level, it nevertheless provoked critics who decried the end of reticence in sexual matters regarding women. They particularly objected to the introduction of sex hygiene instruction in the schools, which the ASSMP advocated. When the Chicago School Board vetoed the inclusion of such a course in 1913, one critic explained their reasoning: "While there are certain things that children ought to learn it is far better that they should go wholly untaught than that the instruction should be given to them outside the family circle. There are some kinds of knowledge that become poisonous when administered by the wrong hands and sex hygiene is among them." Dr. George Whiteside suggested that sex education was inappropriate for girls of a genteel background. "Let us spare the sympathetic sensibilities of girls of the better class," he declared. "Why tell them of venereal disease or loathsome perversions of the sex drive?"[97] Whiteside conceded that instruction should be offered for "girls who must protect themselves, who have no one to look out for them."

Critics charged with some justification that sex education programs could lead to a phobic response among women toward marriage and men. As Mabel S. Ulrich commented:

> I deplore the custom of many "sex lecturers" of dealing out to girl audiences representing all ages, overwhelming statistics as to the probable immorality of fathers, brothers, lovers, and friends. To convince a sensitive adolescent girl that ninety per cent of all the men she has loved and trusted are tainted physically and mentally is a sorry victory for our "cause"—even if it were true.

Miriam C. Gould, a psychologist at the University of Pittsburgh, studied the reaction of a class of adolescent girls to instruction about venereal disease, pregnancy, and prostitution. In the class of twenty-five, eight were "astounded" by a discussion of illegitimate births because they had "supposed it impossible for unmarried people to have children." After learning about venereal infections and their repercussions, the girls responded as follows:

> Three were so disgusted that they have avoided the acquirement of any further knowledge on the subject. Three claimed they were impersonally curious and deliberately sought further information. Ten were impelled to be cautious in frequenting public toilet rooms, in using public drinking cups, in kissing or permitting any other bodily contact with men. Six of these mentioned they thereafter regarded dancing as dangerous. Two were extremely anxious for assurance of their own non-infection. Eleven developed a pronounced repulsion for men, although prior to this they had enjoyed their companionship.

Gould's message was clear: fear of sexuality could have effects which even the social hygienists did not desire. As Talcott Williams concluded, "It is a very serious responsibility to exaggerate the perils of social diseases in such manner as to increase the obstacles to marriage."[98]

The American Society for Sanitary and Moral Prophylaxis insisted, however, on the benefits of their educational programs. Morrow assured the public that the sex hygiene campaign was "not intended to ride rough-shod over conventional propriety or break down the barriers erected by good taste." Physicians asserted that well-informed women would not become victims of the double standard of morality when they entered matrimony. "When the girl reaches the nubile age she will demand a certificate of sexual cleanliness—and it is her right to have it—from the man who seeks to become her lord and master, and too often becomes her inoculator with gonorrheal virus," wrote Dr. Egbert Grandin. Indeed, Morrow contended that women required this knowledge if they were properly to fulfill their domestic duties. Education, he argued, would not violate Victorian propriety but restore "civilized" morality:

> Women—modest, refined, the most womenly of women—are not offended by our plainness of speech, their feeling is not one of outraged modesty, but of indignation . . . that matters which so materially concern their health and life of their children have always been concealed from them by the medical profession.[99]

The efforts to institute sex education during the Progressive years had considerable success. A study conducted by the U.S. Bureau of Education in 1922 indicated that 46.6 percent of all secondary schools offered some form of instruction in sex hygiene. The ASSMP maintained figures on the number of pamphlets they distributed as carefully as if they were for vaccinations. By 1913 the Association and its branches had published and distributed hundreds of thousands of flyers with such titles as "How My Uncle, the Doctor, Instructed Me in Matters of Sex," and "A Straight Talk with Employers and Leaders of Organized Labor." Members of the educational crusade reported that, as a result of their efforts, immorality—presumably sexual activity—was on the wane, especially among the young. Dr. James Pedersen, a leading member of the ASSMP, stated that "immorality in many colleges had been reduced by 20 to 40 per cent." The medical director at Columbia University, for example, suggested that because of the sex hygiene program there the rate of venereal infection never reached more than 4 percent of the student body.[100]

Ultimately, however, the necessity for sexual control underpinned all educational efforts. In the perceived high rates of venereal disease, physicians saw not only dangers to the family, but a more general and ominous collapse of late-Victorian morality. The constellation of sexual values which the social hygienists prescribed—repression, continence, discipline—mirrored the values of middle-class Victorian society and economy.[101] Educational programs were designed less to enlighten than to shore up standards they considered under attack; to return restraint and order to the relations between the sexes. These physicians, trained in a time thought to represent the height of civilized morality, offered no new solutions to the venereal peril. They destroyed the conspiracy of silence—a seemingly radical act—to uphold the conservative sexual mores of their time.

7

Although social hygienists looked to education as the ultimate means of combatting venereal disease, Progressives centered their immediate attention on the repression of prostitution. Physicians and social reformers associated venereal disease, almost exclusively, with the vast population of prostitutes in American cities. They agreed that when a man left the moral path the road usually led to the prostitute, who they argued was the most prolific source of venereal infections. In comparison to prostitution, explained Dr. Ludwig Weiss, "all other modes of propagation [of sexual diseases] are almost *nil.*" Estimates suggested that from 75 to 90 percent of all prostitutes harbored infections. Dr. Katharine Bement Davis, Commissioner of Corrections for New York City, reported, for example, that 70 percent of all women sentenced to the city workhouse for prostitution had either gonorrhea or syphilis. At the Bedford Hills State Reformatory for Women more than 80 percent of the inmates between the ages of sixteen and thirty were found to be venereally diseased. Davis labeled these women "plague spots."[102] These reports of the high rates of infection among prostitutes confirmed for many the notion of two types of women—good and bad, pure and impure, innocent and sensual. Venereal epidemiology was socially constructed upon this bifurcation. Accordingly, an "innocent" woman could only get venereal disease from a "sinful" man. But the man could only get venereal disease from a "fallen woman." This uni-directional mode of transmission reflected prevailing attitudes rather than any bacteriologic reality.

The knowledge that prostitution was not just a moral threat to the civilized sexual code but also a health threat to the family gave the social purity crusade new impetus. Reformers now added the authoritative voice of science and hygiene to the moralistic claims against prostitution sounded in the nineteenth century.[103] Physicians had come to realize an ugly irony: that the double standard of sexual morality—which countenanced periodic visits to prostitutes to spare the "pure" woman from the "animal" passions of the man—actually led to the woman's demise through venereal infection. Indeed, Prince Morrow coined the euphemism "social disease" because the infections were spread through the "social evil," namely, prostitution. These infections, Morrow declared, "link the debased harlot and the virtuous wife in the kinship of a common disease."[104]

In the first decade of the twentieth century virtually every American city possessed a so-called "tenderloin" district where prostitutes openly solicited customers. Bordellos often operated under the protective eye of city and police officials. San Francisco's "Barbary Coast," Washington D.C.'s "Hooker's Division," Chicago's "Levee," and New Orleans's "Storyville" constituted only the nation's most notorious red-light districts. During the late nineteenth century, municipal governments anxious to segregate vice activities officially designated such discrete areas so as not to offend the moral sensibilities of those respectable citizens who wished to avoid this commerce. Purity crusaders had long fought against these enclaves, but without great success. Now armed with the medical knowledge of the impact of venereal disease on the family, as well as new sociological methods to investigate and root out the evil, vice crusaders unleashed a full-scale attack on urban prostitution. "No great wrong has ever risen more clearly to the social consciousness of a generation," noted Jane Addams of Hull House in 1911, "than that of commercialized vice in the consciousness of ours."[105]

Nearly every American metropolis organized vice commissions between 1910 and 1916 to investigate and combat prostitution. These groups relied heavily on expert medical testimony in developing their indictment of urban vice. All reports emphasized the impact of prostitution upon the health of the family. "The effect of vice upon the physical health of the community is receiving at present more attention than any other feature of the problem," noted New York's Committee of Fifteen, the first major vice commission established in 1900. The group concluded that it was the community's responsibility to "disembarrass" itself from venereal diseases by controlling vice.[106] The Chicago Vice Commission, which conducted a nationally publicized investigation a decade later, expressed a similar idea in more lurid prose:

> Prostitution is pregnant with disease, a disease infecting not only the guilty but contaminating the innocent wife and child in the home with sickening certainty almost inconceivable; a disease to be feared as a leprous plague; a disease scattering misery broadcast, and leaving in its wake sterility, insanity, paralysis, and the blinded eyes of little babes, the twisted limbs of deformed children, degradation, physical rot and mental decay.[107]

The vice commissions unanimously condemned the notion of sexual necessity for men as a myth that encouraged vice.

The commissions' reports identified the moral crisis as one peculiar to urban life. The theme of the anonymity of urban existence recurred in their assessments of the prostitution problem, which frequently recounted the plight of the young man who came to the city only to find loneliness and low wages. As the Committee of Fifteen explained:

> The main external check upon a man's conduct, the opinion of his neighbors, which has such a powerful influence in the country or small town, tends to disappear. In a great city one has no neighbors. No man knows the doings of even his close friends; few men care what the secret life of their friends may be. Thus, with his moral sensibilities blunted the young man is left free to follow his own inclinations.[108]

These inclinations, according to the commissions, all too often led to the brothel and ultimately to medical and moral degeneration. Moreover, in cities, where the cost of raising and supporting a family was high, eligible bachelors often postponed marriage, which many doctors now suggested contributed to more frequent premarital associations with prostitutes and a rising incidence of venereal infections.[109]

The commissions insisted that America's burgeoning metropolises provided ubiquitous opportunities for social contacts which could lead to moral decline. Not only were dance halls and theaters suspect, but parks, hotels, and department stores were also cited as providing outlets for debauchery. As Dr. J.H. Landis commented, "The occasional contact of the sexes found in rural districts has given way to practically constant contact in the cities." Landis feared what he called "sexual explosions" in the urban environment. The vice commissions lamented the passing of what they believed had been a rigorous, uniform moral code. Although much of their rhetoric appears anti-urban in retrospect, most of the members of these committees were long-time city dwellers, businessmen and civic leaders, alarmed by the changes they had observed in their midst.[110] Venereal disease, reported in epidemic proportions, seemed to confirm the existence of this more general cultural crisis, the chaotic, alien nature of the modern city.

The vice commissions also examined the reasons why women became prostitutes. Some suggested that they were either enticed or forced into commercialized prostitution through the subterranean "white slave trade." The idea of "slavery" conformed with Victorian notions of feminine purity which held that no woman would enter such a life except under bondage. Muckrakers and purity crusaders frequently drew an analogy between the white slave trade and the cold efficiency of American industry which had recently come to light in press exposés. Borrowing from the anti-monopoly rhetoric of Progressivism, the *Survey* referred to commercialized prostitution operations as "vice trusts" that, they believed, should be "busted."[111] George Kibbe Turner, a well-known Progressive journalist, explained that prostitution in Chicago had been organized "from the supplying of young girls to the drugging of older and less salable women out of existence—with all the nicety of modern industry." He concluded, "As in the stockyards, not one shred of flesh is wasted." The white slave hysteria that swept the nation between 1907 and 1911 culminated in the passage of the Mann Act by Congress in 1910, which forbade the transportation of women across state lines for immoral purposes.[112] Just as the interstate commerce clause had been used to attack the trusts, so too was it invoked to attack vice.

Upon investigation, however, little solid evidence of a fully organized traffic in women ever materialized, and reformers looked to somewhat more complex causes to explain prostitution. As the prominent vice investigator George J. Kneeland noted, "The psychology of the relation of prostitute to pimp is a complicated one, difficult to understand. . . . A spark of affection lives at the heart of this ghastly relation." Kneeland reported virtually no indication of locked doors and barred windows in his detailed studies. But the image of enforced labor remained prominent, especially among feminists who recognized the essentially exploitative nature of prostitution. Maude E. Miner, secretary of the New York Probation Association, though admitting that girls were rarely physically abducted, contended that "through the loss of freedom and will of action, they have been bound to prostitution." Miner concluded, "Their demoralization of character has constituted moral enslavement."[113]

Reformers increasingly looked to the social and economic conditions of the city to explain a woman's turn to prostitution. Again, the anonymity of the city was cited as an important element. Jane Addams noted with sympathy:

> Loneliness and detachment which the city tends to breed in its inhabitants is easily intensified in such a girl into isolation and desolating feelings of belonging nowhere. . . . At such moments a black oppression, the instinctive fear of solitude will send a lonely girl restlessly to walk the streets even when "she is too tired to stand" and where her desire for companionship in itself constitutes a grave danger.

Other observers emphasized that poor housing conditions, particularly in the immigrant ghettos, often led to prostitution. "Who will dare to deny that the thin partition walls and often promiscuous mixing of the sexes in the crowded quarters tend to the demoralization of the young girl blossoming into womanhood?" demanded the prominent New York physician Adolphus S. Knopf. The vice commissions suggested that the transformation of American industry, which brought more women to the workplace, also encouraged prostitution. "Another form [of prostitution] is closely connected with industry," explained the Committee of Fifteen. "A season of non-employment presents them with the alternatives of starvation or prostitution." Moreover, prostitution offered more lucrative rewards to women forced to support themselves and their families than did employment in industry. "Is it any wonder," asked the Chicago Vice Commission, "that a tempted girl who receives only six dollars per week working with her hands sells her body for twenty-five dollars per week when she learns there is demand for it and men are willing to pay the price?" Dr. Ludwig Weiss stressed the problem of the single woman separated from her family, concluding, "The strife of self-support has exposed her to dangers against which she must develop defensive measures."[114]

Although the vice commissions often expressed sympathy for the plight of the prostitute, rarely could they offer substantive assistance. The environmental determinants which they identified as contributing to vice were beyond the scope of the commissions that concentrated on exposing conditions. They gave little if any consideration, for example, to the impact of venereal disease on the health of those women forced to take to the streets. The life expectancy of prostitutes was reportedly very short, for many suffered from the consequences of the sexually transmitted diseases that they were attacked for communicating.[115] Although many of the commissions suggested that women were victims of prostitution, most of the proposed remedies, especially the repression of street solicitation, labeled them as criminals.[116] The vice commissions operated under the Progressive assumption that the revelation of evil would, in itself, have an immediately positive impact.

By the first years of the twentieth century, two opposing strategies for dealing with prostitution had evolved. First, many physicians who believed that prostitution could never be eliminated argued in favor of state regulation. This system, which many French and German cities had adopted, called for registration and periodic medical inspection of all prostitutes to insure their health. Under this plan, known as *reglementation*, houses of prostitution were limited to a specific section of the city and unregistered women, "clandestine" prostitutes, were subject to arrest and fine. Some prominent doctors argued that regulation was the only sanitary, scientific means of controlling venereal disease.[117] In seeming disagreement with Victorian moral notions of perfectibility and self-control, these physicians, many of whom had trained in the European capitals where inspection of prostitutes by public health officials constituted modern hygienic practice, accepted the indomitable nature of the male sex drive and the age-old recognition of the inevitability of prostitution. During the last decades of the nineteenth century, under the influence of these doctors, several American cities proposed ordinances requiring official examinations, and such a system was actually adopted in St. Louis for a brief period in 1870.[118]

The idea of regulated prostitution, however, could not withstand the force of public opinion, and was soon held increasingly suspect by physicians and reformers alike. The complete repression of prostitution emerged as the social reformers' primary goal. When Prince Morrow founded the American Society for Sanitary and Moral Prophylaxis in 1905, for example, he was firmly opposed to regulation. This coalition among reformers on the prostitution problem was probably the result of a growing body of medical literature that suggested the inadequacy of medical inspection—a prostitute could become infected between exams—as well as a desire to attract non-medical reformers to the social hygiene movement. These reformers, veterans of the purity crusades of the late nineteenth century, the settlements, and urban Progressivism, refused to compromise with evil.

They found regulation, quite simply, anathema to the Progressive moral code. First, it suggested a tacit acceptance of the double standard of sexual morality. Second, state regulation of prostitution essentially endorsed the exploitation of women to meet the sexual needs of men. And third, it implicitly validated the notion that the male sex drive could not be controlled, a view subversive of

Progressive ideals of education and reform.[119] As the Committee of Fifteen explained, "State recognition and regulation of prostitution would unquestionably tend to confirm the already common opinion that secret indulgence is an imperative need." In addition, physicians came to realize that regulation threatened their rising professional status by offending public opinion and lowering professional standards. "If there is a lower, more contemptible role that could be played by a medical man than that of official inspector of bawds, I do not know what it is," wrote Dr. G. Frank Lydston. "As compared with such an occupation, that of professional abortionist or the advertising newspaper fakir would be kingly." The vice commissions unanimously rejected regulation in favor of complete repression of prostitution. The Chicago group devised the oft-cited motto: "Constant and Persistent Repression of Prostitution the Immediate Method: Absolute Annihilation the Ultimate Ideal"[120]

Despite the consensus among social hygienists against regulating prostitution, the debate erupted again in New York in 1910. On June 25, the same day that Congress enacted the Mann Act, the New York State Legislature passed the Inferior Courts Act, devised to deal more effectively with prostitution. In addition to establishing a night court for women and requiring the fingerprinting of convicted prostitutes, the act, popularly known as the Page Law, included a provision that called for the medical examination of women found guilty of soliciting. If infected with a venereal disease, the woman would be detained during treatment until she was determined to be noncontagious.[121] This provision—section 79—created a furor within the social hygiene campaign and among women's groups because it was interpreted as tantamount to state-regulated prostitution.

"Is there any distinction between the details of the French system and the details of the Page Law? . . . I fail to see it," declared Columbia University economist E.R.A. Seligman, a member of the Committee of Fifteen. Seligman formulated his critique on the basis of the theory of supply and demand. The solution to the venereal problem, he contended, was not to treat prostitutes only to return them to the streets. Public belief in the health of these women would have the effect of *raising* demand for their services. "The imagined improvement in the quality of the services offered for sale will tend to attract purchasers who would otherwise be somewhat suspicious or on their guard," Seligman explained..[122] He advised measures such as education, which he hoped would lower demand, and better economic opportunities for women to contract the supply of prostitutes.

Supporters of section 79 claimed that comparisons with *reglementation* were spurious; prostitution remained illegal, and the act merely provided for diseased women to obtain medical care. Prostitutes, they contended, had a right to be restored to health.[123] Social hygienists and feminists, however, recognized that the law's penalties fell exclusively on women and viewed this as a tacit endorsement of the double standard of sexual morality. Women were punished for engaging in prostitution, men were not; no law required that infected men be treated. As an impassioned Prince Morrow explained:

[The Page Law] is directed against a particular class of women for the protection of a particular class of men. Not the good citizens who lead regular lives and to whom the prostitute with her cortege of infections carries no menace, but for the protection of the licentious class of men who seek these women for immoral purposes. . . .

The fatal defect of every sanitary scheme to control venereal disease has been that the masculine spreader of contagion has been entirely ignored as mythical or practically nonexistent; the woman has been regarded not only as the chief offender against morality, but the responsible cause of disease; all repressive measures to stamp out the diseases of vice have been directed against the woman alone.[124]

Morrow called this the "double standard of sanitation."

Despite the clear merits of Morrow's argument, a basic assumption lurking behind the attacks on section 79 was that venereal disease among prostitutes served as an effective discouragement to immorality. Fear of venereal disease, according to these reformers, contributed to sexual morality and therefore should not in all cases be removed as a threat—even if at great personal cost to the prostitute. In this light, venereal disease was seen as *serving* the sexual order by deterring "immoral" behavior. Indeed, the debate regarding the Page Law and regulation in general suggested the possibility that venereal disease—usually acquired through a voluntary or "immoral" act—was of a totally different nature than other infectious diseases which found their victims on an apparently random basis. "Venereal disease seeks no man," declared Morrow, "it must be sought in order to be acquired."[125] This belief, that the individual must in the end be responsible for the risk of visiting a prostitute, had the effect of separating venereal disease from most other public health campaigns.

In June 1911 the New York Court of Appeals found section 79 unconstitutional, ruling that it violated due process by making the physician's diagnosis binding on the court. The legal battle had been supported by the social hygiene movement and organized women's groups.[126] Although the rejection of all forms of regulation meant that repression of prostitution became official policy in most cities, on the eve of World War I prostitution still flourished, if less openly.

8

The battle against the Page Law had united the forces of social hygiene and anti-vice reformers. In previous years considerable suspicion had existed between these related movements. Prince Morrow and the American Society for Sanitary and Moral Prophylaxis had long contended that purity crusaders who concentrated solely on the repression of prostitution failed to see the complex nature of the problems posed by venereal disease. Social hygienists believed that the best solution for overcoming vice and disease rested in sex education and public enlightenment. Anti-vice organizations such as the American Vigilance Association, formed in 1912, centered attention on white slavery and the "traffic in women." According to Morrow these groups were "only lopping off one of the branches of the mighty evil."[127] Conversely, purity organizations feared that the social hygiene movement, controlled by physicians and sanitarians, was likely to accept vice as unalterable and to address it solely as a medical problem. Through the vice commissions and the Page Law controversy these two groups were brought together, and reformers began to see the problems of venereal disease and prostitution as inextricably linked.

Calls for a national organization to unite these movements began to be heard. Prince Morrow's death in March 1913 cleared the way for vice crusaders and medical reformers to strike an official alliance. In October, leaders of the American Vigilance Association and the American Federation for Sex Hygiene met in Buffalo to form the American Social Hygiene Association. Grace Dodge and John D. Rockefeller, Jr., two vigorous supporters of the anti-vice crusade, engineered the merger. Rockefeller suggested that consolidation would increase efficiency. "As a business man I naturally appreciate the gain which combination effects," he explained. Charles W. Eliot, former president of Harvard University, agreed to become the first president of the organization at Rockefeller's request. Eliot, however, only served as a titular head. Daily operations were directed by James Bronson Reynolds, a New York attorney active in vice investigations, and William F. Snow, a California physician and public health official. Their joint leadership reflected the organization's foundation in compromise, as well as a residual tension between the two forces.[128]

Rockefeller provided the greatest financial assistance to the Association during its early years, contributing $5,000 per year between 1913 and 1916 and $10,000 from 1916 to 1918, as well as helping to raise the remainder of the ASHA's $60,000 annual budget. Rockefeller's interest in the problems of vice and disease dated back to 1910, when he acted as foreman of a special grand jury appointed to investigate the white slave trade in New York. The jury heard testimony from a wide variety of sources; although evidence was developed that showed that girls had been abducted and sold, no proof of a syndicate was ever demonstrated.[129] His experience on this jury, however, brought young Rockefeller to the center of social hygiene activities.

Rockefeller had come to believe that the hysteria surrounding white slavery did a disservice to responsible concerns about venereal disease and prostitution. After his service on the grand jury, he began to devise plans for a public commission to study prostitution and the "frightful ravages of venereal disease." He soon became discouraged, however, by the significant political considerations involved in the forming of such a group. Instead, he proposed a permanent organization to investigate the problem and formulate public policies. Together with Paul Warburg, a well-known banker, and Starr Murphy, a prominent lawyer, he established the Committee of Three to review potential projects. In 1911 they created the Bureau of Social Hygiene, which Rockefeller explained would be a permanent, non-political organization dedicated to studying prostitution and venereal disease "scientifically," and "continuously making warfare against the forces of evil."[130]

The Bureau emphasized rational, efficient investigations by experts and scientific management as the primary antidote to vice and disease. As a press release explained, "The name 'Rockefeller' stands for a type of efficiency and thoroughness of work."[131] In its first years, from 1911 to 1917 the Bureau sponsored and later published four major studies that were prototypical works of Progressive social science: first, George J. Kneeland's *Commercialized Prostitution in New York City*, a monograph which resembled the vice commission reports without the lurid prose and pat answers; second, Abraham Flexner's *Prostitution in Europe*, a forceful attack on continental systems of regulated prostitution which put to rest, once and for all, debate regarding the viability of *reglementation* in the United States; third, Raymond B. Fosdick's *European Police Systems*, a study which suggested that professionalization of police offered the best opportunity to uproot graft and vice; and fourth, Harold B. Woolston's *Prostitution in the United States*, a comprehensive survey of vice conditions on the eve of World War I.[132] These books provided the informational base that Rockefeller contended was the first step in formulating a public response to vice. Rigorously researched and dispassionately written, they shaped opinion within the social hygiene campaign and encouraged a more "professional" approach to reform.

The Bureau also sponsored a variety of experimental social programs in an attempt to illuminate new methods for civic institutions to adopt in the battle against prostitution. In 1912 the Bureau underwrote the establishment of a Laboratory of Social Hygiene at Bedford Hills, under the direction of Katharine B. Davis, agreeing to allocate up to $200,000. Women sentenced to this reformatory underwent a battery of physical and psychological tests aimed at isolating factors which contributed to prostitution. Through these studies, the Laboratory hoped to develop categories of women deemed capable of reformation. Moreover, the Bureau attempted through this research to develop successful methods for the treatment and rehabilitation of female offenders reflective of an emerging trend toward definition of criminal activity in therapeutic terms.[133]

The Laboratory's research soon came under the influence of eugenicists anxious to demonstrate that most prostitutes showed a genetic predisposition to sexual promiscuity and "psychopathic tendencies." Reports circulated that more than half of all women who became prostitutes were feebleminded and required lifelong custodial care. Charles B. Davenport, the leader of the American eugenics movement, endorsed these findings, noting, "Evidence is accumulating to show that the primary factor is an inherited predisposition toward an exceptionally active sexual life. . . . The heightened licentiousness is favored by an additional germinal determinant that less licentious persons do not have."[134] Eugenicist use of the Bureau's research signaled an important change from the socioeconomic explanations for the causes of prostitution voiced by the vice commissions.

The Bureau of Social Hygiene marked a shift from the moralistic, dramatic objectives of the purity crusades toward an emphasis on instrumental reform that was efficient, scientific, elitist. Scientific, hereditarian notions of crime and disease largely displaced explanations which gave weight to environment and individual choice. Ultimately, the Bureau betrayed a fundamental mistrust of public efforts, which Rockefeller had come to believe rested on the whimsy of politics. Though Rockefeller had few objections to the moralistic elements of

the social hygiene movement, he sought to rationalize the claims of the movement by adding a rigorous social science component. Enlightened philanthropy, he contended, would identify the programs and lead to the scientific
achievements necessary to end vice.

9

In the first decade of the twentieth century a series of pathbreaking discoveries
in German laboratories revolutionized the American medical profession's ability to deal with syphilis. These advances, in conjunction with the efforts of the
social hygiene movement, enhanced the status of scientific medicine in matters
of sexuality and disease. The instrumental ideals of efficiency, prevention, and
cure soon began to influence professional thinking concerning the sexually
transmitted diseases. In 1905 Fritz Schaudinn and Eric Hoffmann, two German laboratory researchers, identified the causative agent of syphilis, a pale,
spiral microorganism, which they called *Spirochaeta pallida*. The following year
August Wassermann and his colleagues, Albert Neisser and Carl Bruck, published an account of their successful efforts in developing a diagnostic test for
syphilis. The exam they devised made it possible to detect the spirochete in
blood samples through the employment of a complement-fixation reaction, a
chemical process based on recent advances in immunology.[135] American physicians greeted the reports of this work with praise. "Where formerly we were
guessing at the nature of a given lesion or condition," explained Homer F. Swift,
"we are now able to state with a fair degree of accuracy whether the condition
is syphilitic or not." Advances in microscopic technique had also moved gonorrhea diagnostics out of the nether world of medical subjectivity.[136] As late as
1912, however, few physicians had the necessary laboratory and technical facilities to conduct these tests.

The therapeutic coup came in 1909 when Nobel laureate immunologist Paul
Ehrlich, working with the assistance of Sahachiro Hata, discovered Salvarsan,
the first effective treatment for syhpilis. Ehrlich had searched for methods of
assisting the body's natural immunologic response to disease. "The antibodies
are magic bullets," he explained, "which find their targets by themselves" In
the laboratory, he sought to create chemical compounds which would serve as
"magic bullets" against specific diseases. The 606th experiment resulted in an
arsenic compound which, when injected into syphilitic rabbits, caused the dramatic disappearance of symptoms, and subsequent research with human subjects confirmed the drug's effectiveness. With the discovery of Salvarsan, also
known as "606" or arsphenamine, Ehrlich initiated the modern age of chemo-
therapeutics.[137]

Physicians greeted Ehrlich's announcement of his work in 1910 with tremendous enthusiasm and a dash of circumspection. By early 1911, a number
of American physicians had experimented with the drug on their syphilitic patients. Though most reported the miraculous effect of Ehrlich's compound, a
number of untoward side-effects also came to light. Some patients suffered from
the agent's high toxicity, and by 1914, 109 deaths attributed to Salvarsan treat-

ments had been recorded in the medical literature.[138] Salvarsan required intravenous injection, a technique involving surgical procedures with which many American general practitioners had little experience. Physicians who could not locate a suitable vein often had the effect of discouraging patients from complying with the required course of injections which treatment demanded. As Dr. John Stokes noted, "Even the poor can scarcely be expected to submit with good grace to repeated barbarities offered in the name of medicine."[139] In 1912 continued research by Ehrlich resulted in a less toxic but also somewhat less effective compound which became known as Neosalvarsan or "914." This agent was widely available in the United States by 1915, and many of the best-trained physicians introduced it into their practices with great success. Universal acceptance, however, probably did not occur until the 1920s, and some physicians continued to rely on mercury.

If syphilis could be properly diagnosed and effectively treated, as physicians now claimed, then it could be placed on the same footing by boards of health as other contagious diseases. Scientific advances opened the way for state and local public health officials to take a more aggressive stand in the fight against venereal diseases and to encourage the growth of the public health field. In the period around the turn of the century, public health had been transformed from a broadly based movement dedicated to environmental reform to a more narrowly defined program emphasizing science, technique, and professionalism.[140] As venereal disease came to be perceived as a scientific problem with a scientific solution, officials centered attention on communicable diseases and the bacteriological revolution that promised their demise. Specific remedies for specific diseases became the hallmark of the modern biomedical approach to public health. This shift, however, resulted in a conflict between private practitioners and new, highly trained professionals who were committed to public health and disease prevention. As public health boards attempted to assert their authority over the venereal problem, this battle over the proprietary right to the responsibility for health care escalated.

Although state and city governments had taken action to combat some infectious diseases, venereal infections had remained outside their jurisdiction, and certainly had not received attention on the federal level. Even after diagnostic and therapeutic techniques had been developed, many physicians and laypeople continued to assert that in cases of sexually transmitted diseases the medical secret must remain inviolate, precluding any involvement by state or municipal officials. "It seems incredible that up to the present syphilis and gonococcus infection are, officially speaking, non-existent, and that as far as the national, and to a greater extent the municipal, authorities are concerned, are deserving only of contempt or complete disregard," noted Dr. Robert Willson in 1912. Increasingly, however, health reformers and public health officials suggested that venereal diseases—like other serious communicable diseases—should be placed under the purview of boards of health. As Dr. Louis Chargin of the New York City Board of Health argued, "Venereal diseases should be classed and dealt with exactly as is any other group of communicable diseases."[141]

Public health officers contended that venereal disease should be considered scientifically and dispassionately as a health threat rather than a moral threat. "It is said to advertise the marvelous effects of Salvarsan, and to place it within the reach of the poor is to place a premium upon vice and to absolve the syphilitic from the just punishment of his sins," observed Dr. Allan J. McLaughlin, a Massachusetts public health authority. "As health officers let us be practical and consider syphilis as a public health problem, leaving the academic discussion of its moral and social aspects to others." Dr. Hermann Biggs, director of the New York City Board of Health and a leading figure in the American scientific hygiene movement, concurred with McLaughlin, explaining, "The moral and social aspects of the problem do not primarily concern the sanitary authorities." The program Biggs devised for New York emphasized laboratory diagnostics and care only for the indigent so as not to offend private physicians who believed public health activities a threat to their practices.[142]

The primary method employed in public efforts to control infectious diseases required that physicians report cases to the authorities. In the last decades of the nineteenth century many municipal and state boards of health demanded that doctors notify them of all patients with serious communicable diseases. This provided officials with the information necessary to locate sources of infection, trace epidemics, and quarantine infectious persons. Moreover, with statistical indications of the rates of disease, local and state governments could better allocate their health care resources.[143] By 1907 Massachusetts had stipulated that some sixteen diseases were reportable, including tuberculosis, measles, meningitis, and whooping cough. Venereal diseases, however, remained unaccounted.

Public health officials soon began to demand that venereal diseases should be subject to these regulations. As William F. Snow explained, "All the general arguments for complete reporting of other communicable diseases apply with equal force to venereal disease."[144] In 1911 under Snow's leadership, California became the first state to take action, requiring all physicians to report cases by number to protect the patient's identity. The New York City Board of Health enacted a regulation in February 1912 that obligated all public hospitals to report venereal cases under their care, and under which physicians were *requested* to report by number. Although anonymous reporting precluded rigorous case-tracing, officials hoped it would deflate the possible objections of practitioners. Moreover, the emphasis on the treatment of indigent cases as the proper domain of public health also sought to reassure physicians. The implicit assumption behind the New York ordinance was that patients who could afford to pay for treatment could be trusted not to spread their infections. In justifying the requirement for institutional reporting, Dr. Charles Bolduan noted, "It may be assumed that the institutional cases constitute the poorer and more ignorant class, and the class most in need of supervision." By July 1913, five states had enacted regulations requiring that venereal diseases be reported. Vermont devised the most unusual plan, calling for the reporting of all cases, as well as providing a twenty-five cent fee to physicians for each case.[145]

Public health authorities quickly found that few physicians cooperated with these requirements. "The ten year long opposition to the reporting of tuberculosis will doubtless appear a mild breeze compared with the stormy protest against the sanitary surveillance of the venereal diseases," commented Hermann Biggs. He estimated that 90 percent of the city's physicians objected to the regulation. Only 1,500 of the city's 8,000 doctors reported treating cases of venereal disease during the first year that the ordinance was in effect, and even this number soon decreased. Despite frequent assurances that the Board of Health had no interest in treating cases already under proper care, private physicians reported only 103 cases of venereal disease to authorities in 1915.[146]

Doctors in private practice contended that venereal reporting held no benefits and, indeed, would ultimately hinder the control of these diseases. Unlike cases in which registered patients could be quarantined during the infectious stages of their diseases, most venereal patients remained ambulatory and treatment could be lengthy. "No man is going to subject himself to quarantine which would expose his immoral conduct and which in most instances would cost him his position, and in many cases involve him in domestic litigation," commented the New York State Journal of Medicine in an editorial protesting reporting. Physicians also frequently suggested that reporting of venereal cases would encourage patients to turn to quacks and unscrupulous druggists for assistance. As a doctor from Buffalo explained, "The treatment of venereal diseases has too long been left in the hands of charlatans and leeches who suck out the gold while they frighten their victims into silence." Most often, critics of reporting, overlooking the claims of anonymity in reporting measures, complained that the regulation demanded the abrogation of the "medical secret." Dr. A. T. Bristow, a prominent New York City physician, argued that "the statute which forbids a physician to divulge the secrets of a patient . . . would prevent the physician from complying with the order of the Board of Health." Hugh Cabot, a urologist well-known for his progressive views, nevertheless harshly criticized venereal reporting. He expressed a central concern, noting, "If physicians are required to report these patients by name, they will in short time, if they are honest, have no patients to report."[147]

Even if physicians did report their cases of venereal disease, facilities for treatment were not generally available. Nothing testified to the opprobrium still attached to syphilis and gonorrhea at the turn of the century so much as the fact that many hospitals and clinics refused to accept patients suffering from these ailments. During the nineteenth century when lay trustees established hospital policy, venereal patients were often prohibited admission on the grounds that they were not worthy of assistance. "There is an old-fashioned feeling in Boston that venereal disease is not a respectable thing to have to do with under any circumstances," explained the Boston Medical and Surgical Journal, "that the victims are suffering for their sins or those of their fathers, and that it is almost flying in the face of providence to assist them." In 1822 for example, the Massachusetts General Hospital excluded all venereal sufferers from admission; from 1851 to 1881, syphilitics were admitted upon the special approval of the board of trustees, but required to pay doubled rates. Revised rules in 1881 again forbade admission.[148] Similar policies denied venereal patients access to medical care in other cities. "It is certainly most discreditable that out of many thousand hospital beds in the city of New York only less than two hundred are available for the care of the venereal patients," observed Dr. Charles Bolduan in 1913. A Philadelphia physician explained that highly contagious cases of syphilis were "treated in some out-of-the-way corner by the least thoughtful and most uncouth junior member of the hospital's surgical staff, with little or no supervision or enforced sense of responsibility." The growing evidence of innocent infections had convinced many physicians of the injustice of these prohibitions. "A school teacher living in a boarding house in New York innocently acquired a chancre of the lip," wrote Dr. Sigmund Pollitzer. "It was impossible to place her in any hospital ward in this city, unless she was willing to go to the City Hospital and mingle with the dregs of the metropolis found in that institution."[149]

Though some physicians had objected to such policies during the late nineteenth century, hospitals remained under the control of trustees anxious to distinguish between patients deserving and undeserving of care. Only when science achieved some competence in dealing with venereal disease did physicians begin to determine hospital policy and overturn these restrictions. From 1905 though 1910, the Massachusetts General's venereal admissions rose from 5 to 45; but in 1911, after the introduction of Salvarsan, 133 were treated, and 194 in 1912. By 1913 the hospital actually recruited venereal patients, and beginning in 1915 all patients admitted to the medical ward of the newly established Peter Bent Brigham Hospital received routine Wassermann tests. More than 12 percent of the first 1,700 patients had positive reactions. At the Johns Hopkins Hospital the noted obstetrician J. Whitridge Willams instituted mandatory Wassermann tests for all women at the prenatal clinic. By the mid-1920s, this procedure had been widely adopted as the best means of preventing congenital syphilis.[150]

Efforts to establish hospital facilities often revealed medical prejudices against venereal patients. In July 1911 New York City allocated funds to construct a venereal ward at the Riverside Hospital on North Brother Island. This facility, although it was connected to the city's tuberculosis hospital, was used primarily to treat convicted prostitutes suffering infections. Dr. Ernest Lederle of the New York City Department of Health argued: "So far as venereal diseases are concerned, the persons who are the most undesirable as hospital patients are frequently the ones who constitute the greatest menace to others if left at large." Lederle urged the construction of special facilities for venereal patients; others suggested the necessity of locked wards for venereal patients who were noncompliant. "Certain of the hospital accommodations to be provided . . . should be under the control of the health authorities and conducted as a 'lock-hospital' to which patients, dangerous to the public health, can be removed, by force if necessary, and retained until no longer infectious," wrote Charles Bolduan.[151]

Physicians recognized the need to make hospital beds available to venereal patients, but members of the profession bitterly opposed the establishment of out-patient clinics and dispensaries by boards of health. Realizing the need for improved venereal diagnostics and treatment, some state and municipal departments of health had begun to provide these services to patients who lacked

resources. Doctors argued that now that they could effectively deal with venereal diseases, public health officials were luring away patients by creating social
hygiene clinics. The New York Academy of Medicine, for example, passed a
resolution objecting to the organization of municipal venereal clinics in February 1913, successfully blocking a board of health proposal. Members of the
Academy cited a limited study by the New York City Medical Society that indicated that 10 to 20 percent of dispensary patients did not qualify for free care.[152]

In cities where private physicians were not as well organized, public health
officials encountered less resistance. Health economist Michael M. Davis developed a particularly well-run venereal clinic at the Boston Dispensary. Davis
castigated members of the profession who objected to the establishment of such
facilities. "We must . . . bear in mind that just because the treatment of syphilis and gonorrhea is in the financial sense profitable from a practitioner's
point of view, we are likely to find an antagonism to the establishment of any
large number of evening clinics," he declared. "Doubtless there will be definite
opposition in the future . . . between the point of view of the practitioner who
sees an immediate personal interest, and the point of view of the public health
officer who sees the public interest. Davis's clinics provided low-cost treatment
and social services for patients to encourage compliance, as well as home instruction to prevent further infection. Such facilities pioneered in the techniques of contact epidemiology, attempting to locate and treat recently infected
individuals.[153] Davis concluded that "the needs of the community must pre-
vail."

Sensitive to professional criticism, many states and municipalities did not
immediately allocate funds to establish facilities for the diagnosis and treatment
of venereal disease. In New York the funds needed to set up a public venereal
diagnostic laboratory were provided by the Bureau of Social Hygiene in June
1914. Although the Board of Estimate had refused to budget the laboratory in
January 1914, Rockefeller agreed to continue to support it through the year.
Under this grant the department of health also created a clinic that provided
only diagnoses and counseling so as not to arouse the wrath of the professional
community. Louis Chargin, a member of the department, emphasized, "Under no circumstances is treatment of any character given." The board of health
encouraged physicians to avail themselves of the diagnostic service, establishing
600 stations at pharmacies and hospitals where needed materials could be obtained and left for examination. In 1914 the laboratory examined almost 58,000
specimens.[154]

The Bureau of Social Hygiene withdrew its support in 1915, contending that
the value of the diagnostic program had been demonstrated and that the city
should now underwrite the continued expense. Although the city did equal
Rockefeller's past contributions, other demands on the laboratory, especially the
need to produce antitoxins to aid the war in France, forced the department to
restrict the venereal program. A survey conducted in 1915 found New York
City clinics deficient in their care of venereal patients; of twenty-seven clinics
investigated, only seven met minimum standards.[155]

On the eve of the United States entry into World War I public health efforts

against venereal disease remained haphazard and inconsistent. Physicians refused to pass their newly gained scientific and sexual authority to public health
officials anxious to lead the fight against disease. Indeed, the failure of private
practitioners even to report cases of venereal disease to public health departments persists today and has proven to be the nemesis of venereal control. Before World War I venereal disease, despite the remarkable scientific progress
made in its diagnosis and treatment, was still distinguished from other infectious diseases because it was sexually transmitted and thus evoked a certain moral
repugnance. In fact, public health campaigns had come under attack for ig-
noring the moral aspects of the venereal problem. Concerned social hygienists
suggested that a purely "sanitary" approach to control of these diseases could
have alarming social ramifications. Even physicians, nominally dedicated to
scientific medicine, expressed concern that with the advent of effective therapy
the value of venereal disease as a restraint against sexual license would be lost.

Salvarsan, the only effective treatment for syphilis, had been quickly accepted into the practice of many American physicians, but also found detrac-
tors in the ranks of social hygiene. Even Prince Morrow at the end of a career
devoted to fighting venereal disease through education and moral reform—and
near the end of his life—refused to grant Salvarsan the status of effective therapy. "It is a preparation of arsenic which does not cure syphilis, although it has
remarkable effects in suppressing certain manifestations," noted Morrow. "Unfortunately, they always come back, and often with a train of disagreeable
symptoms that were not present at first." Morrow betrayed his fear of effective
treatment when he concluded, "So, for the present at least, men and women
cannot sin with impunity." Howard Kelly of Johns Hopkins offered similar sentiments, noting the valuable role that venereal disease played in controlling sexuality: "I believe that if we could in an instant eradicate the diseases, we would
also forget at once the moral side of the question, and would then, in one short
generation, fall wholly under the domination of the animal passions, becoming
grossly and universally immoral." According to Dr. E. L. Keyes, Jr., Morrow's
successor as president of the Society for Sanitary and Moral Prophylaxis, the
moral basis of the movement should remain paramount. "We transcend the
campaign against venereal disease in our aspiration to purify by every means,
moral, religious, hygienic, the morals of the race," he declared.[156]

Tension within the social hygiene movement between Victorian moral norms
and a new secular, scientific paradigm had emerged. Outlining the distinctions
between sanitation and morality, Richard Cabot observed, "Some of our
profession are not profoundly interested in whether people are moral so long as
they are healthy, and because that distinction can be sustained, morality is thereby
discouraged."[157] Social hygiene drew together two prominent Progressive contingents: those demanding a homogeneous moral order and those dedicated to
a new scientific, technocratic vision. The social hygiene campaign, committed
both to health *and* sexual morality, attempted to negotiate the inherent conflict
between these emphases. With medical advances, this friction became increasingly explicit. The debate between moral and scientific contingents, however,
actually reflected a continuum of opinion, with doctors and public health workers

often sharing the precepts of those demanding sexual control, in spite of their attempts to combat the diseases through medical means.

10

In 1913 the social hygiene campaign came to Broadway in French playwright Eugene Brieux's *Damaged Goods*. This play rehearsed the movement's major themes, accomplishments, and limitations. Just as the crisis of the family had generated new professional interest in venereal disease in the late nineteenth century, *Damaged Goods* centered public attention on the threat of sexually transmitted disease to the family unit, and asserted the professional and social responsibility for restoration of the sanctity of the institution of marriage. The play followed the tragic story of George Dupont, who, though warned by his physician that a recently incurred syphilitic infection forbids his forthcoming society marriage, ignores this advice after consulting a quack. His infection is traced as it ruins his brief domestic bliss. George's newborn child, his wife, and the wet-nurse all suffer the mournful consequences of his folly.[158]

The appearance on Broadway of a play that dealt frankly with the impact of venereal disease marked a significant exception to the conspiracy of silence regarding sexuality. In 1905 Anthony Comstock had closed George Bernard Shaw's *Mrs. Warren's Profession*, a play about prostitution, after only one performance. In an effort to head off such opposition, the *Medical Review of Reviews* established a Sociological Fund to solicit contributions from prominent citizens to produce the play. Edward L. Bernays, a pioneer in modern public relations technique, directed these efforts, raising $11,000. After a successful New York performance, the Sociological Fund commissioned a special showing in Washington, D.C., for President Wilson, his cabinet, and members of Congress to acquaint them with the social pathology of venereal disease.[159] *Damaged Goods*, which was, remarkably, not only a play about sexuality but about the possible effects of sexuality, became a symbol of a new sexual openness. A financial success, it spawned a series of dramas on sexual themes.

The play revealed the concerns and tensions that characterized social hygiene in the years prior to World War I. Though noting the opportunities for successful treatment, *Damaged Goods* emphasized a heightened sense of morality and argued that rejection of the double standard was the best means of combatting venereal disease. Unprecedented in its open confrontation of sexual issues, the play nevertheless endorsed the civilized sexual code of the late nineteenth century. Attacking hypocrisy and silence, Brieux's message suggested that patients—not physicians—must bear the ultimate responsibility for protecting the family from contamination. The doctor in the play, who endorses the concept of the medical secret, insists that he cannot defend the family from a man's immorality. "Science is not God Almighty," he shouts at George. Individuals, Brieux argued, must take responsibility for protecting themselves and their families from the ravages of disease. With *Damaged Goods* sexual immorality had been defined as what is today deemed a "voluntary health risk."[160]

Damaged Goods, however, raised another corollary: the modern state could no longer stand idle if individuals refused to act responsibly. The costs to society were simply too great. So all the while stressing the need for personal morality, this generation of reformers at the same time refused to let the problem of venereal disease rest with the vicissitudes of irresponsible individuality. Therefore, they demanded state intervention as a means of encouraging, if not coercing, a sense of individual morality. The doctor in *Damaged Goods* excoriates the legislator (the sorry bride's father) for not facing his civic responsibilities. The "future of the race" depended upon the intervention of the state. This tension between personal morality and public order—a central aspect of Progressive ideology—lay at the heart of debate concerning venereal disease; it would continue to characterize the problem in the years ahead.

Critics hailed the play as a culmination of the attack on Victorian sexual reticence. "Even the hideous subjects of prostitution and sexual disease may be, and have been, treated on the stage . . . with a noble purpose and without the slightest effect of arousing evil passion or satisfying prurient curiosity," commented *Outlook*. John D. Rockefeller, Jr., claiming the play would "awaken a new conscience," contributed funds for its production. "It put to shame and ridicule and to contempt all those people whose mental inertia is far worse than ignorance and whose pathetic habit of turning blind eyes to the truth has been like a dragging anchor on progression," explained Rockefeller. "Is this play decent?" asked *Hearst's Magazine's* drama critic. "My answer is that it is the decentest [sic] play that has been in New York for a year. It is so decent it is religious." Insinuations of impropriety nevertheless persisted. The *New York Times*, though praising *Damaged Goods*, noted politely that "the play deals with a subject which hitherto has practically been confined to medical publications," and obliquely referred to the subject of the play as a "rare blood disease." [161]

With Broadway plays, vice commission reports, white slave exposés, sex education, and the publicity campaign of the social hygiene movement, the venereal problem had achieved a new prominence, especially among the urban middle class. Issues of sexuality intruded in unprecedented fashion into the public consciousness. These discussions opened the way for a transformation in sexual attitudes and practice. H.L. Mencken caricatured the emergence of a "new woman" in 1915:

> Life, indeed, is almost empty of surprises, mysteries, horrors to this Flapper of 1915. . . . She knows exactly what the Wassermann reaction is, and has made up her mind that she will never marry a man who can't show an unmistakable negative. . . . She is opposed to the double standard of morality, and favors a law prohibiting it. . . .
>
> This Flapper has forgotten how to simper; she seldom blushes; it is impossible to shock her. She saw "Damaged Goods" without batting an eye, and went away wondering what the row over it was about. [162]

The emergence of sexuality into the public realm, however, did not go unnoticed by those who looked wistfully to the civility of the past. As Mencken suggested, *Damaged Goods* had also attracted its share of critics who questioned the value of public discourse on issues of sexuality. "I doubt very much that any blithe young libertine tripped gaily into the Fulton Theatre and learned to his consternation that certain painful and disgusting diseases were frequently the result of sexual immorality," argued poet Joyce Kilmer.[163] The prominent journalist Agnes Repplier decried what she called the "repeal of reticence." "Why this fresh enthusiasm in dealing with a foul subject?" she asked. The end of the conspiracy of silence, she explained, had resulted "in the obsession of sex which has set us all a-babbling about matters once excluded from the amenities of conversation." Repplier found the frequent sexual allusions in movies, theater, literature, and the popular press especially alarming. "All these horrors," she concluded, "are offered for the defense of youth and the purifying of civilized society." Even the *Medical Times* expressed concern over these new freedoms:

> With books on sexual topics queer
> We're duly swamped from year to year;
> Imaginative and erotic
> They're yellow 'nough to tinge sclerotic

Noting the profusion of sexual literature, *Current Opinion* declared it "Sex O'Clock in America."[164]

Although those who took comfort in Victorian proprieties found the social hygiene campaign offensive in its openness concerning sexuality, there were also critics who took the movement to task for its emphasis on moral rectitude. The silence had lifted, but the proponents of "civilized morality" continued to speak. Indeed, the emergence of venereal disease into public discourse led these proponents to *demand* adherence to genteel sexual codes. Dr. William J. Robinson, a prominent urologist, attacked those who continued to cite venereal infections as a proper retribution for immorality, a common theme among social hygienists. "It is truly sickening to hear a scientist in the twentieth century make such a statement," he declared. "It is truly a prostitution of the sacred function of science to be guilty of such statements." Robinson castigated social hygienists who sought to invoke venereal disease to control sexuality. Writing in 1910 to Mary Cobb, an important financial supporter of the social hygiene campaign in Boston, he explained:

> You speak the language of the tenth century; I speak the language of the 20th, or perhaps the 25th. You speak the language of gloom and reaction; I speak the language of joy and progress. You speak the language of the shackled theologian; I speak the language of the free scientist. . . .
>
> You believe that the sexual instinct was given to man and should be used by him for procreation purposes only. I believe that such a belief borders on insanity for it limits the man and the woman to but one or at most a dozen acts during their lives. For nobody would care, of course, to have more than a dozen children. You believe that extramarital relations are a sin and a crime. I believe they are dangerous on account of the fear of infection and may be unwise for many reasons, but are not more sinful or criminal per se than the gratification of any other natural instincts, such as eating or drinking.

Attorney and free-speech advocate Theodore Schroeder joined Robinson, accusing the social hygiene campaign of being a "conscious fraud . . . thriving on prudish ignorance."[165]

Even as sober a supporter of social hygiene as E.L. Keyes, Jr., noted the "freakish results" the first decade of the movement had wrought. Keyes expressed concern that social hygiene publicity may have overstressed the dangers of infection:

> Many people today have a very exaggerated idea as to ease of infection and especially as to symptoms of syphilis. Gonorrhea, which used to be likened to a cold in the head, is now-a-days likened to leprosy and cancer; while the innocent victim of acne, shingles, or poison ivy is shunned as an infectious syphilitic. And whereas actually only from five to eight per cent of syphilitics develop grave lesions of the nervous system, every luetic [syphilitic] now-a-days looks upon himself as doomed to locomotor ataxia.

Keyes's father, also a well-known urologist, suggested that one of the results of social hygiene publicity had been the creation of "syphilophobia."[166] The position of Keyes and his father anticipated in many ways the problems that the social hygiene movement would face as the century progressed.

Sigmund Freud's attack on "civilized" morality had come to America, finding supporters such as Robinson and Schroeder. Freud had suggested that the emphasis on fear of sexuality, unbending morality, and strict continence as means of preventing venereal infection had significant psychological and social costs of its own.[167] Among those who came under the influence of Freud's writings was young Walter Lippmann. In 1913 during the same spring that *Damaged Goods* opened on Broadway, Lippmann's persuasive critique of the moralistic tenets of social hygiene appeared in his first book, *A Preface to Politics*. In two closely reasoned chapters, Lippmann dissected the report of the Chicago Vice Commission, which he correctly considered representative of such efforts. He contended that in their blind moralism commission members had developed a program divorced from reality; "In outlining a ripple," he explained, "they have forgotten the tides." The time had come, Lippmann argued, to accept the sex impulse rather than continuing to attempt to deny it outright. "Instead of tabooing our impulses," he urged, "we must direct them." Sublimation, not prohibition, Lippmann argued, held the key to overcoming vice. "The commission did not face the sexual impulse squarely," concluded Lippmann. "The report is an attempt to deal with a sexual problem by disregarding its source."[168] In this broadside against Victorian morality, Lippmann expressed his faith in scientific management as the best means of addressing all social ills. In this respect, he articulated a strain of Progressivism that advocated a rationalistic industrial order rather than the rigidly moral order promoted by the vice crusaders. As Prince Morrow had made clear, morality, not venereal disease, was the campaign's priority. Lippmann justifiably realized that, as long as social hygiene accepted the legacy of the Victorian sexual code, it would never find an answer to the venereal problem.

Although the tensions between a scientific, secular approach to venereal dis-

ease and a strictly moral attitude would persist, a clear shift in cultural authority had occurred. Physicians had accrued prescriptive powers that previously re-
sided primarily with the church. Anna Garlin Spencer's eulogy to Prince Morrow
made this transformation explicit: "I look upon Dr. Morrow as a prophet and
a priest, using that word priest in the highest sense, a dispenser of idealism organized to work."[169] Indeed, in an increasingly secular culture, dedicated to
health, science, and efficiency, much of the status previously allotted to religious leaders had passed to the medical profession. Doctors had become the
arbiters of sexuality in both its scientific *and* moral realms. In this respect, figures as diverse as Prince Morrow and Sigmund Freud met on a common stage.

II

"Fit to Fight": The Commission
on Training Camp Activities

1

Long before the first Americans embarked on their mission to "make the world safe for democracy," the U.S. War Department undertook a major campaign to make the military camps in the United States safe for the soldiers—safe from the twin threats of immorality and venereal disease. The war engendered a sense of both awe and anxiety: awe for the opportunity to reorder and control society; anxiety surrounding the vast potential for disruption. The battle against venereal diseases—unprecedented in magnitude and intensity—reflected both themes. In the charged atmosphere of world war, venereal disease threatened military efficiency and health and, equally important, symbolized moral failure and social decay.

For many Progressives, the war provided a natural culmination of their domestic reforms, an occasion to demonstrate to an international audience the superiority of American ideals and morals. For reformers seeking to define a unified social order and common moral values, the war offered the chance to accelerate their campaigns. In addition, those Progressives who saw in the first decades of the twentieth century the immense potential impact of a new science dedicated to rationality, efficiency, health, and productivity, greeted America's entry into the war with hope.[1] For men and women who would spend the war at home, the venereal disease crusade provided a way to participate in the fight. What began as an attempt to save the health and efficiency of the American fighting man was eventually transformed into a comprehensive program to rid the nation of vice, immorality, and disease. This reform effort constituted one of the most fully articulated ventures in social engineering in American history.

In the military tradition, vice was seen as the inevitable concomitant of soldiery. In 1906 a meeting of the American Society for Social and Moral Prophylaxis was told that soldiers and sailors, lacking the restraining influences of home and family, "appear to be set apart as a class above others to suffer from sexual unrest."[2] The results of this "unrest" were all too well known to the assembled group—immoral behavior and, consequently, venereal diseases. Ten years later, as Americans prepared to join in World War I, social hygienists and Progressive reformers refused to accept the notion that American entry in the war would be accompanied by a dissipation in sexual morals and an increase in venereal disease. Confident in the Progressive tenets of environmental reform and social amelioration, they sought to devise a program that would create a new army, physically fit and morally upright.

While the war in Europe still seemed a world away, the experience of the National Guard and Army on the Mexican border had vividly forewarned American reformers of the complex problems of military health and morals. In March 1916 Francisco "Pancho" Villa had crossed into American territory, raiding the town of Columbus, New Mexico. To pursue Villa, General Frederick Funston quickly assembled an army of 10,000 men.[3] The American Social Hygiene Association, the newly established voluntary watchdog of the nation's sexual mores, soon received disquieting reports of conditions among the troops encamped along the Mexican border. Dr. William F. Snow, the Association's director; Jerome D. Greene, secretary of the Rockefeller Foundation; and Fletcher Brockman of the National Young Men's Christian Association traveled to Washington, D.C., in July 1916 to protest the lax moral environment to Secretary of War Newton D. Baker. The group agreed an investigation was in order, and dispatched Raymond B. Fosdick to go to Texas.[4]

Fosdick exemplified a certain strain of urban Progressivism; he was professional, educated, and pragmatic. Only thirty-two years old when enlisted by Baker, he had already achieved distinction as a lawyer, reformer, and investigator. Although Fosdick's career had had many facets, ranging from investigating graft and corruption in New York City government to protesting unsightly billboards, it was the social settlement movement that had affected him most significantly. After his education at Princeton University, Fosdick had spent a year living and working at Henry Street Settlement on New York's Lower East Side, under the tutelage of Lillian Wald. He later explained, "The emphasis in my thinking, I suspect, went back to Miss Wald and my days at Henry Street."[5] Fosdick had spent the last four years conducting investigations for the Bureau of Social Hygiene. In this capacity, he undertook comprehensive studies of European and American police operations and published two monographs that analyzed the inefficiency and mismanagement of these systems.[6] The group that assembled in Washington thus considered Fosdick an ideal choice to conduct an investigation of the situation along the border. In the years ahead, Fosdick would draw heavily on his Progressive experience.

After five weeks with the troops, Fosdick detailed instances of drunkenness, vice, and debauchery in the towns along the border in a lengthy report to Baker. Prostitutes throughout the Southwest had flocked to the garrisons, and Fosdick found a series of army camps virtually encircled by brothels and saloons. In lurid prose, he depicted the red-light districts of San Antonio, Douglas, and El Paso. "In various stages of undress, and in various postures and poses," he wrote, "women solicit all passersby, openly and daringly, from the front of the 'cribs,' with a constant flow of obscene jest and invitation." In Laredo alone, ten new saloons had opened in the previous month to meet the demand of the soldiers. According to Fosdick, drunken brawls were not an unusual sight, particularly on paydays. "I talked to the young recruits in the militia," he reported, "mere boys—whose first real knowledge of the ways of the red-light districts was obtained from what they saw in merely walking through the 'crib' sections. . . . Such a sight not only demoralizes . . . but leaves a scar on a man's life which he can never efface."[7]

Dr. M.J. Exner, who surveyed conditions along the border on behalf of the YMCA, reported equally disturbing findings. According to Exner, commercialized vice interests assembled to prey upon the military. As an official YMCA report explained, "Where the facilities for prostitution were inadequate, new arrangements were made with a promptness that compared favorably with the German automatic mobilization." Exner discovered soldiers waiting in long lines to visit with women of "very low grade." Saloons operated in spite of dry laws; shacks were erected to house the influx of prostitutes. Based on Exner's reports, the YMCA concluded that conditions on the border marked "the lowest point of shoddiness in the history of American graft."[8]

The situation in Texas resulted in high rates of venereal disease. Among troops stationed near San Antonio, for example, 288 per 1000 reported venereal infections, almost 30 percent. Most officers attempted to control the problem by requiring inspections of prostitutes by medical officers, usually once every two weeks. These physicians then provided the women with certificates attesting their health. Fosdick found this form of regulated prostitution "merely an advertisement for the trade," unscientific and inconsistent, encouraging immorality and enhancing the possibility of infection. Officers also provided their men with chemical prophylaxis after sexual exposure. In some camps as many as 300 men applied for the treatment daily. This procedure proved effective, but Fosdick and Exner discovered its use to be haphazard, and more importantly, considered it only a palliative for a poor moral environment.[9]

It was the traditional military attitude that men required sex to be good soldiers that Exner and Fosdick found most alarming. Though a few officers placed saloons and houses of prostitution off limits, most assumed that "men will be men." "I rarely met an officer who did not take for granted that prostitution could not and should not be abolished," noted Exner. Each divisional and camp commander exercised personal discretion in dealing with the sexual behavior of the troops in his command. In Mexico the army sponsored its own prostitution district. "In these instances," reported Exner, "prostitution was deliberately provided by the officers on the assumption that it was necessary for the contentment and well-being of the men."[10]

Fosdick and Exner attempted to assess the factors that contributed to the demoralization of the troops. Exner, an expert on sexual psychology and education, emphasized the problems inherent in wresting adolescents from the normal restraining influences of their homes and families. Contemporary psychological theory maintained that during this period the "love instinct develops and the sexual desire powerfully asserts itself." To undergo such changes in the military environment, replete with temptations and opportunities for debasement, presented obvious dangers. Observers of camp life identified a tendency to "level down." "It is as a rule the coarse element that creates the atmosphere of the group," noted Exner. "[Soldiers] take a supreme delight in retailing their obscene stories and giving expression to the foul imagery of their minds in vulgar talk or jest." Exner expressed a common Victorian view that all-male groups, lacking the uplifting quality of feminine society, tend to degenerate morally. This, he noted, was particularly true of military life: "The terrific down-pull of the military camp, as of all similar male group life, cannot be easily exaggerated."[11] Exner characterized the atmosphere of the camps as "sensualizing."

Other observers confirmed Exner's view of military life. L.M. Maus, a retired Colonel in the Army Medical Corps, suggested that "life in the barracks . . . is anything but elevating. . . . Considering the sources from which the men are drawn, one could not expect to find the influences of the higher standards of life." Given the class origins of most recruits, Maus held little hope for developing positive camp environments. William Ernest Hocking, the prominent Harvard University philosopher, noted that "the tamer virtues stand in a paler light. . . . The strange comradeship of camp and barracks fans the common and simpler elements of excitement, and send into retirement the sober and reflective self of civil life." Hocking concluded pessimistically, "Given these tendencies, we have to expect . . . that there will be laxity in relations of sex."[12]

The ambience of camp life, and the fact that a contingent of prostitutes surrounded the cantonments, according to observers, produced a sexual powderkeg along the border. True to Progressive ideals of reform, both Fosdick and Exner emphasized the demoralizing effects of the camp and community in their respective reports, suggesting that reform efforts might best be concentrated on environments rather than individual men. "The environment of practically all the camps . . . presented the severest temptations to immorality—an environment which only those who were powerfully fortified by moral principle and will could withstand," wrote Exner. Few of the men stationed along the Mexican border had such reserves of self-discipline. "The soldier is human," Exner concluded, "and men in the unstable period of adolescence, under the unusual moral strain incident to military service cannot be expected to keep clean when prostitution in its most flagrant forms is placed under their noses, with the sanction and encouragement of their officers."[13] Only the amelioration of these conditions, Fosdick and Exner suggested, would alleviate the moral crisis on the border.

Casting his recommendations to Baker as a plea for greater military efficiency and better morale, Fosdick advised that a "strong word" from Washington would have a positive impact on the situation in Texas. The most notorious "crib sections," he argued, should be immediately placed off limits. "The Provost Guard could starve out these vicious areas in a week," he explained. In addition, Fosdick believed it important to seek the cooperation of local authorities to enforce existing strictures upon the sale of liquor and the profusion of prostitution. Although he stopped short of calling for a complete repression of prostitution, this was likely his goal. Already labeled "the Reverend" by officers skeptical of his mission, Fosdick struggled to avoid the image of an idealistic do-gooder.[14]

Secretary of War Baker responded by demanding stricter discipline along the border. "I am entirely satisfied," he wrote General Funston, "that the time has come when the health of the army must be safeguarded against the weakness that derives from venereal disease and excessive alcohol." He proffered "minimum requirements" for the control of prostitution and liquor. Though the army had no legal authority in the communities near the camps, Baker suggested that, if local officials did not maintain "wholesome conditions," the troops could be moved, taking their paychecks to be spent in "cleaner" towns. Anxious, however, to demonstrate to his officers that he was no weak-kneed reformer, Baker explained to Funston:

> I hope you will understand that I have no perfectionist notions on any of these subjects. Having been mayor of a large city dealing with both problems for a long time, I have come to realize that gradual and wise restraint and restriction is both more effective and more permanently helpful than sudden and spasmodic attempts at suppression.[15]

Rather than frame the problem as a moral one, Baker and Fosdick effectively redirected the discussion to the themes of rationality and efficiency.

Although a few officers dismissed these efforts as utopian, Fosdick returned to Texas to find conditions significantly improved and worked to cement his program's gains by canvassing mayors and police chiefs to garner their support in restricting vice and saloons in their towns. Despite his partial success, Fosdick realized that more rigid discipline alone could not solve fundamental problems of military morale. "It does not do any good in dealing with red-blooded young men merely to erect a series of *verboten* signs along the roadside"; he urged, "you must have something positive for them to do." The monotony of camp life and the dearth of organized amusements for soldiers, he believed, contributed to loose morals and the concomitant rise in venereal rates. Fosdick argued for the necessity of supplying alternatives to the red-light districts: organized sports, recreation, movies, and theaters.[16]

As the possibility of American involvement in World War I increased in the spring of 1917, the implications of the border experience took on added meaning. The problems of vice and disease on the Mexican border had been limited, in both geographical and numerical terms. The troops assembled there, moreover, had volunteered for service. A conscript army of American youth would entail greater federal responsibility.[17] Entry into the war would transform the problem of sexually transmitted disease into a national issue of the first magnitude, requiring a centrally conceived program.

Though Fosdick's report to Baker remained confidential, Exner published his account of the Mexican border situation in *Social Hygiene* in April 1917. Exner sought to use the border conditions to raise questions about preparation for the larger conflict. "When the mobilization of a new army seemed to be sure I feared that under the pressure of preparing for war this whole matter might be allowed to rest in the archives of the Government," he explained. "In order, therefore, to bring to bear the pressure of public opinion I wrote my article on social hygiene exposing the conditions which had developed on the border." The article outlined the impact of venereal disease in the army in the most ominous terms:

From the standpoint of military strength and efficiency, such waste is serious; for it means that not only will these men bring back into the social structure a vast volume of venereal disease to wreck the lives of innocent women and children, but they will bring back into it other attitudes and practices which will destroy homes, cause misery, and degenerate society.[18]

Exner represented the consensus of social hygienists when he argued that venereal disease merely represented the physical repercussions of a far more dangerous moral decay. In this regard, he expressed the widespread Progressive anxiety concerning the strength of the family. Exner concluded by calling for a full-scale attack on prostitution.

Exner's position generated considerable apprehension for the physical and social welfare of the troops. Citizens wrote to officials in Washington as conscription approached, urging the government to maintain rigorous standards to protect the morals of the young draftees. As one mother wrote to Secretary of the Navy Josephus Daniels:

If boys of 18 are to be sent out to military encampments now, whether parents approve or not, the parents must have some guarantee that the moral atmosphere will be as high as that to which our sons are accustomed to in their home life. I understand that the moral conditions in our military camps . . . are anything but good, that a large percent of the men in these camps live in accordance with the double standard.

Another mother wrote directly to President Wilson: "We are praying you will make camp life clean for boys [who] are willing to offer their bodies as sacrifice for their country, but not their souls."[19] With the coming of war, organized reformers and social hygienists began a concerted campaign to secure wholesome environments for the American military. The American Social Hygiene Association enlisted its entire staff in preparing for mobilization, and the YMCA created the National War Work Council to develop social programs for the troops.[20]

Baker, aware of the problems that American involvement in the war would raise, needed little prodding from the social hygienists. In early February 1917, after conferring with Fosdick, he had written to General Funston about venereal policy on the Mexican border: "All this seems to me especially important in view of the possibility of our shortly having to undertake the training of large bodies of men—men selected probably from the youth of their country. . . . Normal and wholesome outlets for exuberant physical vitality will be readily accepted as a substitute for vicious modes of indulgence, if the former be made accessible." Only four days before the United States entered the war, April 2, 1917, Secretary Baker wrote to President Wilson indicating the necessity of providing opportunities for recreation in the new army camps. In addition, he sent Fosdick to Canada to study the organization of training camps there.[21]

Baker expected the war experience to build the strength and virility of the American fighting man and ultimately the American people. In a speech delivered in October 1917, he outlined the philosophical underpinnings of his view of camp life and military training. The war, Baker argued, constituted a social disruption of enormous magnitude. Large numbers of young men, many still in their crucial formative years, would be torn away from the positive influences of "normal" social life. Baker believed it was the War Department's responsibility to construct a new, powerful set of restraints which would not only maintain order, but actually heighten the soldiers' moral rectitude. Only in this way could he ensure that the troops would return home "with no other scars than those won in honorable warfare!" Baker sought, therefore, to supply the American soldiers with what he called "invisible armor," to protect them against the "heated temptations" of immorality that the war would present. This armor would be forged by a new set of social habits and a resolve to raise self-discipline above selfish desire.[22]

The Secretary, who had formerly been the mayor of Cleveland, suggested that the camps be modeled on cities, not the disordered, decaying urban areas, but the new, Progressive cities of recreation, parks, and playgrounds. In devising policy for the training camps, Baker recounted an incident from his reformist administration. As mayor, Baker had attempted to clean up the city's dance halls, which reformers had identified as centers of immoral behavior. Under Baker's leadership the city established its own dance hall in the public park, well-lit and chaperoned. The vice-ridden halls soon closed for lack of patrons. The Secretary concluded:

> We learned that where there was a healthily conducted and adequate recreational opportunity, it was impossible for the old downward tendency of young men to continue; that in the presence of that opportunity the natural and spontaneous tendencies of young men asserted themselves. We learned . . . that the way to keep young people from doing bad things is to give them an opportunity to do good things.

"The cities," explained the former mayor, "have come regularly to set out in their budgets of expenditure provision for athletic opportunities and wholesome amusements as the best possible means of combatting the evil tendencies of the congestion of city life." With each of sixteen training camps comprising some 35,000 to 40,000 men, Baker contended, they would be the equivalent of cities. Proper recreation would provide the distractions necessary to avoid idleness, weariness, and monotony, the forces that reformers suggested led to immoral behavior and venereal diseases. "Wholesome recreation [is] the best possible cure for irregularities in conduct which arise from idleness and the baser temptations," the Secretary argued.[23] For Baker, the Progressive years had served as a rehearsal for the programs he now proposed for the training camps.

Baker's counterpart, Secretary of the Navy Josephus Daniels, represented another, complementary strain of Progressive thought in his assessment of the venereal problem and the coming war. Whereas Baker cast his argument in the modern language of rationality and social science, Daniels emphasized morality in words that rang high Victorian. In his lecture to the Clinical Congress of Surgeons of North America, "Men Must Live Straight If They Would Shoot Straight," Daniels urged civilian action to protect the military from the "harpies of the underworld":

There lies upon us morally, to a degree outreaching any technical responsibility, the duty of leaving nothing undone to protect these young men from that contamination of their bodies which will not only impair their military efficiency but blast their lives for the future and return them to their homes a source of danger to their families and communities at large.

Although Daniels emphasized personal morality more than Baker, both men agreed that it was incumbent upon the federal government to make the training camps healthy environments, free of sexual temptation and venereal disease. "Negative work is not enough," concluded Daniels, "We must create competitive interests to replace the evils we are trying to eliminate."[24]

During the spring of 1917, Baker and Fosdick frequently discussed the need for positive social and recreational opportunities in the training camps should the United States undertake a draft. Upon his return from Canada, where he had studied that country's military training procedures, Fosdick propared a detailed memo proposing a commission to oversee such programs in the American camps. He conceived of the commission as a clearinghouse for the various social agencies anxious to do service for the soldiers. "In New York City," Fosdick noted, "no less than seven different agencies are preparing to play some part in connection with this question, and unless their endeavors are centralized and coordinated through some clearing committee, infinite confusion is bound to result."[25] Fearing that the draftees might be overrun by uplifters, Fosdick proposed that a federal agency should direct voluntary efforts for recreation and amusements in the camps.

Fosdick also recommended that such a commission should have the added charge of keeping the areas adjacent to the camps "decent and respectable." In other words, it would work in conjunction with local officials to control prostitution, liquor, and other enticements that Fosdick had discovered on the Mexican border. In order to make this aspect of the program carry weight, Fosdick suggested the need for a central directive from the War Department making it clear that red-light districts and alcohol in the vicinity of the camps would not be tolerated. In March 1917 the New York State Legislature had banned prostitution and liquor near its Plattsburg camp, and Fosdick believed such a policy would have a dramatic impact on a national scale. "That such legislation would eliminate many of the evils that attended the presence of our army on the Mexican border last summer," concluded Fosdick, "cannot be doubted for a moment."[26]

Baker responded by creating the Commission on Training Camp Activities on April 17, 1917, just eleven days after the delcaration of war. He appointed Fosdick as its chairman, and the CTCA soon became popularly known as the "Fosdick Commission." In consultation with Baker, Fosdick chose a group of prominent Progressive social leaders to serve on the Commission, most notably John Mott of the YMCA, Lee F. Hanmer of the Russell Sage Foundation, and Joseph Lee, president of the Playground and Recreation Association of America.[27] With the establishment of the Commission, a two-pronged attack upon venereal disease was born; the CTCA combined elements of uplift and distraction, coercion and repression in its efforts to make the military venereal-free.

The Commission on Training Camp Activities became the central mechanism for the manufacture of "invisible armor." It developed a comprehensive program of recreation, education, and amusements to insure the soldiers' and sailors' health, efficiency, and morality. The moral justifications offered for American entry into the war seemed to intensify the need for the government to provide such activities for the troops. As Fosdick later explained, "The Commissions have surrounded our fighters with such clean and wholesome influences as they conceived a democracy to owe its fighting men." Fosdick emphasized the need for a "rationalizing force" to instill contentment and produce an efficient army. To do this the Commission sponsored programs for singing, libraries, theaters, athletics, and clubs. "It was the first time," he noted, "that a government had ever combined educational and ethical elements with disciplinary forces in the production of a fighting organism."[28]

Most active of all the voluntary agencies in the Commission's programs was the YMCA. The YMCA established "huts" in all the cantonments that quickly became the center of camp social life. Here soldiers could write letters, read, play cards, or listen to music. Bible classes, lectures, and church services, as well as dramatic performances and movies, drew soldiers to the huts. The Knights of Columbus and the Jewish Welfare Board sponsored similar activities. The CTCA had hoped to avoid such duplication, but when the YMCA's National War Work Council refused to appoint a Catholic member, the Commission was forced to invite other organizations into the camps.[29] The CTCA did require, however, that all activities, no matter the sponsor, would be open to all soldiers.

The YMCA also established Hostess Houses, where wives and girl friends could visit under rigorously chaperoned conditions consistant with the CTCA's view of camp life. By September 1917 seventy-six had already been built. Although some officers objected to the presence of women at the camps, Fosdick considered the houses indispensable in "conserving camp morale."[30] Thousands of women reportedly trekked to meet their men before they departed for Europe.

Of all the activities that the CTCA established in the camps, athletics and organized recreation proved most popular among the troops. Dr. Joseph Raycroft, director of physical education at Princeton University, supervised these programs. Every company appointed an officer in charge of games and sports who directed volleyball, basketball, and baseball. Walter Camp of Yale University, known as the father of American football, served on the Commission and created a hand-grenade game. "Never before in the history of this country," declared a newspaper sports editor, "have so large a number of men engaged in athletics. . . . Nothing coordinates the personal faculties needed in warfare like the team-work that goes into organized athletics." At one western camp, sixteen baseball games often took place simultaneously. Boxing, heavily promoted in the camps, reportedly aided in bayonet fighting. The Commission suggested that this "severe muscular activity" would also help repress the soldiers' sexual impulses. Organized sports fostered self-discipline and control according to the CTCA's staff. "Athletics," explained Fosdick, "offers a legitimate expression for the healthy animal spirit which, when pent up, will invariably assert itself in some form of lawlessness."[31]

Observers employed a variety of analogies to describe the introduction of these activities into the training camps. One commentator suggested that the camps had been made into "hard military schools with a country club on the side." Others called them "soldier-cities, or "war universities." The work of the CTCA in the camps, however, most closely resembled the programs of the Progressive social settlements in their ideology, organization, and implementation. Never before had social settlement ideals received such wide attention and application.[32] Fosdick worked very much in this tradition in reserving the camps for the so-called "positive" side of the CTCA's work: the recreation, amusements, and education out of which "invisible armor" would be forged.

2

Just as the settlements provided education in addition to entertainment, so, too, did the CTCA for the soldiers. The Commission, in cooperation with the surgeon general's office, undertook a major program to instruct the troops concerning the venereal diseases. For this purpose, Fosdick established a Social Hygiene Instruction Division under the direction of the American Social Hygiene Association's Dr. Walter Clarke. The Division enlisted the latest techniques of psychology, persuasion, and education to inculcate the men in the ways of sexual continence. In addition to providing a barrage of posters, handbills, pamphlets, and exhibits, the CTCA required that each company receive lectures on the sexually transmitted diseases. "Psychologically, the process of selling soap or shoes or automobiles seem[s] closely related to the 'selling' of conduct," explained Clarke. "The advertisers have contributed unique ideas, methods, and slogans."[33]

The Social Hygiene Instruction Division assumed that families and communities had failed to provide the draftees with necessary information in sexual matters. According to the members of the Division, soldiers either came to camp with grossly distorted views of sexuality, or completely ignorant. Therefore, they argued, experts should provide sex education for the soldiers. "It is up to the government to supply this background not given by their civil life," wrote William Zinsser, a member of the CTCA, "to educate these boys on the vital subjects of reproduction, sex hygiene, venereal diseases, etc., in the teaching of which their parents and home communities have been so woefully negligent." This attitude reflected the Progressive fear that the family was failing in critical areas, as well as a growing trend to look to professionals in such matters.[34] Indeed, instruction by physicians and social hygienists, standardized and federally approved, was greatly preferred to the haphazard or suspect instruction offered at home or in the streets.

In keeping with the basic tenets of Progressive reform, those who directed the social hygiene campaign insisted on the essential mutability of human nature. As H.E. Kleinschmidt, a member of the Division wrote, "Cynics and self-made philosophers have failed to convince us that the sex urge, which is admittedly a primitive instinct, can no more be stemmed than the tide of the sea." Members of the CTCA justified the educational program by arguing that it would not only reduce venereal diseases but also produce better soldiers, and ultimately, better citizens. Joseph Lee called the training camps "our national universities for war purposes." He concluded that "it is our business to see that these men are turned out stronger, in every sense—more fit morally, mentally and physically than they have ever been in their lives." Surgeon General William C. Gorgas believed the program would have a fundamental impact on the health of the army by encouraging continence. "Customs and manners," he noted, "can be controlled almost absolutely by education."[35]

The threat that venereal disease posed for the effectiveness of the military dominated the social hygiene campaign. "That army and navy which is the least syphilized will, other things being equal, win," explained Walter Clarke. Gorgas argued that venereal disease presented a greater menace to the expedient operations of the army than did many battle wounds. "To the commanding general," he wrote, "the loss is greater for a man who contracts gonorrhea than for a man who is shot through the thigh, and even if [he] could lay aside all question of morality, he would probably choose the eradication of venereal disease rather than the prevention of wounds." The troops were not spared this blunt message. As one CTCA lecturer told the men, venereal disease had caused the War Department "more anxiety in many respects than have the bullets and bayonets of German soldiers."[36]

Attempting to avoid the moralism usually associated with sexual instruction, the CTCA emphasized rationality and science in their propaganda. They called their program "educational prophylaxis." The title of the most widely distributed pamphlet, *Keeping Fit to Fight*, expressed the basic theme of the campaign, namely, the necessity of remaining healthy. The language of the appeal was clear and direct. "This is man-to-man talk," the pamphlet began, "straight from the shoulder without gloves." Official CTCA lecturers were cautioned:

> Don't use words that (while good in themselves) have unfortunately acquired prejudices in the minds of many men whom it is particularly desired to influence. This includes words of semitheological connotation, as well as all words with a sentimental or 'sob' tinge.[37]

Although the Social Hygiene Division sought the cooperation of agencies, such as the YMCA, that tended to take a moralistic view of the problem of venereal disease, they feared that such an approach might alienate the rough-and-tumble soldiers, and discredit their efforts. "We all know to what extremes the sexual moralist can go," wrote Dr. William Allen Pusey of the Surgeon General's Committee on Venereal Diseases. "How impractical, how intolerant, how extravagant, even how unreasoning, if not scientifically dishonest, he can be." Though M.J. Exner of the YMCA insisted "that the control of the environment of the camps is up to the government and that the program of moral education is up to us," the CTCA soon assumed responsibility for all sexual instruction within the camps.[38] "The lectures on sexual hygiene and venereal diseases given by the company commanders to their men are not inane, pseudomoral [sic] stuff," explained Pusey. "It is not making saints of them; but it is doing a great deal in saving them from venereal diseases." The CTCA acknowledged ethical arguments for combatting venereal disease, but instead chose to emphasize science and efficiency. As Public Health Surgeon Dr. Joseph S. Lawrence concluded, "It is recognized that there is a moral question involved . . . but we choose . . . to concentrate on the hygienic phase."[39]

Sexual continence, a theme acceptable to both medical and moral contingents, became the precept of all the educational efforts. On April 21, 1917, only two weeks after the declaration of war, the General Medical Board of the Council of National Defense passed a resolution endorsing continence for members of the armed services:

> WHEREAS, venereal infections are among the most serious and disabling diseases to which the soldier and sailor are liable;
> WHEREAS, they constitute a grave menace to the civil population;
> THEREFORE, the Committe on Hygiene and Sanitation of the General Medical Board of the Council of National Defense, recommends . . .
> 1. That the Departments of War and Navy officially recognize that continence is compatible with health and that it is the best prevention of venereal infections.

This resolution represented a totally unprecedented public pronouncement on an issue which had been previously limited to a small coterie of middle-class reformers.[40] The Board also called for the prohibition of liquor and prostitution in the areas around the camps; otherwise, they argued, the demand for continence would be useless.[41] The Council's resolutions and the social hygiene campaign in general made clear that sexual attitudes and practice often were not in accord with middle-class prescriptions.

Encouraged by the Council of National Defense resolutions, the CTCA designed its social hygiene campaign accordingly. The Commission's literature sought to dispel the common notion that men must be sexually active to maintain their health and masculinity:

> It used to be thought that these organs had to be used if they were to be kept healthy. *This is a lie.* If it were true, the boy who exercises them regularly from childhood on should have the greatest sex power—but he is more likely to be sexually dead before he matures. . . . Sex power is not lost by laying off.

The language lecturers used to make this point tended to be even stronger. One medical officer called the argument for male sexual necessity "a grand old dodge with whiskers on it. . . . When I hear a fellow pulling the old health yarn, I'm inclined to keep him away from my sisters." The belief that soldiers could not remain chaste was rejected outright. "Any man with enough nerve and backbone to wear the uniform of a United States soldier," a lecturer declared, "is perfectly able to live a normal healthy life without intercourse throughout the war and afterwards."[42]

The social hygiene campaign assured the soldiers that continence was compatible with "manhood" and "red-blooded virility." The denial of the double standard of morality and demands for premarital sexual chastity for men had been asserted with increasing vigor since the late nineteenth century, particularly in medical circles. Social hygienists now sought to promote these principles *en masse*. "It is not true that the absence of previous sexual experience is any handicap to a man in entering the married state," explained a lecturer. "On the contrary, the man who comes to his bride as clean and as true as he expects that she will come to him will find the most perfect joy in the married state. All the sexual knowledge he requires he can readily secure from his family physician before his marriage." Educational materials frequently reminded the troops that athletes training for competition often restricted all sexual activity. The theory that men possessed a limited amount of energy—and sperm—served as a corollary to the injunction for sexual purity. As one lecturer admonished a group of soldiers, using a string of euphemisms:

> Live strong and clean, and save every drop of your strength and manhood for the supreme experience. You have a right to demand this of yourself. Demand it. Secure it. By refraining from illicit intercourse you will defeat the deadly enemy and preserve your own manhood.[43]

Above all, the CTCA stressed the dangers of the sexual drives and the need for the soldier to control them. *Keeping Fit to Fight* explained:

> Over-exercise or excitement of the sex-glands may exhaust and weaken a man. . . . The sex feelings are so powerful and the risk so great if they are turned loose, that it is common sense not to play with fire.

The risk, of course, was venereal disease. Pamphlets, lectures, and exhibits all advocated continence as the only certain means of avoiding these maladies. One lecturer concluded, "Shun illicit intercourse as you would the Plague."[44]

The instructional program thus not only encouraged the soldiers to engage in wholesome activities and recreation but also to erase sex from their consciousness. Clean minds, the CTCA argued, were the requisite for clean bodies. "Sex organs do not have to be exercised or indulged in, in order to develop them, or preserve virility," counseled one lecturer. "Forget them, don't think about them, or dwell upon them. Live a good vigorous life and they will take care of themselves." According to the official Social Hygiene Division syllabus, from which most officers drew their lectures, "A man who is thinking below the belt is not efficient."[45]

The sexual imagery used in the lectures, however, at times became graphic and must have worked at odds with this goal. Indeed, on occasion the social hygiene orations bordered on the prurient. One overzealous medical officer asked his company, "Does any red-blooded man feel any doubt of his ability to preserve his manhood though tempted by the alluring seductions of voluptuous and beautiful women in the whirl and excitement of the gay metropolis, or the fascinations that may come to you from delicate and devoted attentions in the solitude of remote billets?"[46] The answer was probably far less certain than the lecturer might have hoped.

Fear of venereal disease probably played a more effective role in the CTCA's attempt to encourage sexual abstinence. The social hygiene campaign did not overlook the consequences of contracting a venereal disease in their presentations to the troops. Photographic exhibits explicitly illustrated the most devastating effects of untreated syphilis: twisted limbs, open lesions, and physical deformities. Some lecturers prided themselves on their ability to send chills through the ranks. As one lecturer wrote to Fosdick:

> As I looked into that mass of faces my courage grew . . . to a heated pitch. I stripped the moral issue to the naked bone. . . . I defied them. I schooled them with a world of medical facts . . . on the ravages of venereal disease. . . . I sneered at them for lacking the moral courage to fight the common tendency in armies. . . . I appealed to their regimental pride. Before long they were virtually as pliable as putty. . . . IT WAS THEN THAT I DELIVERED THE GOVERNMENT MESSAGE. . . . I told them that they had to be 100% efficient to win this war.

"No apologies . . . are made for employing the element of fear as one of the restraining factors," explained H.E. Kleinschmidt. "In fact, the fear of disease forms the backbone of practically every preventive medicine educational campaign."[47]

Military physicians described in vivid detail the symptomatology of gonorrhea, syphilis, and chancroid in their lectures, as well as the long-term impact on health. Gonorrhea, the official syllabus noted, could cause kidney infections, arthritis, and sterility. The pathology of syphilis often resulted in paresis, locomotor ataxia, insanity, and sometimes death. One lecturer told the grim story of a football squad which celebrated a big victory by "breaking training." They went "down the line" in a nearby city; seven of the eleven developed venereal infections. "Three of them are now six feet under sod," he told the men, "dead with the most loathsome of diseases, syphilis."[48]

The educational program not only outlined the perils of venereal diseases for the soldier himself; it also stressed what Progressive physicians called "innocent infections." Members of the medical corps reminded the soldiers of the repercussions of infecting their wives or brides-to-be. "Men who supposed they were cured [of gonorrhea], marrying even ten years later," explained a lecturer, "have been known to infect their wives . . . causing complications, resulting in the death of the wife a few months after marrying." These cases, he noted, were familiarly known as "honeymoon appendicitis." More frequent, however, was sterility of the innocently-infected woman or blindness of the congenitally-infected child. "Whether blinded by a red-hot iron or gonorrhea is all the same to the baby," the official syllabus pointedly advised. The Social Hygiene Division did, however, caution over-enthusiastic lecturers not to proclaim venereal diseases incurable: "Don't overstress the horrors—it sometimes creates an undesirable reaction."[49]

Prelectors repeatedly returned to the theme that venereal diseases, unlike most others, could only be obtained willfully. The Army had recognized this idea as early as 1912, when it instituted the policy of stopping pay for soldiers incapacitated with a venereal disease and implemented orders requiring chemical prophylaxis after a sexual exposure. These rulings, though not strictly enforced, gave official sanction to the position that ultimate responsibility for avoiding sexually transmitted diseases rested with the individual. "Not all sickness is a man's fault," explained Walter Clarke, "but the venereal diseases generally are." Another medical officer made the same point more directly when he told the soldiers, "You won't have anybody to blame but yourself if you have to tell the folks back home that when the big drive was pulled off you were back in in the venereal hospital playing pinochle." On several occasions, officers suggested that soldiers who contracted a venereal disease should be listed by name in local newspapers.[50]

The social hygiene campaign concluded that it was the soldier's patriotic duty to remain healthy. At times, however, it became difficult to distinguish between invocations of the flag and appeals to the soldier's sense of guilt. "Does it not amount to aiding and abetting the Germans," a lecturer demanded, "to put yourself by your own wrongful act in the hospital bed where the wounded should lie?" The CTCA equated the contraction of a venereal disease with a national betrayal. *Keeping Fit to Fight* castigated the troops:

> A venereal disease contracted after deliberate exposure through intercourse with a prostitute is as much of a disgrace as showing the white feather. . . . A soldier in the hospital with a venereal disease is a slacker. . . . You lessen the man-power of your company and throw extra burdens on your comrades. You are a moral shirker.[51]

Social hygienists considered yielding to the sex drive an act of selfishness, a demonstration of a lack of self-discipline. They supported the basic Progressive principle that, given the proper education and a sound environment, the ultimate moral obligation rested with the individual.

The CTCA cast the war as a symbolic battle of virile manhood to protect "pure" womanhood. The social hygienists suggested that men should not waste their "manhood" on loose women, but rather devote this limited "energy" to the war effort. Indeed, lectures and pamphlets frequently reminded the soldiers that they were fighting for the right of women to remain virtuous. Accounts of German atrocities in Belgium became standard repertory in the lectures. "How would you like to have twenty Prussian beasts, one after another, indulge their lusts upon your sister," asked one officer. "How would you like to have one American seduce your sister? How would you like to have twenty Americans indulge their lust upon your sister, one after another? Your blood boils and you want to fight the fiends."[52] The only way for the troops to defend the honor of women, the lecturer explained, was to embrace sexual continence for the war's duration:

> We are showing the world a new motive in warfare, a heretofore unheard of motive, and we can show the women of France and Belgium and Italy, a new type of man—red-blooded virile man who preserves his manhood, and will not let a woman not his wife minister to his sex instincts.[53]

The sexual impulse, the educational campaign insisted, was not for selfish pleasure but for marriage and reproduction. The lecturers sought to invent for the troops a concept of virginity and chastity equivalent to that demanded of women; therefore, they frequently employed terms such as "protect" and "intact."

The sexual ideology that the CTCA presented to the soldiers divided feminine society in two. First, there were the "pure" women to whom the war was dedicated—the mothers, sisters, and sweethearts patiently waiting for their heroes to return home. The other group of women was comprised of those who would subvert the war effort by seducing American fighting men. Lecturers used this dichotomy to encourage continence and attack the double standard of morality. A woman's consent did not make intercourse acceptable:

> As a woman values her virtue above all things, so a man treasures his virility. . . . The girl who 'consents', loses her chastity. Her virtue is gone, she is ruined. Suppose the man who went out for his first sexual experience thereby lost his manhood, was ruined, his virility gone.
>
> The man who seduces a girl is committing the gravest possible wrong against her. It may be that this act will entail consequences that would make all her friends and her family say,—"better had she been on the ill-fated *Lusitania* and gone down to the depths of the sea than that this fate had befallen her."[54]

The lecturer concluded that women who surrender their virginity often commit suicide in despair.

If it was the soldier's responsibility to protect undefiled womanhood, it was also his duty to save his own manliness from the tentacles of the fallen woman. The social hygiene campaign stressed that virtually all prostitutes carried venereal diseases. As *Keeping Fit to Fight* warned the troops: "WOMEN WHO SOLICIT SOLDIERS FOR IMMORAL PURPOSES ARE USUALLY DISEASE SPREADERS AND FRIENDS OF THE ENEMY." The pamphlet noted explicitly, "Any man who joins his body with the body of a prostitute or loose girl runs the risk of catching one of these terrible diseases."[55] With such exhortations the CTCA hoped to dispel the attractions of the prostitute.

Despite the vigor of the CTCA's educational efforts, traditional attitudes towards masculinity and sexuality were not easily displaced. When the resolution proclaiming continence compatible with health was approved by the Council of National Defense, Samuel Gompers, president of the American Federation of Labor and a member of the Council, rose in protest:

> What have you been doing? Sold out to the so-called "social hygienists" and the prohibition fanatics, long-haired men and short-haired women? You shall not make the war an opportunity for these complacent so-called "reformers" to accomplish their nefarious work! When have fighting men been preached to on the beneficence of continence? The millennium has not arrived and until it does your pronouncements of yesterday will not be accepted. Real men will be men.

Though the General Medical Board overruled Gompers's objections, his view continued to have adherents in the military. In spite of the directives from

Washington for a celibate army, considerable disagreement among officers concerning the venereal program and sexual morale persisted. Representatives of the YMCA's National War Work Council notified the CTCA that many officers continued to "assume the necessity of illicit relations and base their talks to the men and their instructions on that assumption." The Commission took action against such officers whenever possible. Josephus Daniels had T.A. Berryhill replaced as commander of the Naval Hospital at Mare Island, California, after Berryhill reportedly said that "immoral conditions at Vallejo didn't make a damn bit of difference."[56] It proved impossible, however, to erase completely the conventional military notion that a soldier needed to be a libertine to be an effective fighter.

The propaganda effort culminated in the CTCA's production of a full-length, dramatic motion picture centering on the themes of the social hygiene campaign. *Fit to Fight* attempted to prove the concordance of virility with clean living. The film, the first ever produced by the government, demonstrated the inventive adaptability of the educational program; the CTCA, it seems, employed any available technique to encourage continence. Officers in the Social Hygiene Division placed great emphasis on the film's ability to alter behavior. If, H.E. Kleinschmidt reasoned, effective propaganda constituted "mental inoculation," *Fit to Fight* served this function well.[57]

The film follows five draftees, each representing a particular social background: Billy Hale, a college quarterback who is introduced beating up a pacifist; Chick Charlton, "a gilded youth . . . sneaking through college on one book—his check book"; Kid McCarthy, a boxer given to wine and women; Hank Simpson, an unsophisticated farm boy; and Jack Garvin, cigar salesman and man of the world. This motley quintet find themselves together in training camp, receiving the company commander's lecture on the hazards of venereal disease. Kid and Billy listen attentively, taking his advice seriously; Hank appears embarrassed by the references to gonorrhea and syphilis; Chick Charlton and Jack Garvin waver between boredom and amusement. The next scene shows the five doughboys in a nearby town where they are drinking bootlegged liquor. When they are all picked up by street-walkers, only Billy Hale demurs, preferring "to be considered a mollycoddle rather than accompanying a prostitute." The other four enter a brothel. Hank escapes with only a kiss, recalling his father's warnings of "wild women." But Jack, Chick and the Kid consummate the act. Kid McCarthy, remembering the lecturer's admonition, makes a beeline for the prophylactic station. Jack, however, waits until the next day; Chick ignores the preventive altogether.[58]

The consequences of this urban escapade are not unexpected. Chick Charlton develops a bad case of gonorrhea; he is later shown crippled from the disease. Reporting too late for the prophylactic treatment to be effective, Jack Garvin has contracted syphilis. Hank displays a syphilitic infection on his lip, the result of his kiss from a diseased prostitute. (Clearly, the CTCA wished to discourage *all* contact with prostitutes.) All three will spend the war in the hospital at government expense.

Billy and the Kid, spared infection, still have a score to settle. The Kid taunts

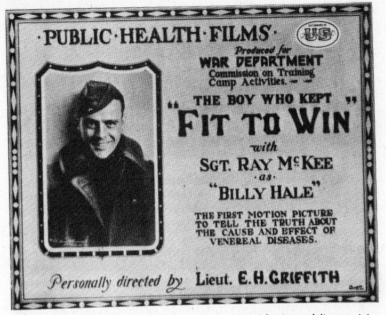

1. A poster for the Commission on Training Camp Activities' first venereal disease training film. Shortly after the war the title, "Fit to Fight" was changed to "Fit to Win." The New York State Board of Censors declared the film obscene in 1919.

Billy for refusing to visit prostitutes. "Ain't yous afraid that yous will have a wet dream tonight?" asks the boxer. With one punch Billy knocks out the Kid, replying that a man is "not a coward because he won't go with a dirty slut." The Kid and the men in the barracks acquire a new respect for Billy's chastity; apparently, they have seen the advantages of clean living for a soldier. The Kid confirms his moral conversion, announcing, "I wouldn't touch a whore with a ten-foot pole." Billy and the Kid become fast friends.[59]

Fit to Fight and the social hygiene campaign in general attempted to define a new male sex role—powerful yet pure, virile yet virginal—perhaps best represented for the Progressive generation in the figure of Theodore Roosevelt. Combining a high sense of moralism with an undaunted masculinity, Roosevelt was typically held as an example of "red-blooded" manhood. His expression of support for the social hygiene program was thus widely distributed to the troops:

> Let them lead clean, self-respecting lives, in the first place because it's the straight, decent self-respecting thing to do; next because it's the only way in which to give the square deal to women of the right type, who, Heaven knows, need the square deal; and finally because they owe it to the country not to ruin their efficiency as soldiers and citizens.[60]

Roosevelt suggested that the battlefield, not the brothel, should be the proving ground of American men.

Reformers celebrated the social hygiene crusade as a victory over prudishness and tradition in the interest of health and morality. The double standard, they suggested, had been dealt a death blow and a new sexual ethic established in its place. Franklin Martin of the Council of National Defense argued that the CTCA had indeed helped to create a new man:

> The new way has not produced a milksop, and on the other hand the 'rounder' in war and society has been eliminated. In his place has come the clean-eyed, strong-limbed, self-respecting athlete with a knowledge of himself and a high sense of moral and spiritual obligation to his fellow men and women.

The results of the educational program, explained the social hygienists, would be far-ranging, perhaps protecting American society from a venereal epidemic after the war. As Walter Clarke concluded: "When the boys come marching home they will know more of the scientific and practical facts of sex hygiene than any similar group of men in the world and they will pass on to the next generation wholesome and sane information regarding healthful living."[61]

The social hygiene campaign combined a high Victorian ideal of civilized sexual morality with a Progressive virility impulse. The CTCA laced this appeal with modern demands from the perspective of science and efficiency. Though few of the ideas concerning sex prescribed by the Social Hygiene Instruction Division were new, the notion of presenting them publicly and officially was totally unprecedented. Indeed, the openness with which sexual matters were addressed in the training camps, the intense propaganda campaign, seemed to vitiate the nature of the injunctions against sexual promiscuity.[62] For reformers dedicated to a rigid, Victorian attitude toward sex and disease, breaking the "conspiracy of silence" had important unintended consequences.

3

No matter how well educated the troops were concerning the dangers of venereal disease, the War Department feared the impact of the visits soldiers would inevitably pay to the cities and towns near the camps. Painfully aware of the allurements such communities held, particularly after his investigation of the Texas camps, Fosdick asked Joseph Lee to enlist the resources of the Playground and Recreation Association of America to plan wholesome activities in the towns near the training camps. Lee established the War Camp Community Service, which became the CTCA's agency for constructive social work in the vicinities of the camps. "It is outside the camps," explained Lee, "that the greatest danger exists."[63]

The War Camp Community Service sought to ensure that the American soldier, "a tree uprooted," received proper treatment from the civil communities. The Service, Lee noted, would meet the enlisted man's "social hunger" by steering him towards a town's better sources of entertainment. The WCCS, working with civilians in the areas around the camps, sponsored clubs and visits, as well as carefully chaperoned dances. Indeed, reformers eager to participate in the CTCA's community activities overran Fosdick's office. "I confess that this canteen business is becoming a veritable nuisance," Fosdick wrote to Lee. "I am besieged by women's delegations and others, asking the privilege of running combination canteens and clubs in the vicinity of Army camps." The CTCA attempted to control the conditions under which soldiers met women, and the clubs and canteens served this purpose well. "Our soldiers and sailors will seek and find female society in any case," observed Lee. "The War Camp Community Service has provided, for the first time in history, that they shall find it in a form that does them not harm but infinite good."[64]

Civic clubs and entertainment could only be successful if organized vice was controlled. Baker worked to forestall a proliferation of prostitution—similar to that which occurred on the Mexican border in 1916—as the nation prepared to enter the European conflict. According to professional investigators, if the government did not take action the soldiers would be left to the designs of organized vice. As the YMCA explained:

> Possibly the most repulsive occurrence in the civilized community in war time is the gathering of the bloodsuckers. Profiteers burr around the honey-pot in countless numbers. . . . The purveyors of questionable recreations know their business perfectly. They are much more alive to the effects of fatigue and monotony than are the well-intentioned citizens at home; they know exactly why their wares are likely to prove acceptable, and until very recent years they have been sure of freedom from competition.

After hearing testimony from Fosdick concerning the conditions in Mexico, the Senate Military Committee drafting the Selective Service Act appended two sections forbidding liquor and prostitution in areas proximate to the training camps. These two riders, sections 12 and 13, became the basis for the most aggressive attack on prostitution in the nation's history.[65] President Wilson gave the Commission on Training Camp Activities the responsibility for enforcing what came to be called the "moral zones" around the camps. Though the Commission publicized its so-called "positive program" in the camps, the battle against prostitution became the central focus of its work. The CTCA was transformed from a clearinghouse for voluntary reformers to an interventionist campaign against vice.[66]

In May, shortly after Wilson signed the Draft Act, Baker wrote to the nation's governors explaining the provisions of sections 12 and 13. If the soldiers were to protect the nation, he argued, they must first be protected from "unhealthy influences and crude forms of temptation." Baker stressed not only the War Department's moral commitment to the soldiers' families and communities but, more importantly, the necessity for creating an efficient army, free of disease. Recognizing the essential need for local cooperation if a national policy against vice and venereal disease was to be established, Baker called on the governors to endorse vigorously the activities of the CTCA in their state and to enforce strictly the provisions of the Draft Act. His letter reportedly had an "electric effect," galvanizing support for the government's repression not only of prostitution but also of alcohol.[67]

Social hygienists justified the ban on liquor as a component of the anti-venereal campaign. They viewed the consumption of alcohol as a major contributing element in the acquisition of venereal infections. Liquor reportedly lowered a man's ability to resist the power of the sexual urges. "The effect of alcoholic liquor is a factor that can not be overlooked in the diffusion of venereal diseases," wrote William Allen Pusey, "because of the inhibition which it produces in those restraining influences that under ordinary conditions prevent man's giving way to his impulses." Military officers suggested that most men contracted their diseases while under the influence of alcohol. "A soldier is not a good soldier if he indulges in alcoholics," explained Dr. Loyd Thompson of the medical corps. "Eighty-five per cent of the men who come to the clinics with venereal disease, new cases, have been using alcohol, enough to make them hilarious or drunk." The provisions of the Draft Act forbidding liquor near the camps were thus considered integral to the CTCA's fight against venereal disease and prostitution. One journalist declared, "John Barleycorn and the Woman of Babylon are partners."[68]

Prostitution, previously a strictly moral issue, was subsumed during the war by a new emphasis on science, hygiene, and health, an emphasis which seemed to be substantiated by recent medical advances concerning the diagnosis and pathology of the venereal diseases. Military and medical experts argued that prostitution constituted the primary locus of venereal infection. "The prostitute," explained one writer, "is undoubtedly the most active single medium for the transmission of infection." Estimates of levels of disease among prostitutes ranged from a conservative 60 to 75 percent to the more frequently publicized 90 percent. As Raymond Fosdick concluded, "The government was not in the futile business of trying to make people good by law, but fighting prostitution because of the fearful menace of venereal disease."[69]

The assault on prostitution now acquired the powerful legitimacy of a public health movement. Medical experts often drew analogies between the prostitute and other carriers of infectious disease. John H. Stokes, a venereal specialist at the Mayo Clinic, wrote:

> No one would seek to deny that commercialized vice is a large factor in the distribution of syphilis and gonorrhea. Medically speaking it can be thought of as the intermediate host or carrier of the Spirochaeta pallida, just as the mosquito is host for the malarial parasite. No rational public action against malaria neglects the destruction of the mosquito and the swamps in which it breeds.

Closing down red-light districts became part of the "hygienic gospel," comparable to the anti-tuberculosis and anti-yellow fever campaigns of the Progressive years. As one federal official explained, "To drain a red-light district and destroy thereby a breeding place of syphilis and gonorrhea is as logical as it is to drain a swamp and destroy thereby a breeding place of malaria and yellow fever."[70] This argument broadened the appeal of the fight against prostitution to include a new educated, professional class dedicated to science, efficiency, and technology.

Moral reformers welcomed these supporters to the anti-prostitution crusade. They insisted on the strict complementarity of the moral and medical viewpoints. For example, J. Frank Chase of the New England Watch and Ward Society, a longstanding anti-vice organization, advocated the establishment of an Army Corps of Moral Engineers to check commercialized vice. Though the metaphor seems mixed, the idea reflected the alliance that was struck between the traditional moral outlook on the prostitution problem and the new emphasis on scientific, preventive medicine. Such an organization, Chase declared, would practice what he called the "science of moral engineering." For Gertrude Seymour of the *Survey*, the question of prostitution demonstrated the concordance of health and social stability: "From every angle the problem focuses at this time on prostitution. From the point of view of public health, prostitution means the greatest focus of venereal disease. From the social angle prostitution must be reckoned with as a menace to any form of stable organization of the home or of the community."[71]

More than any other single theme, however, the offensive against prostitution stressed the connection between threatened health and threatened military efficiency. Social hygienists, reformers, and military officials typically employed dramatic, if over-extended, analogies to make the attack on the red-light districts even more immediate. As J. Frank Chase wrote:

> It is generally recognized that a bad and diseased woman can do more harm than any German fleet of airplanes that has yet passed over London. One woman of such character as effectually destroys a soldier as a German gun would, and more so. A German gun might do much more harm to men in front of it, but it would not leave the wounded as a menace to his associates, as is a man who suffers from "social diseases."

Commandant George of the Mare Island Navy Yard suggested that prostitution in the United States was actually of subversive design. "I believe there is a well defined purpose on the part of the German government to break down the morale of the American troops through liquor and vice," he explained. No matter whom the prostitute worked for, social hygienists hammered one point home repeatedly; she endangered the American war effort. The Western Social Hygiene Association distributed a flyer entitled, "Could the Kaiser Do Worse?":

> If the Kaiser would send an army of German prostitutes into our camps to infect United States soldiers with gonorrhea and syphilis and thus keep them from the front, the nation would wrathfully protest. American prostitutes are estimated to have infected . . . with syphilis alone 445,000 registered men not called in the first draft.[72]

The CTCA took official action by establishing a Law Enforcement Division charged with ridding the cities near the camps of liquor and prostitution, as required by the Draft Act, and appointed Bascom Johnson, counsel to the American Social Hygiene Association, as director of the new division, with the rank of Major in the Sanitary Corps. Johnson had achieved prominence for closing down the infamous San Francisco red-light district, the "Barbary Coast," using the recently enacted California Injunction and Abatement Act.[73] Under his leadership, the Law Enforcement Division's program of closing down red-light districts became the dominant aspect of the CTCA's varied activities.

The Division parceled the nation into sections, one for each camp, and dispatched vice investigators to each. These investigators, usually lawyers, who were to survey and report local conditions in regard to prostitution and alcohol, were recruited from those voluntary agencies that had been most active in the Progressive campaign against vice. They knew the red-light districts well and took encouragement that their efforts had at last achieved federal backing. As Division investigators, they met with law enforcement officials and influential citizens to seek their cooperation in "sanitizing" the cities. Members of the Division lobbied judges to impose maximum sentences upon prostitutes convicted of soliciting. According to an officer of the Law Enforcement Division, the vice investigators "acted as especially effective evangelists for the new gospel of civic decency and military efficiency."[74]

Officials responded to the CTCA's requests for cooperation, generating local campaigns against prostitution, and the segregated districts of prostitution in cities and towns near the training camps soon began to close down. Governor Richard I. Manning of South Carolina wrote to Secretary Daniels assuring him that, because public opinion ran high on the subject, "a vigorous policy will be aroused in suppressing vice." In early October 1917, the notorious red-light district of Charleston fell. The Texas communities of San Antonio and El Paso, which had proved to be centers of organized prostitution during the Mexican border incident of 1916, were among the first cities to eliminate their segregated districts. San Antonio established the "Committee of Five" to keep a vigilant watch over vice conditons. In St. Louis police arrested more than 1,000 women reportedly plying the trade within city limits. The mayor of Pittsburgh fired police officers who refused to act with sufficient vigor to suppress vice. And in California alone, officials closed down more than 300 houses of prostitution. The California State Law Enforcement and Protective League, under the leadership of purity crusader Edwin Grant, boarded up dance halls while searching for organized vice activities.[75]

In some communities, city officials closed the districts simply by ordering all prostitutes to leave town. A medical officer at Camp Sheridan near Montgomery, Alabama, reported that there "were enough prostitutes in town to serve a city of 400,000." He explained, "All have been ordered to leave by Monday, November 12, 1917. The majority have left already." This policy, of course, often caused the influx of prostitutes in near-by cities and towns. Citizens in New Orleans, for example, reported that as red-light districts elsewhere in the South were snuffed out, conditions there worsened. One irate woman wrote to Secretary Baker:

> We have seen these plague spots closed everywhere else, Newport, San Antonio, Alexandria, but to our surprise and disappointment the conditions in New Orleans remain the same. . . . No . . . they are daily growing worse, as the women from these other cities which have been closed are fleeing to our city.[76]

The battle to close Storyville, New Orleans' world-renowned red-light district, illustrated the resolve of the CTCA's attack on prostitution. A Commission investigator described the district as the "Gibraltar of commercialized vice . . . twenty-four blocks given over to human degradation and lust." Citizens demanded that Secretary Baker eliminate the district. "Why is it the Government makes an exception of New Orleans?" asked one angry reformer. "They have made other places clean up." Early in September, Fosdick wrote to Josephus Daniels requesting that he close the district because of its proximity to the navy yard. Fosdick called Storyville "one of the most vicious red-light districts I have ever seen." According to CTCA investigations, Fosdick explained, "sailors in uniform make it a Mecca." The purge of Storyville, he suggested, would have a positive impact on the CTCA's entire program. "If the New Orleans district is closed it will have a far reaching effect on the whole problem in the South," he wrote. "It is the last stronghold of the old regime."[77]

In spite of Bascom Johnson's insistence that Storyville be shut down, and Daniels's appeal to the Governor of Louisiana to do so, the fact that no army installation existed nearby made it difficult for the CTCA to demand its closure. Martin Behrman, the mayor of New Orleans, traveled to Washington to defend the continuation of the segregated district, assuring Baker that no soldiers were ever admitted. CTCA vice investigators had reported, however, that soldiers and sailors had been seen changing into civilian clothes before entering the district. On October 6, 1917, Congress extended the provisions of sections 12 and 13 of the Draft Act to include the Navy. Daniels now reportedly told Behrman, "You close the red-light district, or the armed forces will." On November 12, the citadel of Southern prostitution fell, twenty years after its creation by municipal ordinance. The CTCA celebrated the demise of Storyville, but the district's supporters contended that the action had merely diffused commercialized vice throughout the city.[78]

Although officials sought to persuade local communities to close down the red-light districts near the camps, they did not refrain from employing stronger tactics where necessary. The threat of moving training camps or forbidding the troops from entering cities served as a last resort when local officials proved recalcitrant. Fosdick noted the possibility of exercising such action in Philadelphia, where conditions were reported to be among the nation's most nefarious. During one leave, 500 of 600 soldiers admitted a sexual exposure. Suggesting the city be placed off-limits, Fosdick wrote to Daniels, "Unless the local authorities assume the responsibility which is legally theirs and effectively rid the city of those who prey upon our men, I can see no other way out of the difficulty." Daniels eventually responded by having the city patrolled by Marines.[79] A journalist reported the case of a commanding officer who warned city officials near his camp: "Clear the streetwalkers from your boulevards and stamp out those dance hall-hells or not a man of my thirty-thousand will enter your city." Baker effectively used such intimidation in Birmingham and Seattle to force authorities to take action against commercialized vice. The *Survey* explained that the new efforts to clean up the cities were often motivated by economic realism rather than moral rectitude. Businessmen realized that soldiers on leave had money to spend. As one city official noted, "Our citizens must choose between the big business of these women and their exploiters and the

big business of 50,000 soldiers. Whom will they serve?" The CTCA made its
position on this issue clear; as one member of the Commission declared, "The
Government desires to lead, but it will not hesitate to coerce if necessary."[80]

Shutting down the red-light districts, however, did not completely eliminate
prostitution. If the repression of prostitution stopped when segregated districts
were closed, warned Bascom Johnson, the prostitute would simply continue her
activities in hotels, rooming houses, and apartments, as critics charged had occurred after the demise of Storyville. Moreover, investigators found that prostitutes had devised imaginative new ways to conduct business in response to the
government's action. Taxi-drivers and chauffeurs, CTCA investigators reported, delivered clients to secret locations. "Few city police departments, or
country sheriffs," explained Johnson, "are sufficiently equipped with motorcy-
cle police to patrol the city streets and country roads, and the prostitute may
indefinitely vary the scene of her operations, or the car itself may be used if
necessary." The connection between the automobile and sexual morals, a topic
that would receive considerably more attention in the next decade, was first
discussed during the war. "The automobile prostitute," lamented Johnson, "is
the bane of law enforcement officials." He advocated new federal legislation to
combat these "new and elusive methods of operation." When J. Frank Chase
received reports of such activities, he wrote to Fosdick immediately, "I fairly
gasp at the possibilities for wickedness which this reveals. In my judgment . . .
this is the most subtle form of prostitution of which I have heard."[81]

The activities of the Law Enforcement Division illustrate the Progressive faith
in legislation as a means to desired reforms. Many reformers, in the belief that
the proper combination of laws would destroy prostitution and thereby venereal
disease, lobbied state legislatures to pass a battery of enactments during the war
to penalize "immoral practices." The CTCA promoted such bills by providing
state boards of health with counsel and sample ordinances declaring prostitution, in any of its many forms, illegal. Some states made it a felony for a woman,
knowing herself to have an infectious venereal disease, to engage in sexual intercourse with a member of the military forces. Fornication laws that made intercourse between unmarried couples illegal were also enacted, although they
proved difficult to enforce. Indeed, many of these laws proved impractical, passed
more for their symbolic value than for actual impact. John Buchanan, a lawyer
for the CTCA, suggested, "Why not make it a felony for a woman to commit
fornication with a soldier or sailor anywhere?"[82]

In spite of the many legislative enactments and repressive measures including
the closing of red-light districts, prostitution persisted. Reformers continued to
argue, however, that prostitution could be conquered; it was merely necessary
to pursue the prostitute down the next alley until she gave up or got caught.
To accept the notion that prostitution was part and parcel of American urban
life would have negated the very rationale upon which Progressive reform was
based. When it did become clear that prostitution remained even as the red
lights flickered out, Fosdick was forced to concede, "I do not think we will ever
absolutely eliminate the prostitute, but we do want to make it impossible for
the prostitute to flaunt herself in the face of men on the streets when they are
not thinking about her."[83]

By the time new soldiers reported to the major training camps in September 1917, "moral zones" around them had been firmly established by the CTCA. Altogether, the Commission claimed the destruction of 110 red-light districts throughout the nation during the war. Fosdick suggested that segregated prostitution had "practically ceased to be a feature of American city life." A madam in Troy, New York, complained to one of the incognito CTCA investigators: "The whole trouble now is with the gals; you can't get a girl to work, they're scared stiff. . . . Gals are scarce as hen's teeth; they won't work in a house, the government has them buffaloed." The closing of the red-light districts was hailed by social hygiene reformers, civil leaders, public health advocates, and military officials, as one of the war's greatest victories. George Anderson, a CTCA investigator, described the assault on organized prostitution as "tantamount to a social revolution." Reviewing the CTCA's accomplishment, another official observed, "It is a little difficult to realize that a year ago these places constituted the overshadowing menace to the health and efficiency of the forces of the United States."[84]

4

Venereal disease rates following the closing of the red-light districts indicated that these reforms had had no immediate impact. Though levels of venereal disease in the training camps varied dramatically, they remained high, causing great concern about the health of American youths and their sexual mores. During the year ending August 30, 1918, the surgeon general of the Army reported 126 venereal admissions per 1,000 men, almost 13 percent. Seeking to dispel the popular perception of a profligate army, Secretary Baker rejected the idea that soldiers were particularly prone to sexually transmitted diseases. He suggested this misapprehension had been created because the military collected and published their venereal statistics. Prior to World War I, a venereal disease had constituted a cause for rejection from service. Given the critical need for soldiers and the recently discovered techniques for diagnosis and treatment, the surgeon general quickly abandoned this regulation. Too many draftees harbored chronic infections to dismiss this population from service. "If you were to attempt to get an army without having men who had gonorrhea," noted Dr. Granville MacGowan of Los Angeles, "you would not have an army." Moreover, members of the medical department feared that disqualification for venereal disease encouraged men to solicit infections prior to induction as a means of avoiding service.[85]

The draft revealed the massive endemic nature of the venereal problem in the United States. Though the CTCA's program of recreation, education, and repression of prostitution near the camps would save some soldiers from becoming infected, medical officers soon realized that new soldiers bringing old infections to the camps presented the greatest problem. Military physicians discovered that five out of every six cases of venereal disease had been contracted prior to induction; infections among the new soldiers merely reflected a larger civilian problem. According to several reports, as many as twenty-five percent of the inductees at some camps were venereally diseased. "The amount of venereal disease contracted by the men after putting on the uniform is astonishingly small," explained Drs. William F. Snow and Wilbur A. Sawyer, "while the amount of chronic venereal disease brought to the Army from civil life is a serious burden."[86]

Military physicians and officials concluded that, in spite of the effectiveness of the program to combat venereal disease in the camps, the problem had first to be addressed in civilian life. As Secretary Baker explained, venereal diseases originated in "the laxly governed civil communities . . . where ignorance of conditions and indifference, or something even worse on the part of local authorities, have conduced to widespread infection." Under strict military discipline, military officials argued, the opportunities for infection actually decreased. As one physician concluded after reviewing military medical statistics, "A man is safer in the Army than in civil life." The medical department increasingly looked to civilian life as the focus for controlling the venereal problem in the army. "If it is desirable to protect the young men in the Army from venereal diseases," asked Colonel Victor Vaughan of the Medical Corps, "why should not the young men who are civilians, and, in all probability are soon to become soldiers, be protected from the same disease?"[87]

These findings became the basis for transforming the CTCA's battle against venereal disease into a truly national campaign. No longer would efforts be limited to the areas around the training camps. Arguing that "no citizen is exempt from service in the war against disease," the Council of National Defense established the Civilian Committee to Combat Venereal Disease in December 1917 to elicit public support for the anti-venereal program. As a CCCVD flyer explained: "In a modern battle the artillery clears the way. After the Big Guns comes the individual effort—the bayonet charge, the hand-to-hand conflict. The way is being cleared fo the individual to attack the veneral disease problem." The Civilian committee developed a highly organized propaganda campaign dedicated to generating a nationwide crusade against prostitution and vice. They suggested that every community establish a "Citizen's Committee" to promote law enforcement, sex education, public health, activities for girls, and recreation. "The time is now here," announced the CCCVD, "when ignorance and neglect in these matters indicate lack of patriotism."[88] The citizens' campaign became an effective means for engaging the civilians to do their "bit" for the war effort.

Centering attention on prostitution and its effect on venereal disease, the CCCVD, in concert with the CTCA's efforts in the cities near the training camps, sought to encourage a national attack on vice. "There are now in the United States hundreds of prostitutes who are daily committing what is in effect the crime of mayhem upon hundreds of our country's soldiers and sailors," declared Dr. Franklin Martin in a widely distributed CCCVD circular. "They accomplish the same result by infecting the men with syphilis and gonorrhea." Though the CTCA could close down some red-light districts through enforcement of section 13 or intimidation of city officials, if the assault on prostitution was to be a national success, public support constituted a major requisite. The CTCA called on citizens to "Smash the Line" of commercialized vice in their communities. In red-light districts, the CTCA explained, "venereal diseases have their widest opportunity to spread, insidiously as a poison-gas attack and wreak havoc." The Civilian Committee wrote to sheriffs, mayors, and prominent citizens throughout the nation, urging them to help wipe out prostitution. In all, the Committee sent some 18,000 letters to citizens in 800 communities. "We make it clear to the people we write that a community which does not help to protect the soldiers in its midst is sticking a knife into the backs of those soldiers—no, worse than that!—for a knife cut is easy to handle, whereas the stabs from communities indifferent or hostile to our work are doubly dangerous and criminal," remarked William H. Zinsser, chairman of the Committee.[89]

The CCCVD took measures to augment the powers of public health officials in order to deal with the venereal problem more effectively. The Committee lobbied state boards of health to require official reporting of all venereal infections by physicians, as well as provide free laboratory diagnosis and clinic treatment.[90] The American Red Cross expended $250,000 to establish twenty-five U.S. Public Health Service dispensaries to serve venereally infected civilians. In the first eight months of operation these clinics treated 23,000 patients. The *Journal of the American Medical Association* suggested in an editorial that service in the venereal disease campaign provided "the opportunity for the civilian physician to do his 'bit' effectively." Doctors, they stressed, should be prepared to recognize these diseases and impress upon their patients the dangers of transmission.[91]

The government did not limit its program in civilian communities to protecting soldiers on leave, or even would-be soldiers. Social hygienists and public health officials increasingly emphasized the losses to venereal disease incurred by business and industry; losses that, they suggested, threatened the war effort. Gertrude Seymour, a well-known social hygienist, argued for the importance of protecting the "industrial army," as well as the troops—"the men behind the men behind the guns." William Zinsser noted the relationship between productive efficiency and military success: "In a way never so clearly marked before, it has been brought home to all the nations now participating in the great struggle that *army* really means *nation*; that the 'behind the lines' work is just as vital as the battle-line fighting." The Civilian Committee thus wrote to industrialists urging them to institute anti-venereal programs in their factories. "Have you ever thought what venereal diseases are costing you and your business?" asked Zinsser. The CTCA provided toilet placards and pay envelope inserts with anti-venereal epigrams to interested corporations. In addition, the Committee advocated that employers have their workers examined for venereal diseases and, if need be, treated. Though they suggested that employees found to be infected be given leaves with pay, in all probability such men and women lost their jobs. This, of course, discouraged compliance with venereal examinations.[92]

Social hygienists hoped to encourage a broad shift in sexual mores, to achieve a truly national impact. This required the destruction of the "conspiracy of silence" that had limited public discussion of sexual issues. Zinsser described some of the difficulties the CCCVD experienced in their early attempts to upset this tradition:

Old customs, out-of-date regulations and habits of mind prevented the thinking people of the communities from grasping the significance either of the government's far-sighted and history-making stand, or of their vital part in backing it up. For so many generations have all things pertaining to sex, reproduction, prostitution, venereal disease, etc., been considered "dirty,"—not fit to be touched publicly by the best men and women in our country,—that even the shock of this war seemed unable to break through the barrier.

For example, longstanding rationales for segregated prostitution—particularly the theory that such a class of women protected "responsible society" from sexual lust—died hard. A resident of Columbia, South Carolina, expressed this concern when the mayor closed the red-light district there:

> I'm going to buy a pistol, sir. For twelve years I've lived in this town and never felt the need to protect my two womenfolks. What do you suppose will happen when 40,000 virile, red-blooded young men come here to train for the army and find the segregated district wiped out? I know; and I'm going to buy that pistol, sir, and do it now!

The CTCA felt compelled to point out in its reports that the incidence of rape and assault had not risen in communities that had closed their red-light districts.[93]

According to the social hygienists, the citizens' campaign had generated a revolution in American sexual mores. Never before had issues of sexual morality, prostitution, and venereal disease received so much public attention. Newspapers that had in the past refused to print the words "syphilis" and "gonorrhea" now published full-scale accounts of the government's anti-venereal program. The prudent silence typically associated with these topics had at last, they suggested, been broken. As Franklin Martin explained:

> The arguments of science, clean living, and a great war to which fathers and mothers were to lend their sons aroused public opinion until it was decided to "give the new plan a try-out," and the try-out has been so dramatically successful that a spiritual light has dawned and has illuminated the dark places and driven the greatest evil of civilization to bay.[94]

The CTCA believed that a new, higher standard of sexual conduct, a national morality, was the result of their program.

5

Soldiers nevertheless continued to engage in sexual activity, and the national crusade against prostitution could not prevent them from acquiring venereal infections. As Joseph Lee explained, "Disease is spread not wholly by professional prostitutes but very largely by young girls who have succumbed to the emotional conditions produced by the war." Teenage girls reportedly flocked to the camps in search of excitement, adventure, and love. The soldier, noted the *Survey*, "is a bright mesmeric figure in the dull texture of our lives and quickly touches the romantic sentiments of young girls." CTCA investigators found soldiers and adolescent women surreptitiously entering and leaving wooded areas near the camps. Taxi-drivers allegedly assisted these secret rendezvous, taking couples to deserted areas. "This is one of the forms of clandestine love-making that has become most popular since the war," observed the *Survey*.[95]

Physicians and social workers frequently commented that the professional prostitute had given way to the so-called "patriotic prostitute" and "charity girl." As one CTCA social worker wrote:

> The peculiar charm and glamour which surrounds the man in uniform causes an unusual type of prostitute to spring up in time of war. Girls idealize the soldier and many really feel that nothing is wrong when done for him. One such girl said she had never sold herself to a civilian but felt she was doing her bit when she had been with eight soldiers in a night.

The "girl problem," as it became popularly known, seemed even more ominous to reformers than commercialized vice because it so often included youngsters from respectable, middle-class backgrounds. "Girls apparently of good families drive up in their cars and invite the soldiers who happen to be along the roadside near the camp to come to supper to a roadhouse or the nearest city," explained Dr. Jennie H. Harris. "The results are the usual ones."[96]

Inherent in this assessment was a revised view of sexuality and desire; no longer were young girls seen as essentially passive and sexually anesthetic, but rather as dangerously lustful. By September 1917, Fosdick had received so many complaints concerning the delinquency of young women that he created the Committee on Protective Work for Girls. "We found that venereal disease was coming not from the prostitutes," he told a congressional committee, "but from the type known in the military camps as the flapper—that is, the young girls who were not prostitutes, but who probably would be to-morrow, and who were diseased and promiscuous." Fosdick appointed Maude E. Miner, Secretary of the New York Probation and Protective Association, to direct the government's efforts to prevent delinquency. The Committee sought to protect the girl from the "unusual stimulus of her emotions" and to insure that women demonstrated their patriotism more constructively. The problem of the innocent girl, suffering from the spell cast by the uniform, attracted Progressive reformers to the CTCA's work. "The concentration of a large number of young men in comparatively few places, the tendency of women to flock to the camp towns, the danger of venereal disease, the unsettled social conditions in these towns," explained Henrietta Additon, a social worker with the CTCA, "all forced the government into this much shunned field of social work."[97]

The Committee on Protective Work emphasized education, distributing pamphlets and sponsoring lectures addressed to mothers and daughters (usually separately), warning them of the dangers of the war for purity and health. The lecturers that the Committee sent to schools and churches throughout the country demonstrated a basic distrust of emotion, particularly the sex drive. As one lecturer told a group of mothers:

> Our daughters will come into contact with the soldiers under unusual circumstances. However sensible we know them to be, we cannot expect them to withstand the natural attractions which the glamour of war lends to the soldier's uni-

form. . . . The dangers involved in such developments are obvious, and if such a situation is not delicately and tactfully handled unfortunate results may ensue. . . . The parents' refusal to permit their daughter to meet and associate with the soliders will in many cases at once arouse hostility and promote clandestine meetings—a situation which is, of course, by all means to be avoided *like a plague*.[98]

Lecturers often blamed parental failure for runaways and promiscuity. The "girl problem" spoke directly to Progressive fears of the decline of the family, anxieties that the Committee on Protective Work clearly expressed in its educational program.

The Committee's lecturers and pamphlets frequently warned women of the male's potentially explosive sexual nature. Reports of rapes and assaults in the areas around the camps had circulated, and the Committee played upon these fears. As one lecturer explained menacingly: "Unless he is endowed with unusual willpower, it is not unnatural if he breaks for the nearest town in search of the only kind of feminine companionship he can find—the kind he can buy. . . . Under the slightest provocation their passions rise to the surface as easily as bubbles in a glass of wine." Dr. Katherine Bement Davis, the Commissioner of Corrections of New York City and Miner's successor at the CTCA, believed it important to demonstrate that the uniform did not indicate uniform character. Davis, an expert in the field of sexual psychology, explained:

Young girls thrilled with patriotism, sometimes fail to realize that the uniform covers all the kinds of men there are in the world; men of high ideals, chivalrous instincts who naturally treat every girl as they want every man to treat their mothers and sisters . . . men with lower ideals, who feel that girls should take care of themselves or that they are fair game; or, in the worst instances, men who feel that their own physical appetites must be gratified no matter who suffers.

As the Committee for Protective Work began to develop its propaganda to save young girls from the "lure of the uniform," Fosdick cautioned that this line of argument could go too far. "I am concerned that the mothers of the country should not be scared into feeling that soldiers are beings to be feared," he noted. "We are anxious to get just the opposite reaction."[99]

The Committee suggested that it was the woman's responsibility not to arouse the volatile passions of men. Indeed, it assumed that women would set the moral tone for the war, and thus should play a prominent role in the CTCA's program. Proper dress and deportment, therefore, were required. As one pamphlet explained:

Did you ever stop to ask yourself what might be the effect upon young men of the kind of clothes you wear? The too transparent waists, showing plainly all the underwear beneath, the dresses cut too low in the neck, the gowns that cling too closely to the figure—what are these but suggestions to young men to think only of the physical charms of these young feminine creatures, and of nothing else?

In dancing also, it is possible to stimulate the lower desires and passions if one is not careful both by dress and behavior to avoid everything that is physically suggestive.

National duty required decorum, hygienists often argued. "Girls must be made to realize" declared a lecturer, "that they bear a responsibility to the soldier and that their patriotic duty is to avoid weakening the soldier's devotion to his country's best interests by arousing his emotions to a pitch which will tend to divide that devotion." [100] The educational campaign, which emphasized the need for a higher moral standard, supported these claims by frequent allusions to unwanted pregnancies and venereal diseases.

As part of the educational campaign for women and girls the CTCA produced another motion picture, *End of the Road*. Written by Katherine Bement Davis, the film described the war-time experiences of two seventeen-year-old women, Mary Lee and Vera Wagner. [101] Mary's mother is portrayed as the ideal parent, a confidante and friend, always ready to discuss the perils of adolescence with her daughter. Conversely, Vera's mother is falsely modest, anxious for her daughter to meet a wealthy man to gratify her own ambitions. "Two roads there are in life," began the film. "One reaches upward toward the land of perfect love. The other reaches down into the Dark Valley of Despair where the sun never shines." Not unexpectedly, Mary takes the high road; Vera, the low.

The two girls leave the small town of their childhood to seek their fortunes in New York City. Mary, eager to do service in the war effort, undertakes training to become a nurse. Meanwhile, Vera gains employment in a department store where she meets men of questionable morals over the sales-counter. Mary warns her friend, "I know, Vera, how hard it is to think of the consequences, now when we're young . . . unless we do we shan't find happiness at the end of the road." Mary has learned about those consequences, assisting the world-renowned surgeon, Dr. Richard Bell, as he performs hysterectomies on venereally-infected women. "This is the operation which every year, hundreds of thousands of women must undergo because of some man's criminal folly," explained the film's narration. [102]

The gruesome shots of syphilitic lesions that *End of the Road* displayed made its lesson clear: Most men, especially soldiers, could not be trusted. Women must refuse their demands for sex as Mary does when her boyfriend, leaving for France with the AEF, asks for "a memory [he] can never lose." She immediately replies: "Paul, how could you suggest such a thing?" The price of breaking the moral code, according to the film, was severe: gross physical deformities, stillborn children, even death. Vera eventually contracts syphilis from an unseemly rake who promises marriage and then deserts her; she is, however, successfully treated. Mary travels to France with Dr. Bell to serve the AEF, where during a moment's respite, they exchange marriage vows.

The Committee for Protective Work refused to rely wholly, however, on sexual education and moral exhortation. The CTCA appointed 150 women as protective officers to patrol the nation's streets in search of wayward young women. These officers, usually social workers, were trained to survey a town's social conditions, locate runaways and camp-followers, and return them to their homes. "Take a trolley to the town's amusement park, if it has one," Maude Miner told a group of women seeking to become officers. "Skip the well-lighted parts and visit the outskirts, where darkness is a shield to conduct. You will find these regions alive with men in uniform accompanied by girls." The protective officers drew upon many skills. As Miner commented, "If girls hide in the trenches [in the training camps], as they have occasionally done, protective officers go down and pull them out."[103] These women often served in the capacity of probation officers, investigating arrested girls, arranging for venereal and psychological examinations, and, if necessary, securing commitment to reformatory institutions.

War-time marriages of young girls to soldiers created particular concern among the protective officers of the CTCA. On some occasions, a man accused of raping or assaulting a teenage girl would propose marriage as a means of avoiding prosecution. "We all know how common it is for attorneys, and friends of the defendant's to say to the girl's parents, 'He is a fine young man,' although he may have a venereal disease or a criminal record," explained Arthur Towne of the Society for the Prevention of Cruelty to Children. "Far too often the parents through ignorance, fear, or, old-world information as to the necessity for marriage under certain conditions, will give the daughter in matrimony, only to repent after it is too late." Such forced marriages made explicit the opprobrium attached to the loss of virginity by unwed teenagers. "After one sex experience it becomes harder for them to resist temptation," explained Dr. Rachelle Yarros.[104] A life of prostitution was thought to be the all too frequent result of the fall from purity.

The greatest interest of the social workers employed by the CTCA during the war was not the hardened prostitute—little hope of rehabilitation was held for her—but rather, the young teenage girl, momentarily overcome by the emotional tumult of war. First offenders, "if reached at once," they believed could be saved from lives of prostitution. Reformers engaged in the protective effort increasingly directed their efforts at women who had already fallen rather than those who remained pure. Activities shifted from prevention to reformation, and Fosdick established a Section on Women and Girls under the Law Enforcement Division. This was a subtle admission of the defeat of the moral engineering hoped for by the Committee for Protective Work for Girls, and suggested that the reformers' fears were not ungrounded regarding not only a moral decline generated by the war but also the beginning of a more liberal sexual mores for women, a shift that would only be fully recognized in the next decade.[105]

6

Achieving only uneven success in limiting the soldiers' nonprofessional sexual contacts, the CTCA addressed a new problem in their efforts to prevent venereal disease: the disposition of apprehended prostitutes as cities closed down their red-light districts. If prostitutes merely set up shop in another part of town or a nearby community, as was often reported, the CTCA's anti-vice program would have little impact. Moreover, according to government officials, many of the arrested women harbored venereal infections that required immediate treatment. Fines and short-term jail sentences could return infectious women to the community. Military officers and citizens alike, largely in response to the propaganda campaign of the CTCA, demanded that arrested prostitutes be dealt with more forcefully. Again, prevention gave way to reformation—or, in fact, to containment and to punishment. Quarantine, detention, and internment became the new themes of the attack on prostitution. A Minneapolis lawyer wrote to Fosdick, "Syphilis stalks free, if covert, through our land, and now through our camps, without effort to *quarantine the source*. . . . If it is successfully combatted, it must be done as a war measure." One woman expressed the same idea in a letter to President Wilson, demanding that the government provide for the "internment . . . of all women of careless chastity." She suggested that these women should receive the same "comforts and conveniences enjoyed by interned alien enemies."[106]

In a determined effort to contain venereal infection, the Law Enforcement Division encouraged state legislatures and local boards of health to enact regulations requiring medical examinations of citizens "reasonably suspected" of carrying a venereal disease. The Virginia State Board of Health, for example, empowered all health officers to make examinations of "persons reasonably suspected of having syphilis, gonorrhea or chancroid." The ordinance defined "vagrants, prostitutes, keepers, inmates, and frequenters of houses of ill fame, prostitution and assignation, persons not of good fame, persons guilty of fornication, adultery, and lewd and lascivious conduct" to be "reasonably suspected." Furthermore, the measure provided that no one arrested for any of these various reasons could be released on bail until examined and found free from venereal disease. In San Francisco, the Department of Health provided arrested women with circulars explaining, "You are in quarantine and cannot be released on bail. . . . If you are found ill with venereal disease you will go to the hospital and stay there until found negative. . . . No lawyer or other person can obtain your release." By March 1918, thirty-two states had passed laws requiring compulsory examinations of prostitutes for venereal disease.[107]

The Department of Justice, assisting the CTCA, endorsed the regulations for compulsory examinations of arrested women. Attorney General T. W. Gregory, invoking the doctrine of the police power of the state, explained:

The constitutional right of the community, in the interest of the public health, to ascertain the existence of infections and communicable diseases in its midst and to isolate and quarantine such cases or take other steps necessary to prevent the spread of the disease, is clear.

Gregory issued a series of circulars to the United States Attorneys, outlining legal policy regarding apprehended prostitutes. These memoranda instructed the attorneys to report all arrests under section 13 to local or state health authorities and "to cause medical examinations to be made and to enforce such health laws, regulations, or ordinances relative to quarantine, treatment, and other disease control measures." Most significantly, the attorney general ordered that prosecution should be suspended pending examination, isolation, and treatment by health officials.[108]

The practice of involuntary detention and examination of women arrested on charges of prostitution or vagrancy drew sharp criticism on several fronts. First, some feminists found the idea of the diagnostic procedure itself offensive. "Compulsory exposure of young women," explained Dr. Katharine Bushnell, "deserves the name indecent assault." "You cannot appreciate how a woman feels to have her person exposed to the masturbating hand of a vile doctor," wrote Dr. Bushnell in an angry letter to the U.S. Public Health Service. "How would you like it for your wife?" Second, critics charged that the federal government had officially endorsed the double standard of morality since the program was directed exclusively to the arrest, examination, and detention of women. A man who transgressed the moral law suffered no such punishment. No efforts were made during the war to quarantine infected men. "Why should women be imprisoned for a disease when the man, as responsible, goes scot free," asked Chicago reformer Ethel Dummer. As Joseph S. Lawrence, Chief of the New York State Bureau of Venereal Diseases, observed, "Moralists have always thought that women are the chief offenders." Other critics charged that, because the government advocated holding women through treatment, then releasing them, the policy was tantamount to federally-regulated prostitution. Maude Miner resigned her position as chairman of the Committee on Protective Work for Girls, voicing strong objections to the direction of the federal program. "I could not be satisfied," she explained, "to see the girls' interests entirely subordinated to the interests of the soldier and the only reason for caring for the girls in the detention homes or reformatories reduced to just that." Some attacked the practice on the grounds that overzealous health officers arrested women indiscriminately, searching for foci of infection. Vice raids fell most heavily on working-class women, the unemployed, and the unescorted.[109]

The enactments requiring physical examinations of prostitutes also came under attack in the courts. Some state courts overturned these ordinances because health departments denied women access to bail during testing and treatment. When judges in several states ordered that measures prohibiting bail be ignored by the courts, health officers in these states were forced to suspend all compulsory examinations. A public health official in Richmond, Virginia, complained that since a court ruling there against involuntary examinations "the whole program for the suppression of prostitution and interning of dangerous cases of veneral diseases had broken down and been discontinued." He argued that under such a ruling it would be impossible to quarantine a victim of cholera, smallpox, or meningitis. Though these decisions proved worrisome to the Law Enforcement Division, most courts, invoking the doctrine of police powers of the state, upheld the restrictions on writs of habeas corpus.[110]

The activities of local health officers and police morals squads, as well as federal agents of the Law Enforcement Division and the Justice Department led to sweeping arrests and venereal examinations of women. Defended as a public health policy, the incarceration of women proceeded en masse. Dr. C. C. Pierce of the U.S. Public Health Service justified the procedure on the following grounds:

Conditions required the immediate isolation of as many venereally infected persons acting as spreaders of disease as could be quickly apprehended and quarantined. It was not a measure instituted for the punishment of prostitutes on account of infraction of the civil or moral law, but was strictly a public health measure to prevent the spread of dangerous, communicable diseases.[111]

While many prostitutes were in fact venereal carriers, and while it may have been true, as defenders of the new legal policy argued, that prostitutes were more identifiable than the men who frequented them, Pierce's insistence that the measures were not designed to punish prostitutes seems disingenuous. In fact, for women accused of prostitution during the war, the "red scare" had begun. It was virtually assumed that an arrested prostitute was a venereal carrier; and as such, to be treated as a criminal. The prostitute had become the war's venereal scapegoat, vilified, shunned, and eventually locked up.

The arrest of large numbers of prostitutes—often hundreds at a time—presented a new dilemma for city officials as facilities for incarceration grew scarce. In the past, most courts had imposed fines or minimal sentences on women convicted of soliciting. With the new measures, prosecuting attorneys demanded and often received maximum terms, as well as initial periods of quarantine, if a woman was found to be venereally diseased. Local jails and workhouses, particularly in the South, filled up quickly and were not suited to long-term detention. Moreover, the shortage of suitable institutions threatened to disrupt the government's attack on prostitution. "Policemen will not arrest nor will judges convict if there is no place except an antiquated, insanitary jail to which women, and especially young girls, may be committed," wrote Timothy N. Pfeiffer of the CTCA. "However degraded they may be, they are human beings, and reformation is still a possibility."[112]

Social hygiene professionals worked diligently—to popularize the idea of detention homes—clearing houses for the treatment and study of women arrested for prostitution. Martha P. Falconer, Superintendent of the Pennsylvania State Industrial School for Girls, Sleighton Farm, explained that there was a need for "a place where all arrested girls and women, who are not 'repeaters,' can be held in as normally home-like conditions while awaiting trial." During this period, venereal and psychological tests would be conducted so that "a scientific plan" for the woman's future could be recommended to the judge. Inmates found to be venerally infected would, of course, be treated. If convicted, Falconer argued, girls should be sent to industrial schools for the remainder of their minority; women should be placed in reformatories for indeterminate periods of incarceration. Long sentences would remove the threat of contagion for the war's duration.[113]

Falconer advocated that the government establish four large institutions for vocational training in which to intern convicted prostitutes. These "human reclamation centers" would protect servicemen from the prostitutes while preparing the women to return to "respectable society." "Those who have plied this trade for months and years can not, without general rehabilitation and training, become economically valuable in legitimate work as the result of an edict or a short-term sentence to idleness," explained a government report. Most often, however, internment was justified as a means of reducing the spread of venereal diseases, as well as securing the nation's morals. One government official commented:

> The prevention or reduction of moral and social suicide consequent on prostitution and the protection of society against moral and social murder committed by the prostitute and the roué are functions in part of the detention house and reformatory. These functions are inextricably related to the control of the dissemination of gonorrhea and syphilis through promiscuous prostitution.[114]

The problem of finding a suitable place for women convicted of sex offenses was dramatized in February 1918, when 19 girls under the age of 18 were found guilty under the provisions of section 13 in a South Carolina court. Because the state had no facilities for caring for juvenile offenders, the girls were sentenced to the National Training School for Girls in Washington, D.C. When they arrived, however, the institution was full. The CTCA finally placed the girls in the Massachusetts Reformatory for Women in Framingham. "The difficulty of their disposal," noted a government report, "centered attention of those in the War Department on the lack of institutional facilities for the handling of the camp-girl problem." A survey had determined that only eight states had provisions for detention of venereally infected women.[115]

In late February 1918, President Wilson responded to the social hygiene lobby by allocating $250,000 from the National Security and Defense Fund to establish detention homes for women and girls convicted of prostitution. To administer these funds, the CTCA created a Committee on Detention under the guidance of Martha Falconer. This allocation aided in the construction of eighteen new institutions, as well as the improvement of four already functioning reformatories. These twenty-two institutions were located predominantly in the South where close to 500,000 military men were stationed in 1918.[116]

Congress took action in July 1918, enacting the Chamberlain-Kahn Bill which provided $1 million for a "civilian quarantine and isolation fund" as part of a comprehensive venereal disease program. According to the law, this money would be used in the same manner as the funds allotted by the President, to aid the states in the establishment and construction of reformatories to care "for civilian persons whose detention, isolation, quarantine, or commitment to institutions may be found necessary for the protection of military and naval forces of the United States against venereal diseases." On November 26, 1918, however, the comptroller of the treasury informed the newly created United States Interdepartmental Social Hygiene Board, the agency set up by the act to administer the program, that it had no power to spend federal funds on construction or repair of facilities not owned by the federal government. The Board thus made use of the fund for the maintenance and treatment of women already in the custody of operating institutions. During the years in which the "civilian quarantine and isolation fund" operated, December 1918 to July 1920, $177,089 was allocated to some twenty-seven reformatories and detention houses throughout the United States, less than one-fifth of the total appropriation. The comptroller's ruling had dealt a critical blow to the detention program as envisioned by its originators, forcing the Board to abandon plans for massive construction. If the full $1 million had been available to erect new facilities, many more women would have been interned through the government's program.[117]

In these efforts, protective agents of the CTCA and the Interdepartmental Social Hygiene Board contacted tens of thousands of women and girls suspected of engaging in promiscuous sexual activities with soldiers during the war. Though federal officers found most to be first offenders and placed them on probation, more than 18,000 women were committed to institutions which received federal funding in the period between 1918 and 1920. Of these women, 15,500 reportedly had a venereal disease. This high incidence confirmed for social hygienists their belief that virtually all prostitutes carried venereal infections. On the other hand, this rate could reflect the fact that prostitutes found to be infected in compulsory examinations were subject to conviction and internment much more frequently than those diagnosed free of infection; uninfected prostitutes were usually released, and thus the rate of infection among convicted prostitutes was higher than that within the prostitution population at large. The practice of releasing uninfected prostitutes, in fact, became a source of criticism. As one member of the CTCA Law Enforcement Division complained, "Conviction is too often dependent upon the presence of venereal disease. . . . The magistrate does not realize that every prostitute is a potential, if not an actual, carrier of venereal disease, and that either probation under supervision or reformatory treatment is necessary."[118] For some, the *possibility* of infection had become sufficient cause for incarceration.

Although exigencies of time and funding made a full-scale program impossible, several basic policies nevertheless guided federal activities for the detention of prostitutes. The government required that all women found to be diseased be interned until treated and determined non-infectious. Government-assisted institutions held women for an average of ten weeks during the war. Several institutions, however, admitted inmates under sentence from juvenile courts for the remainder of their minority, or at least one year. Most detention houses and quarantine hospitals where the women received treatment did not permit visitors. Public health officials justified this regulation on the premise that the women were under quarantine; this, despite the well-known fact that venereal diseases could not be communicated through the air.[119]

The need for strict quarantine was taken seriously. Barbed wire and guards secured many of the institutions. Apparently camp-followers, teenagers, and first-offenders were more likely to attempt escape than experienced prostitutes, aware of the necessity of treatment for venereal diseases, and thus the younger girls were guarded more strictly. As a member of the Interdepartmental Social Hygiene Board explained:

> Forcible detention was at no time an integral feature of the program, but it became plain in certain localities, notably those near the more populous military camps, that to erect barbed wire fences around the premises, to employ guards or watchmen, or to resort to both expedients would be necessary, both as protection against intrusion and to insure time for effective work.

Physicians engaged in treating interned women felt that better results were obtained "when patients were literally held in quarantine." Few infected women slipped through; the Board reported that nearly 90 percent remained institutionalized until declared non-infectious.[120]

Social hygienists stressed contemporary theories of rehabilitation and penology in organizing the institutions. First, they continually asserted the importance of segregating young and old, black and white, "less experienced beginner" and "hardened" prostitute. "Since all prostitutes and wayward girls are not of the same class," noted a government report, "no standard type institution could be advocated for each camp community." As C. C. Pierce commented, "The problem of moral contagion [of girls] is as great as that of physical contagion." Second, social workers, expressing a general Progressive anxiety concerning the temptations of urban life, argued that whenever possible reformatories and detention houses should be located in the country. Superintendents promoted farm work as primary therapy. "The work best undertaken by a woman's reformatory institution is agricultural," wrote Martha Falconer, "in view of our country's great need for that development, and the rehabilitating effects of outdoor work on women who are, or have been, venereally diseased." Finally, the government required that women's reformatories be run by women. This ruling was based on the theory that any contact with male society might provoke undesired "excitation" on the part of this "class" of women.[121]

The agents of the U.S. Interdepartmental Social Hygiene Board collected volumes of data concerning the interned prostitutes. These social workers considered their investigations "the first national study of delinquency." As C. C. Pierce explained, "The assembly of large numbers of venereally infected prostitutes offered a splendid opportunity for sociological and psychological investigation of the causes of prostitution in general, and of the type of women that furnished the great bulk of prostitutes." Despite the fact that these studies were not always as scientific as their authors contended—Pierce's sample contained only one hundred women—social workers and physicians considered this research the "laboratory work" of social hygiene.[122] To understand the "social pathology" of prostitution, they claimed, was to understand the causes of venereal disease.

Most social workers endorsed an environmental explanation for the etiology of prostitution. Improper education, failed family supports, and unemployment were typically offered as factors which contributed to "sexual degeneracy." The social workers found what they were looking for. Indeed, their questions and statistical categories are more revealing than the data they collected. Early sexual experiences, for example, were discovered to be common among detained women; the early loss of virginity was considered to be a major step down the road to prostitution. More than two-thirds of the interned women reportedly had histories of sexual relations with soldiers or sailors.[123] Many of the women came from broken homes, or were themselves divorced or abandoned, confirming Progressive fears of the impact of the breakdown of the family.

Not surprisingly, most detained women came from the working-class. According to one study of delinquent women, they had most frequently been employed as domestics, factory workers, and waitresses. At the time of their apprehension, 41 percent had been unemployed. "This corroborates," noted the report, "the generally recognized theory that antisocial conduct is closely linked with unemployment." Rehabilitation programs thus centered attention on developing vocational skills. The professionals who conducted these studies suggested that they provided the information needed for the ultimate reformation and prevention of prostitution. "Without this combination of individual study, and through it recognition of community needs," noted one case worker, "no worker can hope to accomplish the full readjustment of the misfit delinquent and thus shut off one source of venereal disease." [124]

Physicians, however, increasingly stressed the hereditary nature of immorality and prostitution. For example, in C. C. Pierce's admittedly limited study, 91 of 100 women had Binet ages of less than twelve; 41 of these had mental ages of less than ten. Another public health physician, A. J. McLaughlin, presented statistics to suggest that 38 percent of a group of detained prostitutes suffered from feeblemindedness, and another 43 percent provided evidence of "constitutional inferiority." The director of the venereal detention hospital at Newport News, Virginia, Dr. W. F. Draper, noted that "the vast majority [of prostitutes] were of an extremely low intelligence." He complained of not being able to convince the women of the seriousness of their diseases. Upon cure, Draper suggested, most returned to lives of prostitution. He argued for permanent incarceration of women found to be unreformable:

> In cases where the mentality is so low as to preclude the possibility of a life other than one of prostitution, it would be an economy and a humanitarian act to commit such individuals to institutional care for life. They are a far greater menace to the happiness and welfare of society than many murderers who are serving life sentences in our prisons.

Even social workers, more sympathetic to environmental explanations of prostitution and committed to rehabilitation, accepted the evidence of genetic defects. As an Interdepartmental Social Hygiene Board social worker explained:

> It is an interesting commentary on the errors in judgment of which even trained social workers may be guilty before making a social investigation and getting to know the girls, that only 113, or 14.4 percent of the 784 girls admitted for special care to the three detention houses established for so-called younger girls were in the end considered reformable. [125]

According to Thomas A. Storey, executive secretary of the Interdepartmental Social Hygiene Board, the detention of infected women contributed significantly to the protection of military men from venereal disease. He based this assessment on the evaluation of the costs of interning a prostitute versus the costs of hospitalizing a serviceman for a venereal infection. "In three days," explained Storey, "10,000 busy prostitutes, if free, could have produced an expense account for the mere hospitalization of soldiers and sailors that would have equalled the total contribution made by the government for their treatment." Storey estimated that for every fifteen clients served by a diseased prostitute, one would become infected. On this basis he computed that the detention of some 15,500 infected prostitutes had prevented the contamination of over 173,000 military men, which in turn would have cost the government more than $12 million. He termed the detention of prostitutes "a compelling business proposition."[126] Storey's appraisal reflected a growing Progressive penchant for quantitative analysis, as well as the professionalization of reform that the detention program engendered. No longer would prostitutes be taken from the streets to save their souls, but rather to save the efficiency of the military and the tax dollars of the government.

However justified by claims for increased efficiency, the campaign against the prostitute betrayed an underlying hostility towards women, especially those of the working class. These women, most of whom, doctors suggested, were feeble-minded or genetically tainted, would "drain the virility" of American men if left to their own designs, it was argued. Social hygiene reformers and physicians assumed, in effect, that venereal infections could only be transmitted in one direction—that women bore the sole responsibility for the diseases. As Dr. A. J. McLaughlin wrote:

> I would say that about 90 percent of infections are due to women and 10 percent to men. Men take more precautions and are more particular about treatment and prophylaxis. Women are very negligent, and take treatment only for the relief of pain or under compulsion. One woman will infect ten men for every one woman that one man will infect.

Few stopped to consider from whom the prostitute acquired her infection. In a rare instance, however, the conservative *Journal of the American Medical Association* noted this inequity, asking, "For what does it avail to detain the women while the men are permitted to disseminate venereal diseases *ad libitum?*"[127]

7

The intensity of interest in venereal disease that the war provoked was not wholly in response to the demands for an efficient army. The Commission on Training Camp Activities presented a rallying cry for a higher national moral standard. For Progressives obsessed with order and control, the sexual drives raised particular concerns. Venereal disease, the palpable evidence of unrestrained sexuality, became a symbol of social disorder and moral decay—a metaphor for evil. As an American Social Hygiene Association pamphlet, "The Enemy at Home," explained: "The name of the invisible enemy is Venereal Disease— and there you have in two words, the epitome of all that is unclean, malignant, and menacing."[128] The fight against venereal disease became a way of focusing anxieties about the war's meaning and outcome on the home front. In this process, sexuality was transformed into a public issue.

The mixture of persuasion and repression in the CTCA policies reveals a central tension in Progressivism. On the one hand, reformers expressed a pervasive optimism that rationality and education could convince the public of proper behavior. On the other hand, some reformers harbored underlying fears of disorder that prompted them to demand more vigorous interventions—legal instrumentalities requiring controls where education and uplift failed. The CTCA effectively drew upon both Progressive impulses, at the same time minimizing conflict between those who considered venereal diseases from a strictly scientific orientation and those who viewed it solely as a moral issue. Indeed, whenever possible the CTCA suggested the complementarity of both views, thereby strengthening the coalition of support for its programs.

On one point reformers of all stripes could agree: the protection of soldiers from venereal infection would ultimately redound to the nation's benefit in peacetime. As Raymond Fosdick concluded: "To make men fit for fighting—and after—is just plain efficiency plus." The achievements of the CTCA, Walter Clarke observed, would be far-ranging:

> Our men today are not only more efficient fighters, but even of greater importance, they will, upon returning to their families and communities, contribute less damage to the race than would have been thought possible had the United States not asserted itself for the protection against our most subtle enemy. The long trail of disease, dependency and crime will not follow our men after this war as in the wake of wars of other times. The social gains thus achieved can scarcely be conceived. We have no scale with which to measure the distress and the burdens which we trust will be escaped.[129]

For many reformers, the work of the Commission had proved the claim of American moral superiority.

Progressives praised the CTCA as a model of government participation in reform efforts. The *Survey*, the chronicle of official Progressivism, characterized the federal program as unique: "No other nation in the war has attempted anything similar to the work of the Commission on Training Camp Activities. Nothing ever attempted in this country, in similar lines, has approached this plan in magnitude or in completeness of detail." Fosdick considered the CTCA to be "perhaps the largest social program ever undertaken." Combining the reform impulses of the social settlements, the recreation advocates, professional social workers and educators, as well as vice crusaders, the conception and scope of the Commission's activities were unprecedented. For many American reformers, the war became a justification for accelerating and expanding on-going voluntary campaigns against venereal disease on a national level. As William Zinsser explained:

> Uncle Sam . . . decided to fight the thing from the very start. It meant a thing never before attempted by *any country*. It meant that the leading nation of the world on whom all eyes were turned, was to deliver the first great *open blow* against the age old curse.[130]

For some American reformers, the war itself was secondary to the larger battle for moral and spiritual uplift. They credited the CTCA with responsibility for a transformation in national morality.

The crusade against prostitution seemed to typify this broad approach. Reformers prided themselves on the aggressive policy that had brought about the demise of the red-light district, a singular contribution of the federal program.

"No other government in the history of the world has taken the stand on this question that the U.S. Government has taken," wrote an obviously proud Bascom Johnson.[131] In identifying the prostitute as virtually the exclusive *cause* of venereal disease, moral and medical reformers had been able to institute a campaign unique in its definitive breadth. Unlike almost all other diseases, for which responsibility was at least clouded and transmission involuntary, in the case of venereal diseases increased scientific knowledge seemed to affix culpability even more squarely on the prostitute, and reformers congratulated themselves for responding in kind.

On the other hand, the massive arrests and detention of prostitutes raised a basic conundrum of public health: How far could a government go in the name of science and hygiene to abridge the rights of those who might threaten the greater good? Progressives, placing their faith in experts, yielded easily to a scientific rationale. As Hermann M. Biggs, a founder of scientific hygiene in America, had explained two decades earlier, "We are prepared when necessary to introduce and enforce, and the people are ready to accept, measures which might seem radical and arbitrary, if they were not plainly designed for the public good, and evidently beneficent in their effects."[132] The CTCA based its antiprostitution program on exactly these precepts, responding to urgent necessity supported by the claims of medical discovery. Though the prostitute had been anathema to generations of American reformers, only the exigencies of war and the insistence of physicians effected her banishment from the urban landscape. Issues previously seen to be purely of a moral nature now achieved the powerful legitimacy of scientific and health concerns. The "cult of the expert" made acceptable far-ranging policies that conflicted with basic civil liberties, masking fundamentally political issues.

The incarceration and reform of prostitutes as an anti-venereal measure also demonstrated the expansion of the therapeutic realm that occurred during the Progressive years and accelerated during the war. Measures to promote health and control disease, previously circumscribed by the limited abilities of the medical profession to address them effectively, now achieved an extensive breadth. With this transformation, reformers and professionals greatly augmented their domains of activity and influence. Increasingly, social and political programs became subsumed under the all-encompassing rubric of public health. The internment of prostitutes was justified on therapeutic grounds; it was not just to treat venereal disease, but to treat the "illness" of prostitution itself. As Raymond Fosdick had described the work of the CTCA: "The Commission, in short, in its constructive and law-enforcement work, was thus 'one gigantic piece of preventive medicine.' "[133]

On the prostitution front of the campaign against venereal disease, reformers saw the problem of the prostitute as a painful reminder that the Victorian ideal of sex-in-marriage remained only an ideal. As some Progressive women often explained, prostitution rested on the demand of men; if demand could be removed, then supply would contract. The CTCA, therefore, viewed its educational program in behalf of "civilized morality" as equal in importance to its attack on prostitution.[134] Adherence to this moral code—particularly sexual continence outside of marriage—was now seen as a major aspect of the program to prevent venereal diseases. The middle-class reformers who directed the activities of the CTCA thus sought to inculcate this ethic among the troops and thereby to nationalize their morals. In the past, civilized morality served as a means of setting the middle class apart from the working class, which did not always subscribe to such controls. During the war, however, reformers argued that their beliefs and ideals would best serve the interests of the troops going to France. Therefore, they enlisted the unprecedented support of the federal government to teach this rigid sexual code to the doughboys. In so doing, these physicians and social workers usurped the traditional roles of families who, they claimed, had failed to provide proper education in ways of modern morals.

Civilized morality, however, rested on a process of subtle socialization and internalization. To attempt to teach it publicly, to thousands of men, was to sow the seeds of its own destruction. One of the most basic precepts of this code had been that sex should not be discussed outside the home, if at all. With the war, venereal disease provided an acceptable means for the airing of the heretofore forbidden. The "conspiracy of silence," the bedrock of Victorian respectability, became one of the war's first casualties. As William Zinsser wrote:

> Before the war a comparative few had struggled manfully to combat prostitution and venereal disease, both camouflaged under the name of the "Social Evil" for fear of giving offense to the false modesty that existed on these subjects. The war, however, changed all this. . . . Whatever else it will accomplish, it already has been the force that has driven these subjects from darkness into light, compelling attention and focusing public opinion squarely upon a situation that had always been held too lightly and apathetically.[135]

Given the uncertainties that the war provoked, the degree to which a strict moral code was invoked is not surprising. Rigid sexual prescriptions, as well as the vigorous repression of prostitution, indicated the more limited levels of social tolerance that characterized the Progressive period and especially World War I. In retrospect, it is the certainty with which these reformers addressed sexual matters that makes this period seem disjoined from our own. But this confidence appears to have been a defense: it was a denial of the realization that the control and order that they sought might not be so readily achieved in a heterogeneous, industrial society.

The true test of the Commission's program would come in France. Overseas, where temptations could not be repressed by American authorities, Newton Baker's "invisible armor" would be tried. At the conclusion of the film, *Fit to Fight*, Billy and the Kid salute as they steam past Sandy Hook, while their three companions are shown in the hospital, nursing sexually-inflicted wounds. The CTCA had provided Billy and the Kid, physically fit, to the war effort, but their fate in France was far from certain.

III

"The Cleanest Army in the World":
Venereal Disease and the AEF

1

In the United States social reformers could, for the most part, protect soldiers from vice, immorality, and disease; in France, the men would be left to their own designs. To the reformers who directed the social hygiene campaign on the home front, venereal disease among the American Expeditionary Forces would indicate the demoralization of American manhood, in spite of their efforts. They considered the Old World hostile territory for their crusade. The temptations that French towns offered, they surmised, could hardly be compared to those of Charleston or San Antonio, nor could they be repressed so easily. To the military, venereal disease would cause inefficiency that could threaten their ability to wage war. Considerations of manpower and technology would be critical in this war, the first major conflict of the modern industrial age. Though the war enlisted the two most powerful social currents of Progressivism—the desire for a defined moral order and the emphasis on scientific efficiency—in the battle against venereal disease these forces would not always work in concert.[1]

Those committed to Woodrow Wilson's vision of an international moral order saw the war as an opportunity for fulfillment. The idealization of the American soldier, the knight in the crusade for democracy, included rigid prescriptions for upright behavior overseas. Alcohol and sex would thus be taboo for members of the AEF. In this way they would not only demonstrate their allegiance to higher ideals, but would also avoid the taint of venereal disease.[2] The president himself lent his authority to the anti-venereal fervor in words befittingly obscure:

> The federal government has pledged its word that as far as care and vigilance can accomplish the result, the men committed to its charge will be returned to the homes and communities that so generously gave them with no scars except those won in honorable conflict.[3]

Reformers subjected the troops to intense propaganda regarding the moral significance of their mission.

If the war promised to be a demonstration and a test of a new morality, it also held dangers. Venereal disease, if it afflicted members of the AEF, would signal that rather than exporting American democracy and virtue, the doughboys might import old world degeneracy. This fear loomed large as Americans prepared to embark for the conflict. "If by throwing this army into France we defeat the German arms but destroy the moral health of the young men who make up that army," warned a YMCA secretary, "then most assuredly will we have done more to destroy the foundations upon which democracy rests than we can possibly do to protect them." The problems of the training camps and domestic red-light districts paled in comparison to the task of maintaining the health and rectitude of those who crossed the Atlantic. "Is it inevitable," one woman asked Raymond Fosdick, "that our troops (trained here under fine social and moral conditions) must be exposed in Europe to the French policy of 'laissez-faire' in all things sexual?"[4]

World War I, Wilson's "war of experts," erupted as modern germ-theory medicine became integrated into American science. In past wars the Medical Department had fought rear-guard battles, attempting to mend soldiers to return them to the front. This explains the emphasis on surgery in pre-twentieth century military medicine, while endemic disease, though obviously a serious problem, was viewed as an unfortunate yet insuperable aspect of war. By World War I a revamped Medical Department sought to institute newly discovered diagnostic and therapeutic techniques to insure the health and thus the efficiency of American troops. "Sanitary science" transformed the work of military physicians who henceforth undertook responsibility for keeping men fit for action; disease rather than injury was their focus of attention. Medicine assumed a more important status in the structure of military life; manpower and efficiency expressing the themes of its work.[5]

Historically, no diseases had proven as debilitating to military efforts as those transmitted in sexual contacts, and no disease as strikingly ignored. During the Civil War almost 20 percent of those fighting acquired infections. Army admission rates for venereal disease averaged 70.6 per 1000 men during the decade prior to the Spanish-American War. In the late nineteenth century, "a deprecatory, *sub rosa*, hush atmosphere surrounded the subject," reported one military physician. Venereal diseases, though prevalent, were usually ignored among the rank and file; most cases were probably never diagnosed.[6] Indeed, before the discovery of the Wassermann reaction in 1906, the Army maintained no official venereal disease policy.

Developments in American foreign policy, particularly the imperialist thrust that saw American troops stationed in Cuba, Puerto Rico, and the Philippines, forced the Army to recognize the problem. Between 1908 and 1910 venereal disease rates in the Army doubled. In fact, during this period, admissions for venereal disease equaled the total admissions for the next five most frequent illnesses. By 1908 the magnitude of the venereal danger for the Army had become abundantly clear. The surgeon general responded by instituting fortnightly inspections, lectures, limitations on passes, as well as the provision of "preventive medicines," upon request. He outlined his view in his official report for 1910:

> The venereal peril has come to outweigh in importance any other sanitary question which now confronts the Army, and neither our national optimism nor the Anglo-Saxon disposition to ignore a subject which is offensive to public prudery can longer excuse a frank and honest confrontation of the problem.

The rise in admissions for venereal disease from 84.59 per 1000 in 1897 to 196.99 per 1000 in 1910 does much to explain the surgeon general's concern. This vast increase reflected the difficulty of maintaining forces on foreign soil as well as better diagnostics. Army physicians realized that admission figures only accounted for the most troublesome cases, with many others going undetected or unreported.[7]

In 1910 the surgeon general set forth six recommendations for the control of venereal diseases. First, he suggested the introduction of recreation and amusement facilities "sufficiently attractive to keep [the men] . . . away from vile resorts." Second, noting the common connection between vice and drink, he advocated the formation of temperance societies within the military. Third, he recommended the periodic inspection "of the men stripped" in order to provide for the early detection of primary cases; and fourth, he directed that all cases remain under treatment until rendered non-infectious. Fifth, he recommended that lectures be offered, explaining the hazards of the diseases, the dangers of consorting with prostitutes, as well as the compatibility of sexual continence with good mental and physical health. Finally, the surgeon general approved the provision of prophylactic packages for those who, despite official admonitions, exposed themselves to venereal disease. The War Department endorsed the precepts of the surgeon general's program in 1912 by issuing a general order that stopped pay for those incapacitated by venereal disease.[8]

But as American intervention in the Great War approached, the military policy towards the venereal diseases remained less than clear. Reformers active in the domestic social hygiene movement urged the War Department to take action to protect the soldiers while overseas. Despite the intensity of activities within the states to safeguard the troops in the training camps, as General John J. Pershing, commander-in-chief of the American Expeditionary Forces, steamed across the Atlantic aboard the SS *Baltic* in June 1917, he had yet to define the AEF's attitude towards sexual disease. "If we do not at once devise means of continuing the same control in France," warned M. J. Exner of the YMCA, "all that we have now accomplished will largely go to pieces over there."[9]

Unlike the social hygienists on the home front, Pershing had not always been committed to a policy of repressing prostitution. Indeed, while commanding troops on the Mexican border in 1916, he had been one of several generals to institute a system of regulated houses of prostitution for his forces. Although concerned about the moral implications of this practice, Pershing saw no alternative to the problem of a high rate of venereal disease. "The establishment was necessary and has proved the best way to handle a difficult problem," he explained. "Everyone was satisfied." Aware of the general's record on venereal disease, Exner wrote to Raymond Fosdick, "It would be most unfortunate to permit General Pershing to take his contingent to Europe with any possibility of his continuing that sort of policy."[10]

Traveling with Pershing, Dr. Hugh Hampton Young, a specialist in urology at the Johns Hopkins Hospital, outlined the nature of the venereal disease peril for the AEF. Young convinced the Commander, through a series of luridly detailed lectures, of the health hazards regulated prostitution would pose for his troops. Pershing became virtually obsessed with the charge of making the AEF the first venereal-free Army in military history. Felix Frankfurter, in France studying conditions among the American forces, wrote to Secretary of War Baker, "General Pershing is filled with anxiety about the sexual morale of the troops."[11] In the years to come, few subjects received greater attention from the Commander.

Upon Young's arrival in England in June 1917, the chief surgeon of the AEF, Colonel Alfred E. Bradley, appointed him director of the Division of Urology. Young undertook to study the allied efforts to control venereal disease before devising policies for his division. He criticized the British practice of sending all cases to base hospitals in France and England, away from the front. According to Young, this procedure placed a premium on contracting a venereal disease. "After four terrible years of war," he wrote, "some Tommies were frankly glad to get into a venereal hospital and enjoy six weeks or longer surcease from the agony of the front." Some men attempted to reinfect themselves as quickly as possible after the treatment; others reportedly intentionally infected themselves by passing a contaminated matchstick. During his investigation, Young also learned that the French had discovered means of simplifying venereal treatment. On the basis of this knowledge, he revised American therapeutic regimes.[12]

Young found the policies of the New Zealand Expeditionary Forces particularly compelling. Although the French and British commands seemed to be resigned to high rates of venereal infection, centering their attention on treatment, the New Zealand contingent instituted a full-scale program emphasizing avoidance of venereal diseases. They conducted frequent, rigorous inspections for venereal diseases—"dangle parades"—so that infections could be detected and early treatment administered. More importantly, the New Zealand military physicians provided chemical prophylaxis and distributed condoms widely to help prevent venereal infection.[13]

In framing a venereal policy for the AEF, Young combined the pragmatism of the New Zealand command with the moralism demanded by the social hygienists. On one hand he sought to minimize sexual contacts through education, recreation, and repression of prostitution. On the other, he advocated medical instrumentalities such as chemical prophylaxis, frequent inspections, and early treatment to lessen the impact of infections on the efficiency of the AEF. Prevention was the emphasis, be it by moral or medical means.[14] The command of the AEF soon found, however, that aspects of the program did not accord with conditions in France.

2

While the red lights were being snuffed out one by one in the United States, they continued to burn brightly in the cities of France. The French accepted prostitution as an important element of their sexual culture. Aware of the dangers of venereal disease posed by a large population of prostitutes, they attempted to maintain the health of these women and thus protect the health of their clients through a system of *reglementation*. Officials based this arrangement of periodic inspections of prostitutes for signs of infection on the recent advances in venereology and germ theory, many of which had been made at the prestigious Pasteur Institut in Paris. If found free of disease after medical examination, the prostitute received a certificate to present or display to her clientele. If the physician discovered an infection, the woman was committed for treatment. In Paris alone, officials estimated the operation of 40 major houses of prostitution. An additional 5,000 streetwalkers were professionally licensed, but 70,000 women reportedly worked on a clandestine basis without recourse to physical examinations.[15]

Members of the Medical Department of the AEF studying the method of *reglementation* found that French inspections, usually conducted by municipal physicians, left much to be desired. Colonel George Walker reported seeing 59 women examined in an hour at Bordeaux; 15 in thirteen minutes at Cherbourg. Most significantly, examinations did not include microscopic studies and thus could not possibly have detected many asymptomatic infections. Indeed, the Americans argued that the official inspections often had the result of spreading venereal diseases from one prostitute to another. Walker saw the same unsterilized speculum used to examine each woman in line:

> It was truly a doleful spectacle to see these women in line, waiting to mount an examination table for a farcical inspection. It made one fairly shudder to know that representatives of the French government were giving bills of physical soundness to women who were fairly eaten up with disease—permeated through and through with gonorrhea and syphilis—and who not only inevitably broadcasted infection among the French soldiers but among all who were carnally intimate with them.

Although the system of inspections most likely was inefficient, the Americans' predisposition to condemn it was more than apparent. Colonel Walker reported that in five years official examinations of prostitutes had diagnosed only five cases of syphilis—an impossible figure. Although American military physicians granted the potential benefits from inspection of prostitutes, they argued that as practiced in France it was not only useless, but dangerous as well, in that it created a false sense of security among the prostitutes' patrons. Regardless of health implications, official acceptance of regulation was impossible under Progressive moral codes. As General Leonard Wood noted, "I don't think that the mothers of the soldiers . . . would want their sons to go to death from the arms of a prostitute."[16] The Medical Department thus discounted the possibility of relying on the French inspections of prostitutes to protect the AEF from sexual disease.

French toleration of prostitution immediately raised doubts for many Americans concerning the moral rectitude of the nation the doughboys were sent to save. For American reformers the system of regulated prostitution symbolized the debasement of French society. As Charles Eliot, the former President of Harvard University, wrote:

> The failure of the French government to protect their soldiers from these evils is the gravest error that government has committed; for those vices have proved more destructive to the French people since August, 1914, than all the German artillery rifles, hand grenades, poisonous gases and fire blasts. The killed transmit no poison to their families and descendants—the victims of alcohol and prostitution do.[17]

Eliot identified a central theme of the war's venereal disease propaganda: better dead than diseased. In a war fought on moral grounds there would be moral and immoral injuries, moral and immoral deaths.

Americans feared the impact of French sexual mores on members of the AEF. Reports circulated widely regarding the aggressiveness of French street women. Flyers distributed to American soldiers advised:

> You will be accosted many times by public women. Venereal disease is prevalent among them and to go with them invites infection which will not only do you great bodily harm but will render you ineffective for the purpose for which you are in France. Dictates of morality, personal hygiene and patriotism demand that you do not associate with such women.

The caption on a poster expressed the same theme more bluntly: "A German Bullet Is Cleaner Than A Whore."[18]

By the time the first members of the AEF embarked for the conflict, French and British troops had amassed a dismal record of venereal infections. Reports circulated in the United States that as many as 25 percent of some British and French regiments were non-effective from venereal disease. The French had recorded over a million cases of gonorrhea and syphilis since the beginning of the war, and British forces had continually suffered an average loss of 23,000 men for seven-week hospital stints due to sexually transmitted diseases.[19]

For many Americans, the sorry record of the allies in combatting venereal disease confirmed the image of continental debauchery. In previous wars, the American military might have regretfully accepted such casualties, but the combination of the moral stridency of Progressivism and the new consciousness of order and efficiency made losses to venereal disease intolerable. These demands explain the significance of the American battle against sexually transmitted diseases that the war unleashed.

3

The arrival of American troops at French seaports heralded a clash of sexual cultures. The French greeted the AEF hospitably, offering them the run of local amenities, which included, of course, the use of local bars, cafés, and houses of prostitution. Responding to American fears that the *Entente Cordiale* might become excessively intimate, Pershing issued General Order No. 6 on July 2, 1917, less than a week after the first transports landed in France. Indicative of the serious attitude Pershing adopted concerning the venereal problem, the order reminded the soldiers of their responsibility to avoid infection: "A soldier who contracts a venereal disease not only suffers permanent injury, but renders himself inefficient as a soldier and becomes an encumbrance to the Army. He fails in his duty to his country and his comrades." The order called for semimonthly inspections, as well as lectures on the hazards of venereal disease to be given by medical officers, and in addition, required that soldiers report to special stations for administration of chemical prophylaxis within three hours of any sexual contact. Finally, the most radical provision of the order made the contraction of a venereal disease an offense punishable by court-martial. [20]

G.O. No. 6 defined the command's attitude towards sex and disease in the AEF. The order made three points clear. First, the regulation requiring prophylaxis officially recognized that some soldiers *would* engage in sexual activity while in France, despite pronouncements and propaganda calling for sexual continence. Second, the directive illustrated the faith Pershing placed in medical science to minimize the impact of venereal disease on his forces. Finally, the decision to make contraction of a venereal disease a court-martial offense granted these infections a unique place in the corpus of military medicine. [21] The American Army, reflecting ideals of Progressive medicine, considered venereal disease preventable. A soldier need not expose himself; if he did, he need not contract the disease. Therefore, venereal infection constituted a willful, flagrant violation of military discipline. Quite simply, it would not be tolerated in the American Expeditionary Forces.

Just as striking as the provisions for punishment in G.O. No. 6, however, was its silence on the issue of prostitution. The order made no pronouncement on military use of the many *maisons de tolérance,* thus tacitly accepting their service provided the soldier sought prophylaxis following his experience there. Despite the efforts of social hygienists, the classic aphorism that armies required sex still held some weight within the AEF.

The next official declaration on venereal disease—General Order No. 34— sought to avoid the problem of men soliciting infections to forego the perils of combat. Issued in September 1917, G.O. No. 34 required that men with venereal disease be treated within their divisions on an ambulatory basis. Pershing attempted to insure that infected men would not be sent to antiseptic hospitals, while healthy soldiers risked their lives at the front. Edward Hartman of the Massachusetts Civic League felt the order did not go far enough. He wrote to Joseph Lee, a member of the CTCA, to suggest that all venereally infected soldiers should be sent to the front "as promptly as possible." [22]

As the contingent of American troops in France grew in September 1917, all seemed quiet on the venereal front. The admission rate for September was 80 per 1,000; by the end of October it had fallen to 54. The rate rose precipitously to 201 in early November, however, much to Pershing's concern. Reports revealed that new divisions debarking at the port of St. Nazaire accounted for the epidemic. Pershing detailed Young to investigate the situation. [23]

Young found that conditions in St. Nazaire epitomized American reformers' worst fears of Old World degeneracy. After quaffing West Indian rum and Niger gin, the American troops flocked to one of St. Nazaire's six *maisons de prostitution*. "It didn't take much of this rotgut stuff to inflame passions and obliterate all repressions," recounted Young. Each bordello housed only five or six women, with lines of American soldiers winding from doorways into streets. On the average each woman served forty to fifty men a day; one reported a commercial success of sixty-five customers in a twenty-four-hour period.[24]

Under these conditions, the system of prophylaxis broke down. Returning to camp, often intoxicated, the men found the line at the prophylaxis station longer than the one at the house of prostitution, discouraging compliance with the regulations requiring this procedure. Soldiers reporting venereal symptoms overwhelmed the base port hospitals. Young discovered, to his surprise, that the prostitutes in St. Nazaire were carefully inspected and few showed signs of infection. What, then, accounted for the high rates of syphilis and gonorrhea among the American men frequenting these women? "It was apparent," wrote Young:

> that the danger of regulated prostitution was not entirely from the diseases of the women themselves, but also from the fact that by receiving one individual after another without any douching or even arising from their beds, these women came to possess 'septic tanks' filled with almost every type of venereal infection.[25]

Young prepared a full-scale report on activities in St. Nazaire for Pershing. "This is one of the most disgraceful things that has happened to the American Army," the commander told Young. "Drastic measures must be taken immediately." Pershing took the first train to the seaport, where he personally inspected the situation, demanding that his officers follow regulations or suffer the consequences. He ordered that all houses of prostitution as well as saloons be surrounded by military police. Prophylaxis was to be rigidly enforced. Moreover, Pershing took measures to ensure more rapid evacuation of troops from the ports of debarkation. With discipline restored following the commander's visit, St. Nazaire's venereal rate quickly dropped.[26]

The circumstances at the seaport provided the basis for the third and most far-ranging General Order concerning venereal disease issued to the American Expeditionary Forces. General Order No. 77, issued in December 1917, held commanding officers accountable for the health of their troops. "No laxity or half-hearted efforts in this regard will be tolerated," directed the injunction. "The number of effectives in a command is an index of its efficiency and this depends on the efficiency of the commanding officer." The order required reports of venereal rates on board prior to debarkation. All infected men would be detained in camp. Moreover, passes were severely restricted for all healthy soldiers. General Order No. 77 also incorporated Young's recommendation for "closure" of the camps. All encampments, argued the chief urologist, should be fenced, preferably with barbed wire, with a single entrance all men must pass through upon return. A guard stationed at this post would evaluate a soldier's need for prophylaxis.[27] Men returning intoxicated would be given the "early treatment" summarily.

Most significantly, G.O. No. 77 marked Pershing's conversion from his earlier faith in regulated prostitution. His survey of the seaport convinced him of the dangers prostitution posed for the efficiency of his forces. By declaring the regulated houses of prostitution off-limits to his men, he committed the AEF to an official continence. Some medical officers, dedicated to the proposition of the "sexual necessity," expressed their disenchantment with this provision. Throughout the war, despite the vigilance of the Division of Urology in surveying conditions, houses of prostitution sponsored by American officers sprung up in the cities and towns of France.[28]

Regardless of an individual officer's view of the venereal problem, G.O. No. 77 made explicit that AEF policy regarding sexual behavior would come from the top. The directive required each Base Section to report its cases of venereal disease directly to the chief surgeon. In this way any fluctuation in the rates of infection would be immediately realized at General Headquarters. "These reports . . . will be filed at these Headquarters with the personal records of organization commanders, and will be used as a basis in determining the commander's efficiency and the suitability of his continuing in command," warned the edict. Hugh Young, who helped draft G.O. No. 77, considered it "the most far-reaching health order ever issued to an army."[29]

4

Though the American command celebrated General Order No. 77 as a triumph of the will over the wayward, the French military greeted the order with circumspection and derision. The contradistinction of American and French policies regarding venereal disease struck much deeper than a mere military disagreement regarding troop management, efficiency, and civil health. At issue, admitted both sides, was a conflict in sexual mores. Although the immediate debate addressed military strategy, it clearly illuminated larger cultural and social divergencies.

The mayor of St. Nazaire objected vehemently to the provisions in G.O. No. 77 placing the houses of prostitution out-of-bounds for American troops. He argued that if the Americans were provided no sexual outlets the French civil population would be endangered and suggested that reports of rapes and abductions by members of the AEF had risen since the issuance of the order. Particularly alarmed by the presence of black troops, he demanded that houses be immediately opened for these men, or black women be supplied from the United States.[30] The Americans dismissed these reports as mere reflections of St. Nazaire's commercial interests in the prosperity of the prostitution trade.

Premier Clemenceau, concerned about these reports, commissioned a full study of American venereal policy from Inspector Simonin of the French surgeon general's office. The document which Simonin produced vividly represents the conflict between American and French attitudes towards the control of venereal disease. To the French, the American plan represented a strange combination of repression and prudery. "The plan," explained Simonin in his memo, "depends upon anti-venereal education and the distraction resulting from

physical exercises and amusements to turn young men from their sexual pleasures." Simonin pointed out, however, that the French government's intention
to establish houses of prostitution for the American Army "seems very little in
accord with the regulations of the Honorable Secretary of War at Washington
and qualified to surprise him not a little." [31]

The Inspector suggested that the Americans could blame only themselves for
the high rates of venereal disease in St. Nazaire. First, he claimed that many
Americans brought infections overseas from the States, contaminating the prostitutes in France. Second, American orders placing the inspected houses of
prostitution out-of-bounds had given rise to a burgeoning commerce of clandestine and street prostitution, the bane of a system of regulation. Quoting rates
of American infections upon debarkation, Simonin wrote: "In the face of such
figures we may well wonder how many French women were infected from June
to October by these Americans." Simonin also criticized the regulations that
called for court-martial of American soldiers who became infected, describing
this procedure as the "best possible way of inciting them to conceal their disease." [32]

Although the Americans claimed that their methods were based on the latest
developments in sanitary science, the French believed their ally to be unnatural, puritanical, and coercive. "The object of the Americans," concluded Simonin, "is to prevent their soldiers from having sexual relations." He reviewed
American policy in the following terms:

> Beginning with the principle that chastity is possible, they have declared an official
> continence; and they confide to religion and morals the duty of maintaining mo-
> rality in man and keeping him always master of his passions. They depend, how-
> ever, on violent exercise to afford distraction and to diminish the desire for their
> soldiers. [33]

On the whole, it was an accurate assessment.

Such a program, he argued, held dangers for the French system of *reglementation*. First, it contributed to the growth of clandestine trade under which the
licensing of prostitutes broke down. Second, the French expressed skepticism
that the American military officials could actually keep the sex drives of their
troops in check. Already, cases of American rapes and seductions were reported
by French police commissioners. Simonin clearly expressed one assumption
underlying regulation: that if the sexual needs of men are not satisfied, innocent women would be at risk. "America has the noblest moral aspirations," noted
the inspector. "These should be encouraged, but can our ally give similar guarantees of individual morality?" he asked pointedly. [34]

On the basis of Simonin's memo, Clemenceau wrote to Pershing expressing
his doubts about American policy, requesting a reappraisal. The letter demonstrated a total misapprehension of the American commitment to sexual continence. The premier concluded with what he must have considered a generous
offer: to establish "special houses" for the use of the AEF. Pershing, non-
plussed, passed the letter on to Raymond Fosdick, who was visiting France to
survey camp conditions. "They felt," explained Fosdick, "that an army could

not get along without sexual indulgence and that to attempt to carry out such a policy was to court discontent, a lowering of morale and health standards, and perhaps even mutiny." Upon his return to Washington, Fosdick unloaded the letter on Secretary of War Baker, who told him, "For God's sake, Raymond, don't show this to the President or he'll stop the war."[35]

Pershing appointed Hugh Young and Major E. L. Keyes to reply to Simonin's memo. A joint conference on venereal policy took place in Paris in March 1918. Again, the French and Americans articulated their opposing positions, with both sides firmly committed to their respective points of view. Licensing of prostitutes, argued the Americans, violated modern principles of sanitary science because it could not guarantee freedom from infection. Keyes and Young insisted that the United States based its program on scientific hygiene rather than prudery: "The Medical Department of the Army is in no way concerned with the morals of the soldiers; its sole desire is to minimize the incidence of venereal disease," they remarked somewhat disingenuously.[36]

The French, still disgruntled over American policy barring the use of their houses of prostitution, proposed to equip all houses with prophylactic stations. This, they believed, would overcome American objections, as any soldier visiting a prostitute would be required to take a treatment immediately afterward, thus mitigating his chances of infection. But again, the Americans refused, making explicit what was already clear—that their critique of regulated prostitution went beyond the danger of venereal disease to a more general condemnation of organized prostitution. This view was reflected in a memo prepared by Keyes:

> From the moral point of view the licensing of prostitutes implies an alliance between the Government and the pimp. It is also arguable that the emotional relation between a man and a casual prostitute is at least a degree less grossly sexual than is the case in the brothel.

Pershing, acting on advice from the chief surgeon, declined the minister of war's magnanimous offer.[37]

Allied efforts against venereal disease remained uncoordinated. Keyes and Young concluded realistically: "At the present date it would be quite visionary to hope to reconcile the attitude of the French people and the French scientists with the attitude of the corresponding classes in the United States on the subject of sexual hygiene." M. Ogier, a French representative to the conference, characterized the conflict somewhat more bluntly, arguing "that if a man and a woman want to sleep together it was no one's business and no one should interfere with them." As the official history of the YMCA in the war noted with regret, "It was not quite possible to make over the principles of these countries as an enthusiastic American uplifter might have desired . . ."[38] Diplomacy could not bridge the cultural gulf which separated American and French venereal policy.

5

Sexual education, with persistent reminders of the dangers of intercourse, comprised a major segment of the "American Plan," in spite of the Medical Department's declaration to the French that individual morality was of no concern to them. "We refuse to admit," wrote H. E. Kleinschmidt of the Commission on Training Camp Activities, "that man is merely a creature of instinct and not amenable to some measure of mental control."[39] American reformers and physicians insisted that the sexual impulse could be curbed through instruction, exercise, and wholesome entertainment. Distraction and self-control were the means of achieving sexual continence, the expressed goal of American policy.

Contraction of a venereal disease represented a failure of self-control, a central tenet of Progressive ideology. "He whose passions are uncontrolled," argued Dr. Isaac Brewer, "approaches the state of one of the lower animals." The catch words of Progressivism—self-sacrifice, self-respect, self-control—dominated the social hygiene appeal to members of the AEF. Indeed, the latest thinking on the subject suggested that Progressive medicine had shown, once and for all, the complementarity of science and morals. "Scientific research into symptoms and cure goes hand in hand with a new moral appeal—" explained Gertrude Seymour, "not the negative 'warning against sin' so much as a positive attitude of uprightness, a self-control for the individual's own attainment, for his family, community, and race." As Luther Gulick, a YMCA worker, noted, "Morality is an essential part of military efficiency and, hence, is a part of military policy."[40]

Reformers committed to a strict moral code, YMCA volunteers, members of the American Red Cross, and social hygienists apprehended the psychodynamics of war. "Until one comes in contact with a large body of men separated from feminine influence and the social restraints of civilized life, one does not realize how quickly the savage comes to the surface," observed the *Literary Digest*. These reformers sought to combat the spiritual decline and moral breakdown associated with war. "Unless adequate measures are taken," they warned, "a 'sex festival' will be the inevitable result." Worried that men, "fatigued with obligation," would go off on a "moral holiday," many of these activists expressed more anxiety concerning the turpitude of the troops than the danger of combat itself. "Dangerous as the German army is to our soldiers, it is not as dangerous as this enemy left unconquered."[41]

Those who most greatly feared the degeneracy of European culture, especially religious and organized prohibition groups, believed their worst suspicions confirmed when early reports of moral indiscretion by American troops at the French seaports circulated widely on the home front. Because the United States sent troops to France some six months ahead of schedule, the careful precautions to protect their welfare that the Commission on Training Camp Activities devised in the States had yet to be developed for the AEF. As a YMCA observer pointed out, "The only houses open to them were the public houses. The only women they could associate with were the public women." Drunkenness was seen as the first step on the road to the brothel and subsequent infection. The Board of Temperance, Prohibition, and Public Morals of the Methodist Episcopal Church released a statement headed, "Appalling Drunkenness Among the Troops Imperils the Piety of the Army Abroad." The article, published in newspapers throughout the country, accused the government of abandoning the welfare of the soldiers in France. According to the report, 1,046 men of the AEF were arrested for drunkenness after their first pay-day. A vexed mother wrote to Raymond Fosdick, "I would rather have my son exposed to the bullets than to these conditions."[42]

One concerned YMCA organizer wrote to the U.S. Secretary of Commerce regarding the dangers of the commerce on the streets of Paris. "Imagine my surprise," he reported, "when I learned that a force from the Y.M.C.A. had gone to Gare de l'Est on Thursday night last, 300 of the boys came in, the Y.M.C.A. got 40 and the balance went off with 'girls.' " "Now this is a situation," he cautioned, "that may vitiate all the gains from success at arms in this war. Our boys are our responsibility, and we must find a way of protecting them, as well as those at home."[43]

Some YMCA workers took great pride in reporting that they had been approached by beautiful French women, only to reject their advances. At least some of the reformers, however, fell prey to these enticements. "America has as much to fear from the French women of Paris as from Germany," noted an American citizen in France. "The American Red Cross officials will tell you how much more deadly one has been to their organization than the other."[44]

These reformers had followed the AEF to France in an effort to make the "temptations of virtue as great as the temptations of vice." The YMCA led the fight to establish recreational and educational activities, major elements in the social hygiene crusade. Two themes emerged in their work: "cleanliness" and the prevention of "social dissipation." Cleanliness served as a euphemism for the virtual exclusion of sexual allusion from the consciousness of the soldiers. "We recognize the fact that obscene conversation tends definitely and steadily to the promotion of those subjective conditions which make for sexual activity," explained one YMCA theorist. "To be clean in thought and conversation it is important—necessary—to have clean things to think about." The YMCA promoted cleanliness through vigorous exercise and carefully organized amusements. Women volunteers served as a constant reminder to the troops of the girls they left behind.[45]

Those devoted to the troops' social welfare in France feared, above all, the impact of liberties and leisure. Service groups such as the YMCA, the Salvation Army, and the Red Cross centered their attention on filling the soldiers' free time so that the men would not look for amusements on their own. The command, aware of the dangers of undisciplined periods, took measures to restrict the liberties of the troops. All-night leaves and weekend passes provided the greatest opportunity for the men to acquire a venereal infection because the men rarely returned in time for an effective prophylactic treatment. Therefore, the Medical Department greatly limited such liberal passes. In some areas of France all liberties were pared to four hours.[46]

Leaves posed a massive problem for the control of venereal diseases for the Medical Department of the AEF. The command had decided during the summer of 1917 that, for reasons of morale and efficiency, each man should receive a seven-day furlough every four months. Hugh Young had discovered, however, that although the British and French armies only received seven- to ten-day leaves every four to six months, these periods accounted for as much as 70 percent of the venereal infections among their troops.[47] Given the potential to contract a sexually transmitted disease during this period of respite from the rigors and discipline of war, the AEF took great care in choosing and organizing the leave areas.

The YMCA, at the request of the AEF, organized nineteen leave camps that almost all two million members of the AEF visited. The government paid for food and lodgings, and the YMCA covered the expenses for recreation and entertainment. The YMCA filled the seven days with organized sports and dances, sightseeing and movies. YMCA secretaries believed that the quality of these amusements was directly related to venereal rates. A prophylaxis station attendant explained to J. H. McCurdy, director of Recreational Activities for the YMCA in France: "You run a good show out [t]here in the hall. It keeps the boys in and the chippies don't get them." McCurdy concluded, "The strength of the program was definitely related to the proportion of venereal disease."[48]

The YMCA chose leave areas with the venereal problem in mind. Major urban centers, dense with prostitution and bars, were avoided in favor of more provincial, rural locales. Paris, for example, was immediately judged off-limits for men on leave. Conditions varied greatly from one location to another depending upon factors such as proximity to centers of population, cooperation of local governments, and the battery of YMCA activities designed to entertain the men.[49]

The Medical Department required that soldiers be examined for VD before departing for leaves and again upon arrival at the specified area. Officers delivered warnings before sending their men off; some companies demanded signed statements promising upright behavior. The troops also received flyers:

> The United States Government is permitting you to go on leave, NOT in order that you may SOW WILD OATS, but to give you an opportunity to improve your health, and advance your education.
>
> If by misconduct, carelessness or vice, you are not improved in body and mind, you will have defrauded the government and will have wasted an opportunity to improve your station in life.
>
> If you become intoxicated, associate with prostitutes, or contract a venereal disease, you are guilty of a moral crime.
>
> Wouldn't it profit you more to purchase with that money a little gift for MOTHER, WIFE, SISTER or SWEETHEART??
>
> DO NOT LET BOOZE, A PRETTY FACE, A SHAPELY ANKLE MAKE YOU FORGET!! THE AEF MUST NOT TAKE EUROPEAN DISEASE TO AMERICA. YOU MUST GO HOME CLEAN!![50]

In spite of the efforts of the YMCA and their corps of volunteers to keep the troops occupied while on leave, the men often discovered their own recreation in nearby cafés and brothels. The Medical Department soon determined that many men were becoming infected en route to the leave camps. As a result, they established prophylactic stations on board the trains. On several occasions, military police found enterprising prostitutes hiding in the toilets of the trains destined for leave areas. The Medical Department used the number of prophylactic treatments taken by the men while on leave as a general gauge of sexual activity during the furloughs. In the Nimes leave area, 3,934 men who visited applied for 3,712 early treatments. Although some men obviously took more than one treatment, such a high percentage (94.36) indicated a high degree of sexual contacts and thus a significant venereal risk. On the average there were approximately 31 prophylactic treatments given every week for every 100 soldiers on leave.[51]

Medical officers estimated that half of all the cases of venereal disease acquired by members of the AEF occurred during leave periods. Some organizations reported that as much as 75 percent of their men brought back venereal diseases from the resorts of France; a figure noticeably absent from YMCA accounts of the leave areas. Colonel Percy Ashburn, a venereal specialist, clearly expressed the fears of disorder that the furloughs engendered:

> The release from strict discipline and in many respects from military control, the transition from a busy life to a wholly idle one, from one wherein women scarcely entered to one in which their seductions were very appealing, and the pocketful of money which the leave men carried, were sufficient to account for much disturbance of conduct; but, in addition to that, some of the men actually expressed the opinion that the purpose of the leaves was to allow them to have a good time with the girls after a prolonged forced abstinence.[52]

Ashburn concluded that the leaves had a "deplorable effect" on the venereal rates of the AEF.

6

The increased availability of prostitutes in France, despite American attempts to limit this traffic, made chemical prophylaxis a critical element of AEF venereal policy. The Medical Department realized on the basis of their early experience in France that control of sexual contacts, the preferred American method of preventing venereal disease, had limited potential on the continent. Though General Order No. 6 made contraction of a venereal disease a court-martial offense, G.O. No. 32, issued in February 1918, added failure to take prophylaxis after a sexual exposure as a separate offense constituting neglect of duty. Reasoning that some men would—contrary to best advice—expose themselves to venereal diseases, Pershing established prophylactic stations as the last line of defense. Completely convinced of the effectiveness of the treatment, he wrote to the surgeon general: "The prophylaxis, if properly used, is so surely a protection, that any venereal disease arising must be severely punished."[53]

Prophylaxis was a relatively simple procedure, but not a particularly pleasant

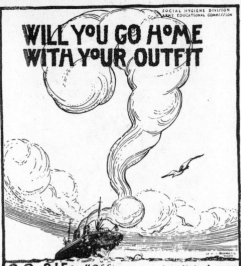

WILL YOU GO HOME WITH YOUR OUTFIT

G.O. 215: "Officers and enlisted men returning to the United States will be subjected to a physical examination previous to embarkation and all those found to be affected with venereal disease in a communicable stage will be detained and placed in segregation camps."

2. A threat unveiled.

3. A joint statement on venereal disease *and* masturbation.

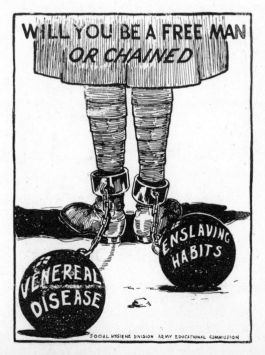

WILL YOU BE A FREE MAN OR CHAINED

VENEREAL DISEASE

ENSLAVING HABITS

SOCIAL HYGIENE DIVISION ARMY EDUCATIONAL COMMISSION

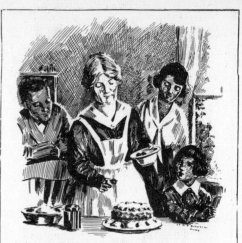

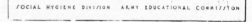

Go back to them physically fit and morally clean

SOCIAL HYGIENE DIVISION ARMY EDUCATIONAL COMMISSION

4. Lest the soldiers forget, a reminder of American family values.

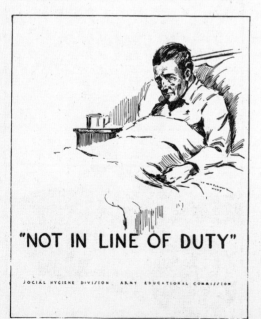

"NOT IN LINE OF DUTY"

SOCIAL HYGIENE DIVISION ARMY EDUCATIONAL COMMISSION

5. Venereal infections, considered by the military to be injuries inflicted "not in the line of duty," could lead to court-martial.

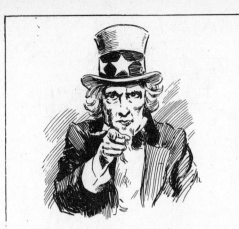

HE STILL NEEDS YOUR *BEST*

SOCIAL HYGIENE DIVISION   ARMY   EDUCATIONAL COMMISSION

6. Uncle Sam joins the anti-venereal disease crusade.

7. The concept of disease broadly applied. This explicit poster may have had just the effect it sought to avoid.

IS *YOUR* MIND DISEASED?

SOCIAL HYGIENE DIVISION ARMY   EDUCATIONAL COMMISSION

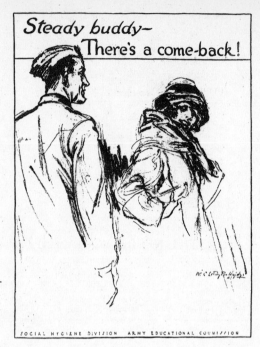

8. Persistent reminders of the dangers of the prostitute.

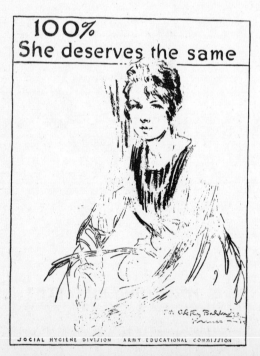

9. The girl he left behind.

one. Pershing ordered each division to establish its own station, easily accessible, sanitary, and private.[54] The Chief Surgeon of the AEF prepared a memorandum detailing the method of prophylaxis devised by the Medical Department. Attendants, appointed to each station, administered the treatments. A soldier reporting for the treatment would first urinate. Then, on a specially constructed stool, he would wash his genitals with soap and water followed by bichloride of mercury, while the attendant inspected. The attendant would then inject a solution of protargol into the penis, which the soldier would hold in the urethra for five minutes, then expel. After the injection, calomel ointment would be rubbed on the penis, which would then be wrapped in waxed paper. For the prevention to be effective the soldier could not urinate for four or five hours following the treatment.[55]

The Medical Department sought to make prophylaxis a respectable procedure. "The point of departure for both attendant and patient is placed in the teaching that venereal prophylaxis, being a major operation like catheterization, is entitled to professional consideration," explained an AEF physician. "The attendant, therefore, must be placed in such a relation with the patient that the latter will see no humor in his position as a 'Professor of Prophylaxis.' "[56] The prophylaxis stool reportedly served this function well, bringing the patient and the attendant into a properly "formal relationship" so that the treatment could be performed with "integrity."

Though the Medical Department expressed supreme confidence in the effectiveness of chemical prophylaxis for preventing venereal infections, statistics indicated that 55 percent of the soldiers who contracted a venereal disease had taken the treatment. This discrepancy caused alarm within the Division of Urology, which conducted an investigation among venereally infected soldiers. Physicians interviewed more than 3,000 men with venereal infections, 60 percent of whom reported having taken prophylaxis. The doctors found, however, that many had taken the treatment after the designated three-hour limit. Moreover, many had been intoxicated and received incomplete procedures. The Medical Department estimated that when properly administered prophylaxis was 99.6 percent effective against syphilis, gonorrhea, and chancroid.[57]

Many sexually active soldiers never took prophylaxis. Between 30 and 40 percent of the men who contracted venereal diseases during the war failed to apply for the treatment. Because lectures and literature placed great emphasis on getting the procedures within three hours, some soldiers believed it useless to report for prophylaxis late. Others, drunk or lost in a French town, simply could not find a station.[58]

Failure to obtain proper prophylaxis was not always the fault of the soldier. Aware that conditions were often unsanitary, lines too long, and the demeanor of attendants derisive, Pershing wrote to the chief surgeon to reaffirm the importance of a well-rendered preventive program: "Prophylactic stations are often not well organized, equipped, or administered, and this fact alone would bring discredit on the treatment rather than confidence in its use." At one station, an observer reported that the attendant used the same syringe for seven men in succession without sterilization; a *faux pas* not unlike the problems the French experienced with medical inspection of prostitutes. Another soldier reported being turned away from a prophylactic station which refused to treat "strangers."[59]

7

The heavy reliance of the AEF on chemical prophylaxis touched off a bitter debate between social hygiene reformers in the United States and members of the Army Medical Department. Those who had worked vigorously to close down the red-light districts in American cities and to educate soldiers about continence felt betrayed by the introduction of this preventive technology into military life. First, they argued, chemical prophylaxis would have the ultimate effect of increasing venereal disease by promoting "illicit" sexual contacts. "In so far as prophylaxis encourages incontinence, and in so far as it undercuts the positive demand for continence on the part of men," wrote an angry Edith Houghton Hooker, "in like measure it defeats its own purpose, that of preventing venereal disease." Secondly, the treatment was viewed as an official sanction for the double standard of morality, the nemesis of the social hygiene movement since its founding in the late nineteenth century. Thus prophylaxis was attacked as an affront to women:

> While the government officially tolerates male prostitution as it does under its present system of prophylaxis, a certain amount of prostitution is of necessity predicated, for a man cannot have promiscuous intercourse alone. It is therefore obviously illogical and ethically unsound for the government to propose a system of repression [of disease] directed at one sex alone.[60]

"To save the country from the pestilence of venereal disease," concluded Hooker, "prophylaxis concedes the necessity of a continual sacrifice of fresh girls to the moloch of men's lust."

In an effort to make chemical prophylaxis more acceptable, medical officers called it the "early treatment," conferring upon it a curative rather than preventive effect. Critics, however, could not be assuaged. As Hooker correctly argued:

> The very term 'early treatment' is a false use of words, for it is impossible to treat a disease if it is absent . . . This abuse of language conduces to an exaggerated notion of the efficacy of prophylaxis and in turn this leads to a false sense of security.

Hooker, the most articulate critic of prophylaxis, condemned every aspect of the entire procedure. "The prophylactic station," she asserted, "reeks of the brothel, for the men there still have the stain of illicit intercourse upon them, and come the self-confessed violators of the moral law."[61]

Proponents of prophylaxis, especially within the military, remained unconvinced that the measure contributed to sexual excess. "The more prophylaxis is urged and talked about, the more will the average man associate in his mind the danger of the disease with the sex relation," explained Colonel George Walker. Prophylaxis, he argued persuasively, protected those men who would expose themselves to disease in spite of the admonitions of those dedicated to a strict sexual morality. "It was recognized," noted Dr. J. E. Moore, a consultant urologist to the AEF, "that a certain proportion of the men (33 percent . . .) were unlikely to be restrained by the influence of religion, home ties, or fear of disease, and that no matter what advice was offered or what penalties imposed, they would expose themselves continuously."[62]

In the debate over prophylaxis, the perception of venereal disease as an illness of individual responsibility became explicit. Those who opposed prophylaxis believed it diminished this sense of responsibility and would thus have a damaging impact on efforts to control sexually transmitted diseases. "Suicide, like venery, is a voluntary act," wrote R. C. Holcomb in response to such arguments, "but should we refuse succor to the unfortunate who willfully commits the act or endeavor to save him from the consequences of his willfullness?" Supporters of prophylaxis argued that it actually heightened individual responsibility. As Colonel Bailey K. Ashford told his troops: "We are getting to pity a man for catching an infectious disease less and less. . . . To get certain diseases today is to confess to a certain degree of plain stupidity."[63]

Both sides cited recent advances in public health to bolster their positions. "There now seems to be an opportunity to place the detection and early treatment of venereal diseases on the same basis as the detection and early treatment of diphtheria, meningitis, and other communicable diseases," wrote Dr. Franklin Martin, chairman of the Medical Board of the Council of National Defense, in support of the provision of prophylaxis. On the other hand, argued Edith Houghton Hooker, any measure that tended to increase exposures to a communicable disease would be treated with extreme skepticism by those dedicated to public health:

> In order to think clearly of the relation of morals to the campaign against venereal disease, it is well to regard continence simply as a sanitary measure. Differently phrased, it is merely avoidance of exposure to venereal infection. This is a fundamental principle in the control and prevention of all other infectious diseases, for example, diphtheria, small pox, rabies, etc.[64]

The weakness in Hooker's argument is apparent: it was simply not possible to equate sexual intercourse with a deliberate exposure to a communicable disease, the motivations for sexual behavior being far more complex than she acknowledges. According to the social hygienists who protested against prophylaxis, those soldiers who exposed themselves to venereal disease should be prepared to suffer the dangerous and ignominious consequences.

On the issue of prophylaxis the alliance of reformers committed to a strict moral order and those committed to a technocratic order came unhinged. The military imperative of efficiency dictated that prophylaxis become the centerpiece of the Medical Department's anti-venereal campaign, scientific exigencies dismissing moral claims. "Let those who regard venereal disease as a divine punishment recall that small pox and other diseases have been at various times, and are even today by some regarded as acts of God," wrote William Lyster of the Army Medical Corps:

If fanatics must interfere in this beneficial work of reducing venereal disease, let them concentrate on an effort to remove the sexual appetite rather than insist on spreading venereal disease, even to the innocent, by abandoning one of the most powerful agents in preventing it.[65]

The debate over prophylaxis became more heated as the military's campaign began to employ a prophylactic packet that was administered by the patient himself. In fact, a packet had been developed for self-administration and distributed to members of the Army on an experimental basis as early as 1910. Several commercial manufacturers produced these "pro-kits" to Army specifications. The packet consisted of a collapsible tube with calomel ointment, carbolic acid, and camphor. During the war, the chief surgeon discouraged the use of the packet, however, for he believed it would replace the stations where a more rigorously controlled and documented procedure could be administered. The Medical Department did supply men with packets when their duties made established prophylactic stations inaccessible.[66] After the armistice, when many members of the AEF received leaves and venereal rates rose rapidly, Pershing responded by ordering that all men be provided with "pro-kits." The chief surgeon estimated that unrestricted distribution would require at least half a million packets, though the Department had only 125,000 available. Therefore the Army continued to supply them only to those distant from stations.[67]

Although chemical prophylaxis was hardly acceptable to many members of the social hygiene movement, the provision of packets to the men seemed to be the straw which broke the moralists' backs. Indeed, in 1915, Secretary of the Navy Josephus Daniels had forbidden the use of individual prophylaxis in the Navy:

The use of the so-called 'preventive or prophylactic packet' is not authorized, and I have been severely criticized in various quarters for my attitude with regard to this measure. The use of this packet I believe to be immoral; it savors of the panderer; and it is wicked to seem to encourage and approve placing in the hands of the men an appliance which will lead them to think that they may indulge in practices which are not sanctioned by moral, military, or civil law, with impunity, and the use of which would tend to subvert and destroy the very foundations of our moral and Christian beliefs and teachings with regards to these sexual matters.

No doubt, Daniels had exposed an important conflict between the new medical technology and late Victorian sexual morality. His edict prohibiting the distribution of the packet could not, however, withstand the demands for efficiency that the war engendered. Raymond Fosdick, concerned with the high rates of venereal disease in the Navy, pressed Daniels to order prophylaxis. When Daniels maintained his steadfast position, Fosdick raised the issue with the young Assistant Secretary, Franklin Roosevelt. Roosevelt signed the order for prophylaxis in Daniels' absence.[68]

The battle against prophylaxis was, for the duration of the war, a lost cause. The demands for an efficient military force were too intense, and faith in the ability of soldiers to refrain from sexual contacts did not run high among military officers, in spite of their official pronouncements. In one respect, the critics of prophylaxis were probably correct: for members of the AEF, the prophylaxis stations must have symbolized the command's tacit acceptance of active sexual behavior. Only an estimated 30 percent of the men who fought in France maintained the officially prescribed continence while overseas. Although the Army never released any official statistics, the total number of prophylactic treatments administered to members of the AEF must have surpassed several million. Without exception, medical officers attributed their ability to control sexually transmitted diseases to the prophylactic stations.[69]

8

Despite the prodigious efforts of the Medical Department to keep the Army free of venereal disease, these infections had a tremendous impact upon American forces. At home and abroad during the war, almost seven million days of active duty were lost to venereal diseases, the most common illnesses in the service next to influenza, which struck in epidemic proportions. A total of 383,706 soldiers were diagnosed with either syphillis, gonorrhea, or chancroid between April 1917 and December 1919. The economic losses to the government were considerable. A case of venereal disease cost the Army about seven dollars per day for approximately thirty-three days. Thus venereal diseases during the war cost the government almost fifty million dollars.[70]

Although the military worked to close red-light districts and demand continence of soldiers encamped within the United States, venereal diseases remained a serious drain on manpower and efficiency. Some 12.7 percent of the over two million men in the Army stationed in the United States were admitted to sick report with a diagnosed venereal disease. Indeed, soldiers serving in the United States accounted for 76.6 percent of the venereal infections in the entire Army during the war. Several factors explain the high rates within the States as compared to levels in the AEF. First, careful inspections prior to embarkation for France kept most venereally diseased soldiers in the United States. Second, provisions for discipline and prophylaxis were more stringent in France. And third, French inspection of prostitutes may have served to prevent some infections among members of the AEF. The Medical Department of the Army insisted that the high rates of infection resulted from the fact that five of every six cases were brought into the Army from civilian life by the draft.[71]

Of all the American military forces mustered during the war, the AEF registered the best record for avoiding venereal diseases. In explaining these low rates, in which only 3.4 percent of the men were admitted to sick report with a venereal infection, the Medical Department emphasized the sexual deportment of the troops. Educated in the ways of continence, with vice and temptation shut off, argued the Army physicians, the doughboys had remained relatively "clean." Percy Ashburn laid great stress on American propaganda in aiding the members of the AEF to avoid sexual contacts: "Well reared boys and men in general desire to do what they know to be right; and when it is difficult to do so a little encouragement was certainly afforded by the campaign of propaganda." Education and repression, no doubt, had an impact on reducing VD among the AEF, but Ashburn was forced to admit that chemical prophylaxis had been the key to keeping the rates of infection low. He calculated that prophylaxis had "reduced the liability to venereal disease to about one-third of what it would have been otherwise."[72]

The venereal disease situation in France nevertheless became serious enough by the summer of 1918 that the Medical Department established special camps to segregate the infected men. Of the approximately two million men in the AEF, 18,000 missed action each day because of venereal disease. The Medical Department designed the camps as a means of restraining infectious venereal patients who did not require hospitalization. In this way non-effective days could be kept to a minimum and the men could not spread their infections. Regulations required that all men work while being treated. Flyers distributed to the doughboys warned: "How about a job with a Labor Battalion? Would you like to join one? Then keep clean." The camps reduced the days spent in the hospital as well as time spent away from an organization. No patient could be released back to his company before being declared non-infectious. Medical officers believed that the punitive nature of the camps encouraged men to avoid infections through continence and prophylaxis. As one officer in the Medical Corps noted, "The moral effect of segregation has undoubtedly been felt." A sign that hung over the camp at Gievre announced: "This is a Venereal Camp. These Men are Helping the Hun."[73]

The Army reported exceedingly high rates of venereal disease among "colored" troops. In such statistical breakdowns, it usually appeared that blacks contributed to the venereal role five times as much as whites. Among the white troops in the United States, just over 10 percent contracted a venereal disease, though a remarkable 58 percent of the black soldiers were diagnosed with alleged sexually transmitted diseases. Although percentages of venereal disease among blacks may well have been high, it is probable that many Army physicians were predisposed to diagnose many ailments among black troops as sexually transmitted. Moreover, many blacks with venereal diseases were accepted for service, though whites were excused. This policy was based on the assumption that virtually all blacks had venereal disease. High rates also reflected the poor quality of health care in the United States for most blacks, many of whom had never been examined by a physician prior to their draft physicals.[74]

Because of the high rates of venereal disease among blacks in the AEF, many divisions ordered compulsory prophylaxis for all black soldiers regardless of exposure. In Base Section No. 1, for example, a wire stockade was erected around the camp and the black stevedores were forced to enter and leave through a designated checkpost. Passes were limited to four hours and all returning men were required to undergo chemical prophylaxis. Venereal rates reportedly fell dramatically, encouraging several other divisions to institute this measure. When blacks did acquire a venereal infection they received from ten to thirty percent fewer days of hospitalization than did white patients.[75]

The question of black rates of venereal disease suggests only some of the difficulties of assessing venereal statistics. Debates regarding the extent and nature of venereal diseases would be fought throughout the twentieth century on statistical battlefronts. Figures based on whimsy, wishfulness, and predilection stood as the foundations for positions regarding the method of combatting the sexually transmitted diseases. The military statistics kept during World War I point to several of the problems of venereal disease record-keeping—a continuation of the debate waged several years earlier by Prince Morrow and Richard Cabot.

9

The allied victory renewed fears of lack of discipline and moral indiscretion. With the battle won, soldiers who had remained true to the standard of continence might no longer accept its rationale. Moreover, some Americans believed that French women would surpass the bounds of decency in expressing their thanks to their American saviors. As Pershing wrote to the chief surgeon, "I have watched with concern the gradual rise in the rate of venereal disease in the A.E.F. since active operations ceased. Steps must be taken at once to check this, as I am determined that a very high standard in this respect shall be attained." Indeed, the increase in venereal admissions as the troops were granted more leaves and liberties had been more than gradual. In September 1919 a yearly admission rate of 766.55 per 1,000 was reported. A Medical Department circular announced that the American forces in France were "fast approaching a venereal rate of 1,000 per 1,000 per year."[76]

Medical officers and social hygienists had expressed great concern throughout the war about the problem of infected soldiers returning to the United States. As an editorial in the *Journal of the American Medical Association* warned:

> One of the greatest disasters of war is the spread of infections that occurs through . . . the disbanding of troops at the close of war. Epidemics following wars have often caused greater loss of life than have the actual casualties of war itself or diseases occurring among the troops during the prosecution of the war. This applies particularly to the venereal diseases.

The potential for bringing venereal diseases back to the United States invested the campaign against them with an importance almost as large as the war itself. "The nation which controls and dries up the race poisons of venereal disease has the best chance of surviving during the coming ages," wrote Lieutenant Walter Clarke of the Sanitary Corps. "The fight against venereal diseases is a long campaign for a clean bill of health for the children and grandchildren of the boys now in the trenches."[77]

The threat of what Progressive physicians called "innocent infection" was repeatedly invoked in an attempt to urge continence prior to the AEF's demobilization. As a proposed bulletin of the Medical Department stated:

> Our Civilization being what it is and founded upon the family with but one wife and mother, the purity of blood and of family depending upon her chastity, it needs no religious teaching that to expose her to disease which would affect her children is not only unfair to her, but is also a crime against civilization.

To meet this danger, General Headquarters issued G.O. No. 215 in November 1918, requiring venereal inspections before embarkation for the United States. Infected men would remain segregated in France until determined non-communicable. "The people of America know this," warned a standard lecture to the troops, "and will want to know why you did not return with your company."[78] A pamphlet distributed to some members of the AEF in advance of the return voyage asked a series of pointed questions:

Can you look straight into piercing eyes
And swear you've kept the faith;
That through all war's hell you've guarded the trust,
And you've brought no red souvenir of lust
To betray and tarnish that faith?

The German is licked, but this old war has one more kick in its hind leg. Look out for it!

You don't want to go back to the old home town with a curse on you.

You wouldn't go out on purpose and pick up a dose of clap or a case of syhpilis. Sure! But, maybe, before you swing aboard for Coney Island and points west, you'll find a neat little welterweight queen tugging away at your arm with a mon cheri smile and—well, you know: she'd do anything for her American hero.

And she would too—that's the hell of it. She'd do the one thing for you that would give you a shifty eye and a game conscience and a dirty body—and who's a hero then?

A surgeon in the Medical Corps, anxious that returning soldiers might infect their wives and children, recommended that families be notified of such illness.[79]

Although the command opted not to institute this plan for reasons of discretion, members of the AEF whose arrival in the United States came to be delayed suffered the consequences. The press suggested that only venereals had failed to gain clearance, though men were detained in France with a variety of communicable ailments. Broken engagements, crushed sweethearts, and marital tensions followed these reports. One healthy infantryman arrived in the States to find a letter from his fiancé. He explained:

My sweetheart expresses sympathy for me in my condition and wishes me well. But she does not think she would care for a husband who could not respect the girl he had asked to be his wife.[80]

10

In spite of the persistent fears of a profligate army, most reformers celebrated the venereal record of the AEF as a triumph of Progressive morality. They offered the venereal statistics collected by the Medical Department as evidence that the men had returned spiritually and physically purified by the war experience. "Our fighting force to-day is not only the cleanest body of fighting men the world has ever seen," noted one observer, "but the cleanest group of young men ever brought together outside a monastery." Medical officers and social hygienists also heralded the American campaign against the sexually transmitted diseases as a massive victory for social engineering. As Raymond Fosdick concluded, recalling Woodrow Wilson's charge to the troops:

> The victory over Germany is won. When the members of the American Expeditionary Forces return to their homes they will come 'with no scars except those won in honorable conflict' because America has been far-sighted enough, idealistic enough, to undertake to fight an unseen enemy, and win, in the face of tremendous odds, a victory over it as notable, in proportion, as the victory forced from the Central Powers.[81]

Though reformers during the war had been apprehensive about the return of a libertine army spreading venereal disease, they now argued the danger was to the undefiled crusaders returning home. "Will America debauch our Army when it comes back?" asked Luther Gulick of the YMCA. In anticipation of the troops' homecoming, Secretary of War Baker telegraphed the governors, cautioning them to redouble repressive measures in their states so as to protect the doughboys; "laxity," he advised, "would be a disaster to our soldiers and their families."[82]

Other difficulties were suggested concerning the soldiers' return to civilian life. Amid celebrations of the Army's purity, some took a more skeptical view of the war's impact on the troops. Colonel George Walker feared that American boys had been corrupted by the French. Walker, a prominent member of the urological department, felt compelled to include a chapter on "Sex Abnormalities (Perversion) in France" in his monograph on venereal disease in the AEF. "Whatever the origin of the twisted impulse," he wrote, "it creates but one effect, a subtle state of demoralization that is far more dangerous to society as it is presently constructed, at least from the Anglo-Saxon viewpoint, than mere immorality could ever be." Walker sent investigators to cafés to interview prostitutes who reported, almost without exception, the American soldiers' newly developed preference for the "French way," a euphemism for oral sex:

> When one thinks of the hundreds and hundreds of thousands of young men who have returned to the United States with those new and degenerate ideas sapping their sources of self-respect and thereby lessening their powers of moral resistance, one indeed is justified in becoming alarmed.[83]

Walker, dedicated to a scientific view of the venereal problem, seemed to lament the impact prevention had upon morals. As far as he was concerned, the AEF had won the battle against venereal diseases, but lost the war to the contagion of immorality infecting France.

Certainly the troops' exposure to continental sexual culture must have punctured American provincialism. Even if the doughboys did not submit to the allures of French women, the omnipresence of sexual possibility forced the men to confront their own sexuality. As one young lieutenant in the AEF wrote:

> Walking through dark streets, ever-present women. So mysterious and seductive in darkness. . . . A fellow's got to hang on to himself here. Not many do.[84]

YMCA reformers and social hygienists who proclaimed the war's impact in undermining the double standard of morality concerning sexual matters had fallen prey to their own propaganda. As the institution of chemical prophylaxis had made all too clear, low venereal rates no longer meant a continent army. The doughboys returned for the most part free of venereal diseases, but the war's legacy for American sexuality was a mixed one.

The venereal disease campaign during the war forced a general consciousness of sexual behavior unprecedented in American life. The public crusade against the red-light district and the frequent press accounts of the venereal menace brought the discussion of sexual matters to a new prominence, shattering the Victorian "conspiracy of silence," at least for the time being. Yet inconsistencies in defining a sexual code persisted. The American vilification of prostitution and extramarital sex during the war brought the double standard to its official nadir, but the late-Victorian demand for a single, rigid standard of morality had fewer adherents as well. The place accorded sexuality in American life remained unclear.

The efforts directed against venereal diseases during the war clearly established the relation of modern medical science to sexuality. The new effective therapeutics, the Wassermann reaction, arsphenamine, and chemical prophylaxis, lent legitimacy to medicine's role in sexuality. Increasingly, medical doctors would define and prescribe sexual behavior; and the profession would become the locus of authority in sexual matters.

The physician's status also grew with the war-time emphasis on preventive medicine. By the early twentieth century the need for the conservation of human resources had become clear. Health was an important aspect of this conservation, and the draft had manifested the problem of neglecting public health. The new stress placed on preventive medicine during the years preceding World War I indicated a redefinition of the role and function of health care.[85] Industrial and military order would best be served by avoiding illness altogether. Prevention thus became the key element in the Medical Department's battle against venereal disease during the war.

The efforts directed against venereal diseases in the course of World War I serve to define what has come to be known as "Progressivism." The Progressive impulse had two concentric circles of emphasis: morality and efficiency. The call for a strict moral order placed responsibility at the individual's doorstep. Thus the language of Progressivism, clearly reflected in the anti-venereal exhortations delivered to the troops, demanded *self*-discipline, *self*-denial, *self*-sacrifice, and *self*-control. Reformers stressed education as the primary means of shaping individual behavior. Thus members of the AEF received their first officially sanctioned lessons in sex education from medical officers.

Progressives, however, also feared individual weakness. So they looked to instrumentalities of social engineering to insure the efficiency and order that the twentieth century required. Thus they were willing to institute measures, interventionary and technocratic, from propaganda to punishment, to guarantee their view of the social order. In the case of venereal disease, those dedicated to the moral order and those dedicated to the industrial order discovered common ground upon which to base their work.

Within the military, and particularly among the AEF, the instrumental impulse of Progressivism became paramount. Though accepting the basic tenets of moral reform, medical officers refused to be hindered in their efforts to prevent venereal diseases. The institution of chemical prophylaxis, more clearly than any other issue, served to divide reformers committed to strict morality and those concerned with manpower and efficiency. Moral reformers argued that the oft-invoked "cleansing influence of war" should be achieved through moral and not chemical means. The question was thus boldly posed: Which was a greater threat to society, venereal disease or immorality?

The efforts to inculcate sexual morality among the members of the AEF made evident that a rigorous sexual code, at least for some, would persist well into the twentieth century, shaping attempts to control venereal disease by demanding "proper" behavior. For others—particularly in the medical community—influenced by biological and psychological theories about the determinants of sexual behavior, the demands of science outstripped the last vestiges of the rigid moral argument. Tensions between these two poles would define the debates regarding venereal disease control in the years to come.

IV

"Shadow on the Land":
Thomas Parran and the New Deal

1

In November 1934 the Columbia Broadcasting Company scheduled a radio address by New York State Health Commissioner Thomas Parran, Jr., on future goals in the area of public health. Parran planned to review the major problems confronting public health officers in their battle against disease. But the talk was never delivered. Moments before air-time, CBS informed him that he could not mention syphilis and gonorrhea by name; in response to this decision, Parran refused to go on. Listeners who had tuned in to hear the address heard piano melodies instead. Parran, reacting angrily to being censored, pointed out the hypocrisy in the standards for radio broadcasting. In a press release issued by his office the next day, he commented that his speech should have been considered more acceptable than "the veiled obscenity permitted by Columbia in the vaudeville acts of some of their commercial programs."[1]

Fifteen years earlier, during the anti-venereal crusade during World War I, the conspiracy of silence had appeared to be defeated. Newspapers and magazines had dramatically publicized the problem; Congress and the military addressed it forthrightly. In the following years, however, the anti-venereal campaign had faltered. After the radical interventions that the war brought on—not only in politics and economics, but socially as well—America returned to a "normalcy" that also pervaded public health efforts.

The 1920s, despite their apparent frivolity, marked less of a watershed in the area of sexual morality than has often been assumed. Though among the young there was a distinct increase in sexual activity, a strong crosscurrent of demands for moral rectitude and gentility persisted.[2] While women took champagne baths at speakeasies and couples went on jaunts in roadsters along country lanes, respectability was reasserted in many quarters. It is important to remember that if the twenties marked the decade of bathtub gin, so, too, was it the decade of prohibition. In spite of the new openness towards sexuality, the sexually transmitted diseases were drawn once again behind a veil of secrecy. Until the 1930s the venereal problem would go largely unheeded.

During the New Deal, Thomas Parran would commit the nation to the eradication of venereal disease by dramatically bringing these infections to the center of public consciousness. Indeed, rarely, if ever, in the twentieth century has a public health campaign created such a public furor. In this process, venereal disease once again would be redefined. Parran, barred from the radio in 1934, found his picture on the cover of *Time* in 1936.[3] His was a mission whose success, however, would never be complete. Parran's efforts reveal the tension between scientific and moralistic approaches to the venereal problem as well as the strengths and limits of New Deal reform.

2

In 1921 Congress failed to renew the Interdepartmental Social Hygiene Board's appropriation, despite the protests of Progressive reformers and social hygienists. The Board, created by Congress in 1918 to protect the troops from the dangers of venereal disease, had developed a comprehensive program. Many predicted that the end of the ISHB would result in a moral debacle. "Are we to keep up and finish the fight?" asked Dr. Rachelle Yarros. "Are we to make this idea that man can and must abstain from promiscuous relations a permanent contribution in morals and health, or is it to be only a war measure?" The League of Women Voters, the Women's Christian Temperance Union, the Parents-Teachers Association, and the National Federation of Women's Organizations all lobbied in favor of the Board's continuance, but to no avail. Neva R. Deardorff of the *Survey* explained their concern: "The question that citizens and parents of service men have a right to ask Congress is whether it is less worthwhile now to protect boys and girls than it was a year ago." By October 1922 the ISHB, the war's most ambitious experiment in social engineering, had been dismantled. The Program of Protective Social Measures—the anti-prostitution crusade designed to insure a single standard of morality—was transferred to the Department of Justice.[4]

The demise of the Interdepartmental Social Hygiene Board marked the first critical sign of the decline in efforts to combat venereal disease after the war. The Board came under attack from several fronts shortly after the armistice was signed. The Venereal Disease Division of the Public Health Service argued that the Board constituted an unnecessary duplication of their activities; this, despite the fact that the Division's budget was merely ten percent of the Board's. The most powerful critic, however, was the American Medical Association, which claimed that the ISHB had overstepped its mandate, invading the province of public health, and more importantly, the medical profession. With the wartime emergency weathered, an AMA editorial argued, the nation should return to more traditional means of disease prevention. "The Board," declared the AMA "has shown an inability to distinguish between measures for the proper regulation of public health and those intended for the control of public and individual morals." Although elements of the AMA's response were justified, their ongoing concern about the growth of "state medicine" informed their critique.[5] The excesses of the ISHB notwithstanding, the failure to renew government funding for venereal disease control marked a significant shift away from the notion of federal responsibility for health and disease prevention that the war had encouraged.

The reaction against the war's vigorous social hygiene campaign, however, transcended Congress. As if to add insult to injury, the film "Fit to Fight"—the centerpiece of anti-venereal propaganda during the war—was declared obscene in New York State by the Board of Censors, a ruling upheld by the Circuit Court. New York City License Commissioner John F. Gilchrist told the court: "The fact that a small body of specialized medical opinion supports the picture . . . does not free a given picture from the vice of violating the standards of morality." Governor Al Smith's top adviser, Belle Moskowitz, also testified against the film, noting, "Only a wrongly conceived scientific zeal could consider it fit for indiscriminate use." In Pennsylvania the State Board of Censors banned any film that mentioned the words "venereal disease." Catholic lay organizations bitterly protested the public release of "Fit to Fight" throughout the nation. The more conservative social hygienists and purity activists centered their attack on the film's advocacy of chemical prophylaxis: "If you can't be moral, be careful."[6] By 1922 the Public Health Service had withdrawn all its anti-venereal films. The arguments of expediency framed during the war now held little weight; public health gave way to concerns about public morals.

The fate of chemical prophylaxis against venereal disease in the years after the war is the best indication of this shift in attitudes. During the war the administration of this treatment had greatly reduced the rates of venereal infection among the American Expeditionary Forces, as well as troops stationed in the United States. With the armistice, however, opponents of this procedure fully mobilized and forced public health officials to draw back. State boards of health now suggested that the use of prophylaxis was "not practical," although treatment could easily be administered without medical assistance. The American Social Hygiene Association remained strongly opposed to the use of chemical prophylaxis as a venereal disease control measure, charging that its institution would lead to a drastic increase in promiscuity and disease.[7]

Public health officers recognized the benefits of prophylaxis for preventing disease, but in most cases succumbed to the sentiments of the ASHA and other critics. In 1924 the Venereal Disease Division of the Public Health Service polled state health officials on their positions regarding prophylaxis. Most suggested that public opinion did not permit its use. "It might be disastrous to our work to distribute information on venereal prophylaxis and we cannot afford to take chances of possibly closing these doors of entrance to the public mind," wrote Dr. Roy K. Flannagan of the Virginia State Board, despite his firm belief in the efficacy of the procedure. Shortly after the war, the Pennsylvania Health Department had undertaken the widespread provision of prophylactic packets as part of their anti-venereal program. But the failure to produce a verified decline in cases coupled with objections from moral reformers brought the project to a quick conclusion.[8]

The debate over prophylaxis revealed an ongoing tension in approaches to the venereal problem. Dr. George Bigelow, commissioner of public health for the State of Massachusetts, directly confronted the issue, asking, "Why not through this means [prophylaxis] wipe [venereal diseases] off the slate as of community significance, and stop the sneering reference to us as a 'syphilized people?' " Bigelow provided an answer: "As I see it, the reason is because we are cowards, we health officers, and dare not face the charge that we are using public funds to make promiscuous intercourse safe." Bigelow's forthright approach demanded a response; it issued from the very top of the public health bureaucracy. "It must be borne in mind that persons most in need of protection are usually the more irresponsible groups in a community and under the circumstances often would not have sufficient foresight to provide the protection which Dr. Bigelow recommends," countered Surgeon General H. S. Cumming, expressing a frequently cited argument.

The surgeon general's reply had actually been drafted by a young lieutenant in Cumming's service, Dr. Thomas Parran. Parran, appointed chief of the Venereal Disease Division in 1926, argued that the distribution of information concerning prophylaxis might have a deleterious effect on his anti-venereal program. "It is believed," he explained, "that such propaganda reaching all ages would have an ill effect which possibly would counterbalance the cases prevented."[9] Parran repeatedly insisted that his resistance to prophylaxis did not rest exclusively on moral precepts. "Not only are large groups of 'moralists' opposed to this method of prevention," he noted, "but there are some thoughtful scientific men who take the position that the evil results of a campaign in promoting promiscuous sexual intercourse will more than counterbalance the good of prevention."[10] But it was the power of public opinion coupled with a general decline in state activity that negated the possibility of widespread education and provision of prophylaxis.

Parran, who had joined the Public Health Service at the beginning of World War I, had directly witnessed the decline of federal support for venereal disease control efforts. Born in 1892 on a Maryland farm where his ancestors had first settled in the seventeenth century, Parran received his medical degree from Georgetown University in 1915. Two years later the Public Health Service commissioned him an assistant surgeon; for the next decade he performed a variety of services in this position, investigating epidemics and administering sanitation programs around the country. By the time he was appointed to head the Venereal Disease Division, he had established himself as a leading figure in the public health bureaucracy.[11]

When Parran took over the reins of the division, however, the halcyon days of public efforts to control venereal disease had long passed. Although the Venereal Disease Division won the bureaucratic battle for exclusive jurisdiction over these infections from the Interdepartmental Social Hygiene Board, it nevertheless lost the war. Congress reduced appropriations for work in this area so significantly that it had become, in Parran's words "a dying operation." Yearly spending had dropped from $4 million in 1920 to less than $60,000 in 1926. Dr. O. C. Wenger, director of the USPHS Venereal Clinic in Hot Springs, Arkansas, complained, "With our present appropriations, Federal and State and private, we might just as well try to empty the Pacific Ocean with a teaspoon."[12]

With the onset of the Great Depression, funding for venereal disease control became even more scarce, the Venereal Disease Division little more than a holding operation. It was thus with few regrets that Thomas Parran left the federal government in 1930 when the governor of New York, Franklin D. Roosevelt, appointed him state health commissioner. In March 1933, as the depression hit bottom and FDR assumed the presidency, Parran wrote to his successor at the Public Health Service, Dr. Taliaferro Clark: "I am very pessimistic about the future of worthwhile governmental activities of all types."[13] The venereal problem, once the subject of national debate and federal efforts, had receded from the public consciousness.

3

Rather than attributing the persistence of venereal diseases to the decline in public health measures, many social hygienists argued that the prevalence of infection derived from the "new morality" of the 1920s. The increasing sexual candor of the decade alarmed them rather than impressed them as an opportunity for bringing the seriousness of the venereal disease problem into the open. Critics of the so-called "sexual revolution" feared that a freer sexuality would lead to license—and more infections.[14]

Social hygienists responded to the incursion of Freudian thought in America with a combination of fear and loathing. "The advent of Freudianism has been attended, together with a few benefits, by numerous evils," declared Dr. Paul E. Bowers, a consultant to the Public Health Service. He suggested that the "perverse sex emphasis" of Freudian psychology and the ensuing fad of psychoanalysis were bound to "lead to promiscuity in those social levels where we ordinarily expect to find the highest types of sexual ethics and culture." Up-to-date social hygienists tended to emphasize the theory of sexual sublimation, which argued that the sexual drive could be converted into productive activity or work, while they discounted Freud's attack on genteel strictures against sexuality. At the All-American Conference on Venereal Disease—a convocation called by the USPHS shortly after the war to set venereal policy for the 1920s—the assembled group of physicians and public health officials attempted to confront the implications of Freudian theory for their program. After considerable debate, they endorsed a resolution:

> Resolved, that although there is danger that a superficial and erroneous interpretation of the Freudian psychology in regard to the repression of the sex instinct may be detrimental to the successful development of the program for the control of venereal diseases, a more thorough-going, complete and scientific interpretation tends to aid such a program in that it places the emphasis upon the practical means for guiding the sex instinct into socially useful and constructive activities.[15]

Clearly, the social hygienists considered themselves to be professional sublimators. Already the American pattern of the convenient selection of Freudian thought could be seen at work.

To those who sought to control venereal disease by controlling behavior, the activities of American youth were viewed with particular alarm. The new, faddish dances, from the toddle to the black bottom, were cited as both a moral and a medical threat. "It is certain that the dance of today, as performed in the majority of places, does not have a tendency to diminish or regulate the normal

Rules and Regulations for Public Dance Halls

1. No shadow or spotlight dances allowed.
2. Moonlight dances not allowed where a single light is used to illuminate the Hall. Lights may be shaded to give Hall dimmed illuminated effect.
3. All unnecessrry shoulder or body movement or gratusque dances positively prohibited.
4. Pivot reverse and running on the floor prohibited.
5. All unnecessary hesitation, rocking from one foot to the other and see-sawing back and forth of the dancers will be prohibited.
6. No loud talking, undue familiarity or suggestive remarks unbecoming any lady or gentleman will be tolerated.

POSITION OF DANCERS

1. Right hand of gentleman must not be placed below the waist nor over the shoulder nor around the lady's neck, nor lady's left arm around gentleman's neck. Lady's right hand and gentleman's left hand clasped and extended at least six inches from the body, and must not be folded and lay across the chest of dancers.
2. Heads of dancers must not Touch.

MUSIC

No beating of drum to produce Jazz effect will be allowed.

Any and all persons violating any of these rules will be subject to expulsion from the hall, also arrest for disorderly conduct.

By Order of
CHIEF OF POLICE

---

10. Regulations such as these posted in Lansing, Michigan, dance halls around 1920, made explicit the fears that the new dances and new morals of the post-war decade could lead to sexual license.

sex urge," commented Dr. Bowers. Indeed, he concluded, "The reverse is quite true in many cases." Henry Ford, the self-styled cultural critic, added his voice to the chorus of concern, suggesting that in contemporary music "monkey talk, jungle squeals, grunts and squeaks and gasps suggestive of cave love are camouflaged by a few feverish notes." In response to such criticism, the American National Association of Masters of Dancing developed a series of rules and regulations to prevent moral declension on the dance floor. The Association recommended prohibiting "vulgar, cheap jazz music" which "almost forces dancers to use half steps and invites immoral variations." After considerable (and graphic) discussion of a variety of gyrations to be discouraged, the organization cautioned its teachers "not to teach any movements that cannot be controlled."[16]

Although many social critics such as Henry Ford looked with horror upon the new dances, it was, in fact, the automobile that many identified as the principal cultural culprit. The automobile provided the dangerous combination of mobility and privacy that invited new sexual mores. "Since the 'red light' district is practically a thing of the past, the entire situation has changed," explained Dr. O. C. Wenger. "The automobile has replaced the room of the prostitute." Prostitutes reportedly complained about competition from "amateurs" as male sexual initiation more frequently took place in the back seat than the back room.[17] As more young women engaged in premarital sex, the prostitute became something of an anachronism.

In retrospect, all this may seem somewhat far afield from the problem of venereal disease, but such matters were followed with avid interest by the American Social Hygiene Association and the Venereal Disease Division of the USPHS during the 1920s. A circular distributed to dance hall managers under the signature of the surgeon general noted: "The unregulated dance hall became a source of worry to authorities because of the number of infections originating from contacts made at such amusement places."[18] As the ideal of premarital sexual continence eroded, social hygienists directed their efforts to the restoration of this code. Those interested in controlling the incidence of venereal disease during the twenties centered attention on sexual mores rather than medical approaches.

All too often, accounts of the shift in sexual behavior during the 1920s have failed to detect the essential conflict surrounding the change. Though it is true that the "revolution in morals" led to a new openness of discussion and activity regarding sexuality, these changes met sharp criticism. As a growing number of men—and women—rejected the notion of chastity, the conservative middle-class reformers who dominated the social hygiene movement watched with anxiety. Moreover, the reaction against the liberalized sexuality of the 1920s was not merely voiced by prudish Bourbons. Leaders of the social feminist movement of the prewar years often found the "new woman" of the 1920s to be capricious and indulgent. Charlotte Perkins Gilman, for example, asserted that women were following "the solemn philosophical sex-mania of Sigmund Freud." She deplored the indecency of the flapper, noting that women were accepting the "masculine" assumption that "the purpose of sex is recreation."[19]

Social hygienists who had ultimately been more concerned with preserving sexual ethics than preventing disease could not countenance the changes they observed. In their reaction, however, they would move further from the center of American life. As sexuality did emerge more openly in the 1920s there was nevertheless also a palpable disinclination to examine with any care the less pleasant aspects of this transformation. The wartime venereal disease campaign had been an aberration; these infections could only be directly addressed in times of crisis. The war had demanded unprecedented interventions by the federal government that, it was argued during the 1920s, should properly be abandoned. In peacetime, public mores held no place for the apparently unseemly subject of venereal disease. In this respect, America had returned to the Victorian era; the conspiracy of silence regarding these diseases had been reconstituted.

4

Although the 1920s witnessed little progress in combatting sexually transmitted diseases, the staggering dimensions of the problem had nonetheless been clarified. Increased reticence, declining government commitment, and a continued insistence on solving the venereal problem through moral uplift rather than medical means all combined to ensure that these diseases reached epidemic proportions. The Public Health Service conducted a series of surveys of cases under treatment in an attempt to project levels of infection. By the early 1930s the most frequently cited figures suggested that approximately one out of every ten Americans suffered from syphilis. Each year, citizens of the United States contracted almost half a million new infections—twice as many cases as tuberculosis and a hundred times the number of cases of the dreaded infantile paralysis. Gonorrhea, statistics showed, proved to be even more extensive, with close to 700,000 new infections annually. Among blacks, the poor, and the young, rates of venereal infection reached disproportionately high levels.[20]

The long-term pathology of these infections, in the past often hidden under other classifications, now became more apparent. Syphilis could affect the cardiovascular system, leading to a variety of serious heart ailments. According to one study, 18 percent of all deaths from organic heart disease could be attributed to syphilis. If it reached the nervous system, syphilis could cause insanity, paralysis, or blindness. Reports suggested that as many as twenty percent of all mental institution inmates suffered the consequences of tertiary syphilis. Of the deaths occurring in these hospitals each year almost 9,000 were tied to advanced syphilis. In addition, syphilis remained a leading cause of miscarriage, congenital defects, and sterility; each year 60,000 children were born with congenital syphilis in the United States. Only one indication of the seriousness with which the medical profession regarded the impact of syphilitic infections was the fact that life insurance companies refused to issue policies to any persons known to have been infected.[21]

These remarkable statistics, numbers indicating personal, familial, and social tragedies, stood in the face of the fact that medical science had a good deal to offer the individual infected with syphilis. Even in these pre-antibiotic years, the epidemic levels of venereal disease could not be attributed to the limitations of medical knowledge. The discovery by Paul Ehrlich of Salvarsan in 1910 gave physicians a treatment that offered victims of syphilis a definite benefit although physicians still debate whether it offered a complete cure. Admittedly, the arsenical compounds with which physicians treated syphilis entailed some risk and the course of injections was lengthy and unpleasant, but most patients could be rendered non-infectious through these means and avoid the disastrous consequences of late and tertiary syphilis. [22]

Despite the consensus regarding the effectiveness of arsphenamine within the profession, therapy for syphilis remained subject to considerable debate and conflict. Correct dosages, length of treatment, definitions of cure, as well as accompanying medications were bitterly contested among even the most noted syphilographers during the 1920s. "Syphilography . . . in 1925 was a chaos of different dosages, of private preference for different variations of the arsenical compounds," explained Thomas Parran. "There were many piece-meal case studies but not accurate data upon which the scientist could judge the relative efficacy of these methods." [23] Parran hoped to remedy this situation by promoting clinical research.

In 1928 a group of young philanthropists, influenced by the impact of syphilis upon several of their friends, offered to establish a fund to encourage laboratory and clinical research to expand and define scientific approaches for dealing with the infection. The stigma attached to syphilis had not only precluded public discussion of the problem, but had discouraged funding for research work as well. Few prominent philanthropists wanted their names tied to these diseases. With the assistance of the American Social Hygiene Association and the Public Health Service, a group of distinguished scientists were brought together to establish the Committee for Research in Syphilis. Charter members included William H. Welch of Johns Hopkins and Hans Zinsser of Harvard. Surgeon General H. S. Cumming appointed Parran to the Committee to represent the USPHS and he was elected chairman. W. Averell Harriman, who provided the Committee with $100,000 on an anonymous basis, served on the Board of Directors. [24] Despite sizable grants to prominent syphilographers and research scientists, the stock market crash brought the promise of the Committee for Research in Syphilis to a quick end.

The CRS, however, had led to the formation in 1929 of the Cooperative Clinical Group, which consisted of the directors of the five leading university syphilis clinics in the United States. This group was able to stay afloat, pooling data and information in an attempt to establish uniform treatment regimens for a variety of syphilis-induced ailments. Between 1931 and 1940 these investigators published some fifteen papers documenting a preferred course of syphilitic therapy. Among the areas investigated were syphilis in pregnancy, neurosyphilis, and cardiovascular syphilis, as well as a number of technical therapeutic problems relating to the length of treatment and infectiousness. The CCG marked the first such cooperative venture in the history of American medical research, and the success of the group set a valuable precedent for future joint ventures in American clinical medicine, laying the basis for the now orthodox cooperative clinical trial. The findings of the CCG, moreover, had immediate utility for physicians treating syphilis. Reports were generally published in *Venereal Disease Information*, a journal issued by the Public Health Service. By 1934 *VDI* had become the most widely circulated of all government subscription publications. Members of the PHS summarized the accomplishments in venereology: "Since World War I, there has been more scientific work accomplished and more progress made in our understanding of syphilis, both in the laboratory and in the clinic, than in any other disease of equal importance."[25] And yet, despite these gains, syphilis and gonorrhea flourished.

5

According to the American Social Hygiene Association, the disruption in traditional family roles created by the Great Depression generated criminal and juvenile delinquency, immorality, and higher rates of venereal disease. Men searching for work, as well as women leaving home to assist in the support of their families, implied neglected children, social chaos and increased disease, in the opinion of the Association. Moreover, the Association speculated that, as men lost jobs and women sought to support their families, prostitution would increase during the depression.[26] Syphilis and gonorrhea were seen as the consequences of social instability and decay, the manifestations of an essential failure of traditional social controls. Again, the propensity to view these infections as symptoms rather than diseases became clear. Any disturbance to the familial status quo, in this view, could lead to higher rates of infection.

In one way, without question, the economic crisis did lead to greater prevalence of infection: fewer individuals could afford the required treatment. The depression greatly increased the numbers of individuals seeking free care for venereal disease; demand at public health clinics rose by at least 20 percent between 1929 and 1933. According to estimates of the New York State Division of Social Hygiene, fully one-half of all newly infected cases now sought treatment at public expense. Health economists Leon Bromberg and Michael M. Davis argued that eighty percent of the population could not afford the cost of adequate care for syphilis from private physicians. Treatment for an uncomplicated case of syphilis required repeated visits to a physician for injections of arsenical compounds alternated with injections of bismuth to reduce the chance of toxic reaction. Sometimes this necessitated weekly appointments for more than a year. The cost of such treatment with a private physician in the early 1930s averaged between $305 to $380, but could range as high as $1000.[27] Even public clinics often charged as much as $80 for a curative level of therapy. These costs were often multiplied by the fact that typically more than one member of a family needed treatment if an infection was diagnosed.

The expense of treatment often caused infected individuals to forgo a complete regimen, risking relapse and continued contagion. According to one study, more than 80 percent of all syphilis patients failed to complete the arduous therapeutic course. As Dr. Albert Keidel, a venereal expert at Johns Hopkins, explained: "I believe that one of the chief reasons for failure to continue is the high costs of medical care, and that the element of costs prevents not only the proper treatment of many patients, but even the recognition of the syphilitic condition." Tragically, some doctors refused to continue treatment when patients failed to pay their bills. "It is indefensible," declared Keidel, "to treat the patient until his funds are exhausted and then drop him." Some physicians argued that failure to act responsibly in the conduct of venereal cases would lead to state controls on the profession, if not to socialized medicine. "The medical profession must at this time provide cheaper and better medical treatment or else this will be taken out of our hands and we will be directly facing state medicine," noted Dr. J. Frank Schamberg.[28]

In addition to the high costs of treatment, the poor quality and scarcity of public clinics also discouraged individuals from seeking medical attention. Many hospitals continued to refuse admission to patients with venereal infections, tacitly endorsing the assumption that these individuals were morally tainted and less deserving of care. Public clinics devoted to the treatment of venereal disease were noted for their unpleasant and crowded environs. A study conducted by the Bureau of Social Hygiene reported grossly inadequate facilities with long lines of individuals waiting for injections. Even pay clinics set up for the exclusive treatment of venereal infections at costs below those of private practitioners were often shunned by the diseased; the powerful stigma of venereal infection discouraged their use. As Albert Keidel explained: "The classification of syphilis as a venereal disease and the fact that it is associated in lay and medical minds with the sexual act make it impossible for a pay clinic for syphilis or for venereal disease in general to attract patients as can similar institutions with more general medical aims."[29] Once again, social attitudes constrained medical practice.

When patients turned to private practitioners they often found themselves being treated by doctors inadequately trained to diagnose and treat venereal diseases effectively. Most physicians did not consider the sexually transmitted diseases to be a particularly interesting or status-oriented clinical specialty. According to some public health officials, syphilis was treated like the "illegitimate child" of medicine, tossed between dermatology and urology depending upon the manifest symptoms. Syphilis and gonorrhea were given minimal time in the average medical school curriculum. Dr. N. A. Nelson attributed this to stigmatized views of these diseases, attitudes shared by public and profession alike:

> Unfortunately in years past the medical profession has been influenced, and the lay public has been, by the feeling that syphilis and gonorrhea are venereal diseases and therefore, are disgraceful diseases; and that the average practitioner who would stoop to treat those diseases was to be classified as a dishonorable doctor and a disgrace to the community, which has led to the neglect of teaching those subjects to students in the medical schools.

Failure to provide sufficient education, of course, led to poor practice. "There is, I think, no use in blinking the fact that, by and large, syphilis is badly managed by the average practitioner," concluded Dr. J. E. Moore, who emphasized the high proportion of missed diagnoses. This explained, in part, the critical fact that only one in ten cases of syphilis received treatment during the early stages of the disease when a cure was possible.[30]

In an attempt to escape the stigma of venereal infections, many individuals turned away from orthodox practitioners to quacks and patent medicines promising quick cures. In a poll of almost five hundred men in San Francisco, randomly selected on the street and asked for advice about venereal care, only 41 percent recommended seeing a doctor; most suggested home remedies, nostrums, and quacks. Another study found that 63 percent of Chicago drug stores offered over-the-counter "cures" for all venereal diseases. Although one of the attractions of unscrupulous practitioners was the prominently advertised promise of confidentiality, a number of stories circulated about quacks who not only bilked their patients but blackmailed them as well.[31]

The reservoir of untreated and inadequately treated infections thus grew, generating a national health problem of immense proportions. The high costs and poor quality of most treatment exacerbated the problem. Finally, the powerful stigma of the sexually transmitted diseases limited both the public and the profession's ability to respond effectively. As N. A. Nelson concluded: "It is inconceivable that an intelligent program can be developed for the control of the genito-infectious diseases by those who adhere to the traditional notion that infection is, in itself, evidence of sexual misbehavior."[32]

6

The traditional argument—that venereal victims got what they deserved, and therefore should not receive assistance—came under attack during the 1930s as public health officials like Thomas Parran began to calculate the larger social costs of these diseases. Estimates suggested that more than $15 million was spent annually for the ambulatory care of venereal patients (in both private and public clinics). The cost of not treating syphilis went even higher as the complications of the disease developed. Experts argued that syphilis cost taxpayers between $40 and $50 million each year for the institutional care of the insane, paralyzed, and blind.[33]

The cost of venereal disease, however, extended beyond that of taking care of the ill. During the depression years, physicians and public health officials placed increasing stress upon the cost to American industry in diminished productivity, industrial accidents, and workmen's compensation. As Dr. Morris Fishbein of the American Medical Association explained:

> In industries the costs of venereal diseases are tremendous. It has been estimated that from 8 to 10 million workers lost 21 million working days each year at an average of $4 a day as a result of infection with these conditions. The cost may well be more than $100,000,000 annually.

Thomas Parran calculated that such losses were the equivalent of every American man between the ages of 15 and 45 missing a half-day of work each year.

According to the American Social Hygiene Association—well-known for its somewhat liberal use of statistics—losses from syphilis and gonorrhea came to more than $285,000,000. (They did not provide the basis for this figure.)[34] These projections reflected the general concern during the 1930s about restoring and maintaining the nation's industrial capacity. If venereal disease could be shown to have great economic costs, public health officers reasoned, the government and business would be more willing to bear the financial burden.

Officials appealed to enlightened capitalistic self-interest in their campaigns for expanding public health facilities for venereal disease. In this mode of thought, men became machines; venereal disease a deadly, but more importantly, a costly corrosive. As Parran explained to a group of businessmen:

> This is a day of intensive organization, of specialization, of expert talent, of complicated machinery; and most industrial plants see to it that their machinery is constantly inspected and kept in the very best running order. But all too many of us rely on the natural course of events as regards the most important element in the success of that business, namely, the human machine.

This argument had formed the rationale for "welfare capitalism," which spawned medical departments in major industries during the 1920s. During the depression, however, many industries considered health programs an unnecessary expense, particularly with the great surplus of available labor. Parran concluded that protecting workers from venereal disease constituted good business practice. In an especially cold turn of phrase, Parran made his message clear, noting: "As employers of labor, as businessmen of a community, it seems to me that you have a peculiar opportunity for enhancing the human machinery which is at your disposal."[35]

The costs of venereally infected workers could often be hidden beyond the loss columns of the business ledger. Industrial accidents were often attributed to syphilis, with its dire impact on the neurological and cardiovascular systems. Public Health officials frequently reminded businessmen of the costs of workmen's compensation for injuries incurred by syphilitics. Even more ominous, however, were the dangers of accidents not only to workers but to the public. A number of major train wrecks during the 1920s, for example, were attributed to advanced syphilis in the engineer. Officials typically cited workers who traveled as being at greater risk for infection (due to unstable homes and few communal ties). State health departments enjoined railroad operators to ensure that their workers were free of infection, and many railroads began to require that all employees be examined.[36]

Some corporations responded by creating anti-venereal programs for their workers. The American Social Hygiene Association offered a consultant service to businesses seeking to educate employees about the menace of venereal disease. E. I. DuPont de Nemours and Company established a full program for venereal detection among its workers beginning in 1934, under which all new employees received Wassermann tests as well as all old employees who agreed to be examined; only ten percent refused. Four percent of all employees were found to be infected. At first, DuPont did not provide treatment for these individuals, choosing instead to refer them to private physicians. They soon found, however, that these men often did not complete their treatment; the company then undertook to provide therapy for them. Though DuPont promised not to dismiss employees found to be infected, this was not always the case with other companies that examined their workers. Applicants for employment found to be diseased rarely were hired. Often companies whose employment benefits paid for the care of almost all serious illness specifically excluded syphilis and gonorrhea, maintaining the view that these diseases only afflicted the immoral and willful. All too often, workers already strapped by paying for expensive syphilitic treatment would find themselves out of work if their employers gained knowledge of their infection. In many such cases the patients had long become non-infectious, yet the contagion of stigma persisted.[37]

The issue of the costs of venereal disease to business nevertheless had considerable impact. Much as the notion of extra-genital infection was used during the Progressive years to suggest that venereal infections could reach any segment of society, now the calculus of social costs suggested that no matter who became infected, all society would bear the financial burden. This argument, of course, reflected heightened concern during the depression about increasing industrial capacity while lowering the costs of business. Public health officials sought to make the business community their ally in the fight against these infections. As Dr. Ray D. Dixon of the Detroit Venereal Clinic concluded: "When we can convince the business world that the venereal diseases are an obstacle in its path of progress the venereal problem will be in a fair way of becoming solved."[38]

7

Before the problem of the venereal diseases could be addressed, however, the restraints upon public discussion had to be lifted. These taboos not only kept Parran off the air, but more generally handcuffed public health efforts in the years after the war. Newspapers and magazines that had broadly publicized the wartime anti-venereal crusade now looked askance at the venereal problem. As Judge Anna Moscowitz Kross later commented, "We spoke of social diseases, we spoke of social evils. None of us dared even think of uttering the words syphilis and gonorrhea."[39] The essential medical problems raised by the diseases were obscured by the emphasis on rectitude.

Criticism of the reticence surrounding the venereal problem emerged only in the 1930s, with blows falling most heavily on the American Social Hygiene Association. Though it was the central voluntary organization dedicated to the control of venereal disease, it had opted for a moralistic, circumspect educational campaign that emphasized the menace of prostitution and promiscuity. Medical and public health approaches to alleviate the problem, however significant, had remained secondary. In the 1930s, the tenets of the ASHA regarding sex education, for example, were held up for ridicule: "The Sex Hygienists, with their irrelevant gabble about dahlias and philo-progenitive bees, only make the essential mystery more mysterious, and hence more baffling." Michael M. Davis, the eminent health economist, wrote to Parran decrying the ASHA's conservative approach: "If after the war the ASHA had only had the courage to deal with the problem boldly, as you have, instead of always treading softly, we should have been a lot further along."[40]

By the early 1930s, a number of critics, influenced by the liberalization of sexual mores during the 1920s, cited the prudishness of the social hygiene movement as a central cause of the high venereal rates. As one writer in the *American Mercury* noted:

> Unfortunately . . . in Puritanical America, babies are still brought by storks, decent people copulate only in wedded antisepsis, and the pubic region is mentionable nowhere except in alleys and medical colleges. If the existence of sexual diseases is at all recognized, the approved method of dealing with them is by anointing the population with ecclesiastical oils and moral salves. But since pathogenic germs are more sensitive to chemicals than to homilies, they have managed to multiply with little interference.

Principles of decorum were, as some critics observed, hypocritically defined. Newspapers, for example, generally refused to print the words "syphilis" and "gonorrhea," but these same publications carried advertisements for feminine napkins, hemorrhoid nostrums, and hernia supports, many more explicit than those found in today's publications. When the New York State Department of Health sought to change the name of the Division of Social Hygiene to the Division of Syphilis Control, a title that specifically defined its mandate, state legislators balked. "I may be old-fashioned, reactionary, and a Bourbon," remarked one state senator, "but I say this word is not decent and should not be spread among the children and the youths." This gentility, however, had its impact on public health measures directed against the venereal problem. Health officers suggested that in honoring public sentiment, constraints were placed upon their activity. As public health expert Haven Emerson explained: "We have hinted, and hidden, and yet hoped for results; and still this malign infection flows almost unrestrained through marriage as through brothel, in childhood, in maturity, in age."[41]

Physicians and public health officials in the 1930s went on the attack against the moralistic precepts of social hygiene, an attack that Thomas Parran was to lead. Doctors urged that the time had come to reject euphemism, reduce moralism, and address the venereal problem on the level of science and medicine. Although Parran sought not to alienate those social hygienists who had previously worked against venereal disease, he nevertheless hoped to redirect priorities within the movement:

> It is true that the control of syphilis and of other venereal diseases would be accomplished if the ideal of a monogamous sex relationship were universally attained. Efforts toward this ideal are eminently commendable, both on account of their influence on the prevalence of disease and because of the sociological results in-

volved; but it should be possible to control syphilis by direct medical measures long
before any considerable change in the sex habits of the population normally can be
expected. . . . Greater progress . . . will be made by concentration of effort on
the medical aspect of control rather than through continued scattering of effort in
an attempt to carry out the 'ideal program' of the social hygienists for moral prophylaxis.[42]

In Parran's view, the public health establishment—medical experts—should now
assert their authority over the venereal problem.

A number of physicians contended that the very names used to describe these
ailments tended to make them more difficult to deal with from the perspective
of public health. The metaphorical meanings attached to the venereal diseases—the connotation of immorality, evil, infidelity, taboo—actually ob-
structed medical efforts. Because these infections were considered apart from
other communicable diseases, as unique infections limited to the immoral, traditional public health approaches had been overlooked. As Herman Bundesen,
commissioner of health for the City of Chicago, explained: "When you treat
syphilis as you treat smallpox, then we will control syphilis as we control smallpox, and not until then." Not only did euphemistic expressions such as "social
hygiene" and "social diseases" come under attack, but the term "venereal disease" as well. Physicians frequently pointed out the nature of so-called "innocent" infections: congenital syphilis, familial infections, extra-genital transmission—to demonstrate that the diseases were not always communicated through
"venery." An editorial in the *Journal of the American Medical Association* noted:
"One of the principal obstacles to the conquest of syphilis has been squeamish-
ness about facing the problem and the unfortunate classification of syphilis as
a venereal disease. It is, of course, a venereal disease only in part." Doctors
sought to strip venereal disease of its immoral connotations. "Do we think of
syphilis as a 'venereal' disease?" asked Nels A. Nelson. "If we do, how do we
propose to convince the public, to which venery is synonomous with lasci-
viousness, that syphilis is altogether not a venereal disease?" As a replacement
for "venereal disease" Nelson offered "genito-infectious diseases" which, not
surprisingly, failed to attract a following. Even the conservative American Social Hygiene Association came to advocate the abandonment of the term "venereal disease." "Scarlet fever acquired from a prostitute is not called a 'venereal' disease," noted medical director Walter Clarke in a somewhat labored
argument, "but gonorrhea acquired from a woman by her lawful husband is
called a venereal disease."[43] In the 1970s, "sexually transmitted diseases"—
STDs—became common medical parlance in yet another attempt to take the
venereal out of VD.

The debate over how to identify venereal disease reflected two related themes.
First, it signified an attempt to reduce the moral stigma attached to these infections in order to make it possible for physicians to deal with them more dispassionately, in a manner similar to the way other infectious diseases were approached. Second, it revealed a larger conflict over the jurisdiction of these

ailments. Passed from the theologian to the social reformer, the concern over venereal disease, it was argued, should henceforth be placed exclusively in the domain of the physician. This, of course, reflected a more fundamental transformation regarding sexuality in American culture.[44]

8

Soon after his appointment as surgeon general by President Franklin D. Roosevelt in the spring of 1936, Thomas Parran resolved to bring the venereal diseases to national attention. In July Parran outlined the extent of the venereal problem in an article entitled, "The Next Great Plague To Go," tearing away the veil of secrecy. Although the medical profession had been directing increasingly greater interest in their journals to the problem, Parran's article, appearing first in the *Survey Graphic* and then in *Reader's Digest*, was among the first to reach such a broad audience. At a time when most newspapers and magazines still prohibited the mention of syphilis and gonorrhea, Parran's message reached some 500,000 subscribers to the *Reader's Digest*. In this article, the surgeon general reviewed facts well known among his medical colleagues in simple, direct prose. The time had come, he argued, to bring the problem into the open; without this essential step, syphilis would continue to have a serious, detrimental impact on the health of the American people. "First and foremost among American handicaps to progress against syphilis," Parran observed, "is the widespread belief that nice people don't talk about syphilis, nice people don't have syphilis, and nice people shouldn't do anything about those who have syphilis." Parran ascribed this view to hypocrisy, pure and simple. "Scratch a scamp who is too sanctimonious to say syphilis and, usually, you find an ex-syphilitic," he remarked.[45]

"The Next Great Plague To Go" contained a number of illustrations, graphically depicting the dimensions of the problem of syphilis in the United States. These pictographs of critical statistics, designed by Rudolph Modley, included the ages of those most likely to become infected, the impact of treatment and the effect of syphilis on pregnancy, as well as comparative rates of infection. These illustrations dramatically communicated to readers the extent of the problem and the necessity of committing the resources of public health to the eradication of syphilis.

Parran brought a scientific, bureaucratic approach to the venereal problem. As a career public health officer, he came from a tradition different from that of the social hygienists who had heretofore directed most anti-venereal efforts. Parran made clear that it was not the limits of medical science that explained the high levels of syphilis within the United States. As a veteran of the modern public health movement, he had witnessed the precipitous decline of major communicable diseases, including tuberculosis, diphtheria, and typhoid, through the techniques of isolation, case finding, treatment, and immunization; techniques for the most part available and yet not employed in the attack against syphilis. "Syphilis does a hundred times as much damage annually as polio-

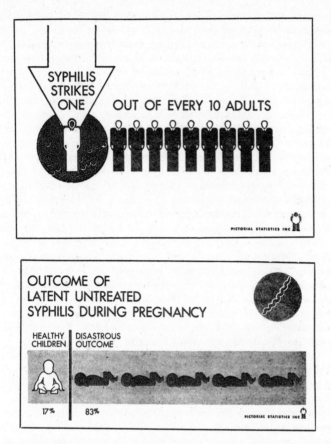

11. Thomas Parran, "The Next Great Plague To Go," *Survey Graphic* 25 (July 1936).

myelitis," noted Parran, "yet we can cure most of it. We still do not know how to cure poliomyelitis, only how to mitigate it."[46]

Parran advocated a five-point program for controlling syphilis largely based upon traditional public health precepts. First, and most important, was the need to find cases of the disease. For this purpose, Parran called for free diagnostic centers where individuals could obtain confidential blood tests. For high-risk populations, especially the young and blacks, the surgeon general suggested "Wassermann dragnets" that could administer hundreds of tests. The rationale behind locating these cases, of course, was to bring infected individuals under immediate treatment. Prompt therapy for the diseased constituted the second of Parran's recommendations; delay after infection made treatment much more difficult and less successful. Third, Parran argued that all contacts of infected patients must be identified, located, tested, and treated if infected to stop the perpetual spread of the disease. In order to prevent congenital syphilis, Parran offered as his fourth recommendation mandatory blood tests before marriage and early in all pregnancies. Finally, he called for public education concerning syphilis; without knowledge of symptoms and treatments the great chain of infection could not be broken. Although these techniques were not new, Parran's public proposal generated demands for a comprehensive program. In the surgeon general's judgment, public efforts to combat syphilis had until this time been "scattered, sporadic, and inadequate."[47]

Parran modeled these proposals on the programs of several European nations that had taken concerted action to bring venereal diseases under control after the war. Great Britain reduced its rates by half through the establishment of government supported clinics. In little more than a decade, new admissions to British venereal clinics dropped from 40,000 to 20,000 annually. The Scandinavian countries, in particular, devised public health measures that were remarkably successful in stemming the tide of venereal infection. In 1935 at the suggestion of New York Mayor Fiorello LaGuardia, Parran led a commission to Norway, Sweden, and Denmark to investigate their venereal programs. In Sweden, where the population of 6,100,000 approximately equaled that of upstate New York, there were only 431 cases of syphilis in 1934. If this rate of infection were applied to the United States there would have been 8,620 new cases annually; instead, the Public Health Service estimated there were 420,000. Sweden's rate had fallen by ten times in just fifteen years. Denmark and Norway reported similar declines in the years following World War I. All three nations provided public clinic facilities of high quality, required reporting of all cases by physicians and compulsory treatment. In addition, Sweden had devised rigorous measures for the investigation of all sources of infection.[48] Although he was aware of the fundamental political and cultural differences between these nations and the U.S., their abilities to deal effectively with the venereal diseases had a major impact upon Parran. He returned from abroad confident that similar, well-organized and supported public health measures would meet with success in the United States.

Explicitly missing from Parran's program was the traditional moral call to arms. Though he sought to avoid offending the social hygienists, Parran downplayed the moral argument. "After careful scrutiny of our reform efforts to date," he explained, "I have come to the conclusion that it is much easier to control syphilis by making Wassermann tests routinely for the age groups needing it, and seeing that treatment is obtained by all people who require it, than it is to alter the way of life of a people." Indeed, Parran's approach to the problem of venereal disease marked an attempt to wrest control from the social hygienists with their emphasis on behavioral reform. Shortly after the publication of the "Next Great Plague To Go" he noted, "In an effort to emphasize the fact that syphilis is a contagious disease and should be treated as such, I deliberately minimized the morality issues. . . . We doctors and health officers have been derelict in doing the things which obviously are our first responsibility in the control of syphilis." At the very heart of Parran's effort was an attempt to transform the discourse of venereal disease. As Parran indicated upon submitting his manuscript to the *Survey Graphic*: "So far as has been possible in dealing with a subject held intrinsically lurid by most people, I have avoided the lurid description and overstatement."[49] Significantly, the surgeon general personally shared many of the moral precepts of the social hygienists, but he resolved not to let this hinder the public health battle.

By the fall of 1936 the popular press had responded to Parran's challenge by broadly publicizing the problem of venereal disease. In October *Time* featured Parran on its cover to accompany a story on the extensive public concern about the venereal problem. "The ice of journalistic reticence," had been shattered, the magazine declared. "To break down this taboo in the U.S. and tackle syphilis scientifically rather than morally is the high and burning purpose in the official life of Surgeon General Parran." Articles explicitly calling attention to syphilis and gonorrhea appeared in such newspapers as the New York *Herald Tribune*, the St. Louis *Post-Dispatch*, and the Chicago *Tribune*. In all, some 125 papers broke precedent, carrying articles outlining the problem of dealing with the sexually transmitted diseases. In 1937 the Pulitzer Prize Committee accorded an honorable mention to the New York *Daily News* for "the most disinterested and meritorious public service rendered by any American newspaper" during the year 1936. The Committee specifically cited the newspaper's "campaign covering venereal diseases and prophylaxis."[50]

Monthly subscription journals proved to be a more difficult barrier. Paul De Kruif, the well-known science writer, attempted repeatedly to place an article on venereal disease in the staid *Ladies' Home Journal* without success. He explained to Parran that "certain of the lady sub-editors are abstinate [sic] in their belief that this is a subject too hot for a great fireside lady's magazine to touch." But editor Bruce Gold soon relented, and in August 1937, the *Journal* carried an article on syphilis jointly authored by De Kruif and Parran. The *Journal* now became the leader among women's magazines supporting the campaign to control venereal disease. A self-congratulatory full-page advertisement in the New York *Herald Tribune* declared: "The *Ladies' Home Journal*, believing that a publishing force can and should be a great social force, is proud to have played its part as the focal point for this great social revolution."[51]

The massive reaction to his article surprised Parran. Indeed, the surgeon general seemed somewhat embarrassed to find himself the center of so much attention. "The facts seem so commonplace to persons like you and me," he wrote to a medical colleague, "it seems remarkable that the public should be so much interested." Those active in the battle against venereal disease when it was, by necessity, fought *sub rosa*, shared the surgeon general's astonishment. "After all the years of choke tactics one feels positively embarrassed to read a present-day news sheet," noted Dr. John Stokes with a touch of irony. Parran's initial article in the *Survey Graphic* was repeatedly cited as the impetus for this emergent crusade. "The article will go far towards making the 'hush-hushers' end their mental sit-down strike," remarked the *New Yorker's* "Talk of the Town."[52]

Interest in Parran's campaign reflected, in part, an important shift in popular notions of science and medicine that occurred in the 1920s and 1930s. Parran typified for many the dispassionate, rational medical scientist, dedicated to the public welfare, above moral and political concerns. A public that acclaimed Sinclair Lewis's medical hero, *Arrowsmith*, and Paul De Kruif's *Microbe Hunters* saw in Parran the eiptome of a new medical spirit.[53] Physicians and public health officials were increasingly viewed as highly skilled technicians, applying a science of miracles. The anti-venereal movement drew heavily upon this positive perspective. Just as Martin Arrowsmith's research had foundered on the rocks of politics and bureaucracy, public health officials emphasized the fact that they had the necessary scientific knowledge to wipe out syphilis but were prevented by prudishness and lack of funding.

In 1937 Parran published a book detailing the themes of his campaign against syphilis, *Shadow on the Land*. The book attracted a wide audience and soon became a bestseller. Clearly, a significant shift in public opinion concerning the venereal diseases had occurred. Paul Kellogg, editor of the *Survey Graphic*, wrote to Parran, "Newspapers throughout the country carried the nib of your challenge. We broke the taboos of a women's magazine of three million circulation; and the whole movement you were initiating took on new drive." Parran, eager to solicit federal aid for his campaign, noted this transformation in a letter to President Roosevelt: "During recent months there has been a great change in public attitude toward syphilis, particularly in the willingness of the newspapers to open their editorial pages and editorial columns to a discussion of this important public health problem."[54] Science and medicine, it seemed, had overwhelmed the forces of reticence.

The Gallup Poll, only recently initiated, recorded the impact of Parran's campaign. When asked by the pollster: "Would you be in favor of a government bureau that would distribute information concerning the venereal diseases?" over 90 percent answered yes, the largest majority Gallup had registered on any question put by his Institute of Public Opinion. The poll also found overwhelming support for free clinics and premarital venereal testing. Indeed, over 70 percent favored punishing those syphilitics who failed to take a full course of treatment. The very fact that Gallup questioned people about the campaign testifies to the new importance of venereal diseases in the public mind.[55] Parran's campaign had opened a flood-gate; the battle against venereal disease had been legitimized. The surgeon general had paved the way for government action.

9

Defining venereal disease as the most pressing of all public health problems, Parran devised a "New Deal" for its victims, one that he hoped would rid society of its dangers within a generation. In December 1936, Parran called a national meeting of state and local public health officials and venereal experts to set an agenda for the fight against venereal disease. The National Conference on Venereal Disease Control concluded that available facilities could serve only a quarter of those patients needing treatment. Delegates to the meeting advocated a national commitment, especially the allocation of federal funds to support anti-venereal work. "Public health is purchasable," explained the surgeon general, "as has been proved in the past when aroused public interest has stamped out plague after plague which once ravaged the population as syphilis does now." Officials took hope that support might be forthcoming when Franklin Roosevelt became the first president to address the question of sexually transmitted diseases directly. FDR sent the following message to the Conference:

> The recent increase in public interest in the problem before the conference is extremely gratifying. . . . The federal government is deeply interested in conserving the resources of the country by all appropriate methods. The attainment of your objectives would do much to conserve our human resources and would reduce considerably the present large costs for the community care of the disastrous end-results of the venereal diseases.

"No President," noted *Time*, "had ever said or written so frankly."[56]

Under Parran's direction the PHS expanded its programs and services, broadening what had in the past been a tangential role in American life. Parran put public health on the map of national priorities; during his tenure, food and drug regulations were extended, the National Institutes of Health dramatically expanded, and the federal government became committed to the battle against infectious diseases. The Social Security Act of 1935 made this explicit; through Title VI the PHS was provided with $8 million to disburse to the states for health care. This was the first money the state boards of health had received from the federal government since the years immediately after World War I.[57]

The distribution of Title VI funds reflected Parran's overriding concern about the venereal diseases. Ultimately more than 10 percent of this money was channeled to the fight against syphilis, the largest percentage allocated to any communicable disease. These funds served as a major impetus for venereal disease control work. States used the money to establish diagnostic facilities, clinics, and epidemiological programs. "The worthwhile attainments of the States now adopting new measures for venereal disease control," explained Raymond Vonderlehr of the PHS, "will without doubt serve as an increased incentive to the rapid expansion of this work."[58] The Social Security appropriation alone increased the budgets of state health departments by an average of 10 percent.

The crowning achievement of Parran's campaign against venereal disease, however, came in May 1938 when Congress passed the National Venereal Disease Control Act. Senator Robert LaFollette of Wisconsin and Congressman Alfred Bulwinkle of North Carolina, the sponsors of the bill, offered the legislation as an amendment of the World War I act that created the Interdepartmental Social Hygiene Board and the Venereal Disease Division of the Public Health Service. This made explicit the relation between the unprecedented activities during World War I and the New Deal.[59] Just as the war had demanded the expansion of the federal government, so now the crisis of the depression had brought forth the need for a more powerful centralized State.

Supporters of the legislation emphasized the national nature of the venereal problem. As Herman M. Baker, president of the Indiana State Medical Society, declared: "These germs do not know state lines and you have simply got to handle the thing as a problem that is national in scope." LaFollette reiterated this point to his Senate colleagues:

> It is obvious that if this battle against syphilis is to be won, it must be fought on 48 fronts. A program must be carried on in every state. The germ that causes syphilis does not respect state lines. It does not take into consideration the financial ability of states or communities.[60]

Although some states had developed successful public health programs for dealing with the venereal diseases, facilities continued to vary considerably from state to state; Parran's publicity had served to make clear the national dimensions of the problem and the need for a national solution. This theme was consistent with the manner in which the New Deal sought to address other problems. Just as they could not handle directly unemployment and relief, the states simply could not bear the burden of what was clearly a national crisis. This realization laid the foundation for the expansion of the federal government to provide new services and attack issues heretofore viewed as within the domain of the states. The National Venereal Disease Control Act marked—as did other New Deal welfare legislation—a shift in notions of federal responsibility for ameliorating social problems.

The Act provided for federal grants to the state boards of health to develop anti-venereal measures. As part of the requirements of the legislation, each state submitted to the surgeon general a comprehensive summary of current venereal disease control activities as well as plans for improving services on both the state and local levels. Money could then be allocated by the PHS to set up diagnostic and treatment facilities and train necessary personnel. In addition, the Act called for research into the treatment and prevention of the diseases. As originally written the bill provided for the allocation of $271 million over a thirteen-year period—a national blitz against the diseases. But the bill was soon revised to a more realistic $15 million over a three-year period: $3 million in the first year, $6 million in the second, and $7 million in the third year when health departments would be in a position to spend additional appropriations to greatest benefit. In the first year, the Act mandated the PHS to spend $600,000 to conduct field studies, and develop educational programs for public health officials.[61]

Individuals testifying before Congress in support of the legislation consistently stressed that the expenditures that the bill required would ultimately save the nation greater expense. As Herman Bundesen, commissioner of the Chicago Health Department, noted: "It costs more money not to do the job than it costs to do the job." Legislators clearly found such logic compelling. Thomas Parran explained to a group of senators, "We are paying for syphilis now, whether we control it or not. We are paying for it in our relief rolls; we are paying for it in our institutions for the crippled, the blind, and the insane." When the surgeon general expressed concern that FDR was not providing sufficient support for the bill, his ally in the campaign, science writer Paul De Kruif responded: "The President does not yet see this simple arithmetical relationship: that the more you spend fighting a communicable disease, the more you save." De Kruif concluded: "This one thing I know: that his strongest allies would be the financial overlords of our country. Against this enemy there is the one chance of a true, united people's front—of all the people, haves and have-nots."[62]

The anti-venereal battle did indeed have broad appeal. Heightened consciousness of venereal diseases had opened the way for legislation. The publicity of the preceding years helped to create a groundswell of support. Parran recounted the history of these efforts before a Senate committee:

> As I see the problem broadly, during the past 10 or 12 years we have built the foundation. Then, we moved ahead on to the first stage: that is, the stage of public education, the stage of talking about it. I would like to point out to you that we cannot talk syphilis out of the United States; the spirochete does not listen to us. Men and munitions are needed on a national scale to deal with this problem.

Education, however, had generated support for these measures, and groups such as the National Junior Chamber of Commerce, the American Legion, and the General Federation of Women's Clubs now came forward in support of the bill. Fiorello LaGuardia, mayor of New York, commented on the new awareness of the venereal diseases in his testimony supporting the legislation: "Now you remember some 15 or 20 years ago when ladies met they would ask, 'Have you had your blood pressure taken?' and talk about their blood pressure. Now, they ask about their Wassermanns."[63]

Even the American Medical Association, noted for its attempts to keep the government out of medicine, offered no resistance to the anti-venereal legislation. Apparently the AMA decided its priorities rested with the battle to defeat provisions under consideration for national health insurance. Fee-for-service, the bedrock of the American medical profession, was not threatened by the Venereal Disease Control Act. Moreover, venereal diseases had never constituted a particularly lucrative element of medical practice. Preventive medicine and public health programs, especially those devoted to specific infectious diseases, did not usurp the economic position of the profession as would the more comprehensive proposals. As Dr. Hugh Hampton Young, the eminent Johns Hopkins urologist, explained to the House committee: "I myself am opposed to socialized medicine, but I think that this [National Venereal Disease Control Act] is different, and I think so long as it can be accomplished in this clearly outlined method, dealing with this kind of disease, I think it has its place."[64] Young noted that only the PHS could properly coordinate the activities of local institutions, clinics, and hospitals to achieve results against the venereal diseases. In addition, he pointed out that private physicians needed state assistance to provide the facilities for sophisticated diagnostic work. He compared the campaign against venereal disease to those that had been waged against other epidemic infections like yellow fever and typhoid.

Other physicians frequently suggested, however, that venereal disease control programs might well become the entering wedge for socialized medicine. "It may be frankly said," wrote Dr. John Stokes, "that at no point in the entire practice of medicine does the profession in the United States face more directly the issue of so-called socialization than in the case of the venereal diseases." Some doctors argued that if they were to maintain their stature in the care of venereal diseases they must provide better care to venereal patients, even those who could not afford their full fees. "If the private practitioner wishes to maintain his control of this field he must raise his standard to that of the public service," Stokes concluded. A number of physicians advocated the establishment of pay clinics as the proper alternative to public medicine. "The straws are in the wind," commented the prominent syphilographer Dr. J. E. Moore. "Failure to solve it means that the problem will be taken from the hands of the medical profession by outside sources with state medicine as the forced alternative."[65] But few physicians shared these concerns; most seemed willing to concede the venereal diseases to the state so long as their larger economic interests remained secure.

Only organized religious groups raised any significant objections to the bill. One of the few individuals to offer questions concerning the propriety of the legislation was William F. Montovon of the National Catholic Welfare Association. First, Montovon suggested that the legislation would allow the state to usurp the role of the medical profession. "I think everybody would accept the statement that we do not want to make the medical profession dependent upon the State," he explained. "Everybody is desirous of preventing the extension of State medicine to interfere with the present work of the private physicians and private clinical agencies, particularly medical schools." Montovon's primary doubt was about the moral issue that the bill represented. In his view, the proposed bill could actually have a deleterious impact on sexual ethics. "The moral standards must reach a point where the relationship which exists between the sexes is on a higher plane," he declared. In a veiled reference to chemical prophylaxis and the use of condoms, the two principal venereal preventives, he noted, "Now, if we are going to unload on the population a lot of gadgets and contraptions, and ideas for protecting themselves against contamination, we are not going to remedy or solve the problem that will follow the enactment of this legislation." The social hygienists also expressed some concern that in the new emphasis on attacking venereal disease through medicine, science, and public health, their larger goals concerning sexual mores and family life would be lost. Dr. William F. Snow cautioned: "While it seems important once more to concentrate attention and effort on the medical and public health division of the [American Social Hygiene] Association's work, there should be no lessening of our determination to continue the established education and protective divisions of the Association's program. . . . Education is the method by which we may ultimately expect to make permanent gains through the promotion of normal, unaffected attitudes and practices in relation to sex."[66]

Though tension persisted between moral and medical approaches to the problem, the voices of apprehension could not match the rising chorus of support for a national venereal disease program. On May 24, 1938, after its overwhelming approval in both the House and the Senate, FDR signed the National Venereal Disease Control Act, calling it "a major piece of social legislation." Raymond Vonderlehr, chief of the Venereal Disease Division, told reporters that the Act "makes possible a continuous scientific, coordinated attack which undoubtedly will materially reduce the incidence of syphilis and gonorrhea in the United States within the next decade."[67] The federal government was now committed to the alleviation of this previously taboo problem.

The legislation had a substantial impact upon the problem of venereal disease in American life. By 1940 the effects of programs that the federal funding helped to establish could be partially measured. Clinic facilities for the treatment of venereal disease had grown from 1,750 in July 1938 to almost 3,000 in July 1940. Moreover, the improvement and expansion of existing treatment centers had also served to make therapy more accessible. The $15 million appropriation helped to provide private practitioners with diagnostic and epidemiological services, as well as with free drugs when necessary to assist in the treatment of disadvantaged patients, and in some cases for all their patients regardless of income. As a result of the increase in facilities and public subsidies, the number of patients receiving the minimum required therapy jumped from 15 to 58 percent. Another indication of the value of the legislation was the fact that the number of blood tests performed to detect syphilis increased by some 300 percent between 1936 and 1940; funds from the Act helped to make the necessary diagnostic facilities available. "Since the detection of syphilis is to a large extent dependent upon mass blood-testing," noted Vonderlehr, "this increase in laboratory tests for syphilis is perhaps the best index of the effort which has been made to discover and bring to treatment infected individuals."[68] More cases now came under treatment during the early stages of the disease when therapy proved most effective. The "shadow on the land" had begun to lift.

10

Many states took action to join the federal campaign, passing legislation designed to protect the family from venereal infections. By the end of 1938, twenty-six states had enacted provisions prohibiting the marriage of infected individuals. Although by the end of World War I almost half the states had statutes whose ostensible purpose was the prevention of venereal disease in marriage, these laws typically had little impact. Most merely required a note from a physician or, remarkably, for the groom to sign an affidavit assuring that he was free of infection. As a physician, let alone a layperson, cannot identify a syphilitic infection without laboratory exams, such oaths really constituted character references; a premarital moral ritual with little benefit for health. Some of the penalties for failure to comply with these laws were severe—in Oklahoma and Michigan it was a felony with fines and imprisonment—but they were almost never enforced.[69] Moreover, these requirements rarely applied to women, reinforcing the sense in which they were truly half-measures.

Without the requisite of scientific diagnosis—the Wassermann test—these laws had reflected social convention and educational precepts more than any epidemiological reality. In 1935 Connecticut passed the first law requiring a blood test and physical examination for all prospective brides and grooms; if one party

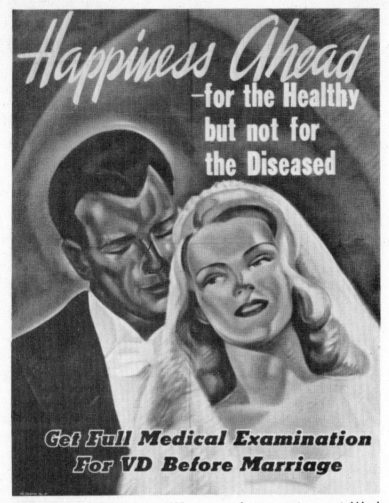

12. Beginning with Connecticut in 1935, many states began to require premarital blood tests.

was found to be infected a marriage license would not be granted until the individual was found to be non-infectious, a process that could take a number of years. Women's magazines became the strongest advocates of these enactments, frequently publishing articles and short stories detailing the tragic consequences of syphilis in the family. "Premarital tests aim at averting tremendous economic loss . . . as well as avoiding needless anguish and suffering," explained the *Literary Digest*.[70] Several states, however, continued to require only the examination of the bridegroom, arguing that a mandatory test affronted "pure" women. This, of course, compromised the laws' effectiveness in finding infections and protecting the family; in addition, it reflected a somewhat anachronistic view of the "double standard" of morality. Only the widespread acceptance within the medical community of serologic examination made the laws feasible; indeed, many physicians noted the advantage of this newly required, mandatory visit to their offices.

Although public health officials typically suggested that one in ten Americans carried a syphilitic infection, statutory blood tests revealed a much lower rate. In New York City during the first year in which the law took effect, premarital testing exposed only 1.34 percent positive for syphilis. Officials accounted for this figure by suggesting that individuals who knew of their infections postponed seeking marriage licenses until determined to be non-infectious. This may well have been the case, but it seems more likely that the low rates of infection reflected the fact that some claims of prevalence had been inflated, or that the premarital exam was not the optimal locus for screening. When the tests did reveal infections, officials assumed with some justification that new, unknown infections had been discovered. As William F. Lorenz of the Wisconsin Board of Health explained: "In every instance, those . . . individuals had no knowledge that they had syphilis; otherwise they would not have taken the chance of stigmatizing themselves by applying for a marriage license and then having the license refused them."[71]

According to some reports, many applicants for marriage licenses sought to evade the premarital tests. After Connecticut passed its law in 1935, and before the New York State Legislature had taken action, weekend marriages in New York counties bordering Connecticut rose by 55 percent. Moreover, the number of marriages in some states reportedly declined after premarital exams became legally required. After the New York law went into effect in July 1938, there was a 41 percent decrease in marriages, which many commentators attributed to the new statute. In New Jersey some state legislators expressed concern that premarital laws that restricted marriage to the healthy could lead to an increase of free love, illegitimacy, and common law marriages.[72] Although no organized opposition to the bill emerged, it passed by only one vote.

In addition to provisions for premarital exams, public health officials also supported legislation requiring pregnant women to undertake prenatal tests to prevent congenital transmission of syphilis. Congenital infection of the newborn often had disastrous consequences; children born with the infection often died or suffered from a number of serious repercussions including blindness and paralysis. As already noted, some 60,000 infants were born yearly with syphilis, most of whom died shortly after birth. As early as 1916 Dr. J. Whitridge Williams, the noted obstetrician at Johns Hopkins Hospital, required all women at his prenatal clinic to receive a routine Wassermann test. Williams found in investigating 700 fetal deaths among 10,000 deliveries at the Hospital that 26 percent could be attributed to syphilis. Early, continuous treatment of pregnant syphilitics, he demonstrated, prevented the infection of the infant in almost all cases. Williams's findings nevertheless went largely unheeded for the next two decades. In 1938 New York and Rhode Island enacted laws requiring prenatal blood tests for all pregnant women. These laws soon became virtually universal in the United States.[73]

New York's law, popularly known as the "baby health bill," was signed by Governor Herbert Lehman in March 1938. The law required all persons caring for women in pregnancy to submit a blood test to an approved laboratory. At the time of the bill's passage only half of New York City's practicing obstetricians made such tests as a matter of course. Many doctors reportedly suggested that the recommendation of the test might offend their patrons. According to one study, women who attended public clinics, where serologic exams were routinely performed, were less likely to give birth to syphilitic babies than moderately "well-to-do" women under the care of private physicians.[74]

The prenatal laws had a powerfully positive impact on the incidence of congenital syphilis within the United States. Indeed, unlike the premarital laws, which turned up few new cases, the prenatal legislation led to the decline of congenital transmission even before the advent of antibiotics. A study of the impact of the prenatal exams in California, for example, showed that the infant mortality rate for syphilis fell from 6.50 per 1000 in 1938 to 0.15 in 1945; cases of congenital syphilis dropped from 1.60 to 0.54 in the same years.[75]

The American Social Hygiene Association and public health organizations heralded both the premarital and the prenatal laws as a major triumph in the battle against venereal disease. "If these laws are administered satisfactorily, there can be no question about the great benefit to the people and the nation," the ASHA commented. "We may indeed see the day when syphilis is 'outlawed.' "[76] The assumption behind these measures—clearly expressed by the ASHA—was that through these statutes syphilis would eventually be conquered. This, in turn, reflected a view of sexual relations not substantiated in practice. Everyone, they assumed, would pass through the sieve of marriage and pregnancy; all infections would then be discovered and treated. These laws marked the dramatic incursion of the state into public health and the family. Unlike the National Venereal Disease Control Act, which sought to provide services to venereal victims, these laws marked the expansion of government into family life. Only statutory tuberculosis testing has rivaled these massive screening programs for a communicable disease in the twentieth century.

In addition to these laws, the other significant public health innovation of the 1930s—case-finding—also marked the expansion of public health into areas previously considered to be in the private sphere. Public health officials now emphasized the need to identify a venereal patient's sexual contacts. These individuals would then be apprised of the possibility of infection, tested, and, if need be, treated. Only in this way, officials argued, could the geometric progression of infection be stopped. "Contact epidemiology," a traditional approach to communicable disease, was now applied vigorously to the venereal diseases. As Thomas Parran commented:

A physician would not consider treating a case of smallpox without investigating fully the source of infection. He would either undertake this himself or report to the health department to make the investigation. On the other hand, one does not feel any such responsibility in cases of early syphilis. Yet the tracing of the source of syphilis is no more difficult than tracing the source of smallpox and is just as important. As a matter of fact, it is easier, for the person knows more definitely the source from which he may have acquired the disease.[77]

This assessment, however, was essentially naive, for syphilitic patients often did not wish to reveal the names of their sexual contacts.

Public health officials and social workers devised techniques to encourage patients to identify their sexual intimates. The University of Pennsylvania Hospital, through a grant from the Milbank Foundation, worked to develop "persuasion" methods to get the cooperation of venereal patients. "The clinic, by friendly sympathy, persuades the syphilis patient to disclose the identity of his recent sexual intimates," explained social worker Louise Brown Ingraham. Through these interviews, case workers reported that 80 percent of all contacts were located, although their ability to quantify this rate seems doubtful. "The approach dips deep into the heart of the individual and society, slowly bringing into the community a realization of the ominous presence of syphilis and makes possible a more intensive medical attack," noted Ingraham. Case workers in the field, following up reports of contacts, coined the term "shoe-leather epidemiology" to describe the unflagging rigor with which they sought out potential venereal victims for examination and treatment. Physicians advocating the need for "public health sleuths" repeatedly told stories of massive epidemics originating from a single source, developing into a pyramid of infection.[78]

The ultimate impact of case-finding remains difficult to evaluate. The search for infections required sensitive and difficult probing; it demanded that an individual discuss intimacies with strangers, secrets which could wreak havoc in the infected person's life. Contact epidemiology clearly brought many unsuspecting individuals into treatment before they could spread their infections to others. But the knowledge that information regarding contacts would be sought by public health professionals also had the effect of encouraging some individuals to seek the aid of quacks or private practitioners who guaranteed absolute confidentiality. Indeed, most private physicians have resisted public health requirements that they report individuals suffering from venereal disease to public officials so that contacts can be approached.[79] Venereal disease posed the fundamental dilemma of individual privacy versus the public good, a conflict that remains largely unresolved.

The notion of finding cases through screening and bringing infected individuals under treatment nevertheless became the basis for the modern campaign against syphilis initiated during the 1930s; nowhere was it pursued with as much vigor as in Chicago. With the assistance of the Chicago *Tribune*, which provided necessary publicity, the local, state, and federal health bureaucracies developed a comprehensive plan to rid the city of syphilis. The Works Progress Administration, and Title VI of the Social Security Act provided funds to undertake a massive effort to uncover and treat cases of syphilis beginning in 1937. In July more than a million questionnaires were mailed to Chicago families to ascertain their interest in such a campaign. More than 261,000 persons indicated their desire to receive a free blood test.[80] At the height of the program, ten to twelve thousand individuals daily were tested in what Parran had called a "Wassermann dragnet."

The Chicago project contained all the elements of a full-scale crusade against syphilis. There was widespread publicity encouraging individuals to be tested. On August 13 a syphilis parade marched from the Loop to City Hall carrying signs declaring, "Friday the thirteenth is an unlucky day for syphilis." An airplane with an anti-syphilis banner circled the city, newspapers carried announcements, and the radio filled the airwaves noting locations for free exams. Even the Federal Theatre Project got into the act with the production of Arnold Sundgaard's "living newspaper," *Spirochete*. The "fictionalized-documentary" reviewed the history of medical treatment for syphilis, attacked the conspiracy of silence, and urged on the Wassermann campaign. During intermission, theater-goers were invited to be tested in the lobby. Paul De Kruif, writing to Parran about the plans for the program, exclaimed: "If nothing else it is the most audacious and spectacular public relations move that has ever been made in syphilis. It will enormously increase syphilis consciousness." *Spirochete* later opened in Boston, Seattle, and Philadelphia.[81]

Officials expanded diagnostic facilities to meet the tremendous demand the publicity generated. Between 1937 and 1940 over 31 percent of the city's population received Wassermann tests. The "dragnet" uncovered and provided treatment for some 56,000 individuals infected with syphilis—all at public expense. The program had particular benefit for the city's black population, for whom health care facilities had been grossly inadequate in the past and among whom rates of infection ran especially high. In fact, more than 60 percent of all cases treated came from Chicago's black wards. Under the program, the number of cases of syphilis under treatment in Chicago increased by 300 percent.[82] The fact that Chicago had the lowest syphilis rate of all major cities during the selective service physicals for World War II revealed the program's striking impact. With funds, facilities, and the support of the press, a major attack on syphilis could be waged to great effect.

All public health programs directed against syphilis, from Chicago's dragnet to statutory prenatal exams, rested upon the ability of the profession to detect cases accurately—in other words with the Wassermann test. Many colleges initiated campaigns to test their students. At the Illinois State Fair of 1938, free blood tests for syphilis proved to be a big attraction. The Wassermann test and subsequent variations were, no doubt, extremely helpful in determining cases of syphilis and furthering efforts to track down infections, but these exams were often subject to error. Some physicians indicated that between 2 and 14 percent of all Wassermann tests produced false positives, and thus should be frequently repeated. Dr. John Stokes explained: "They [serological tests] are not the infallible things that the laity especially is inclined to think they are." In fact, some contemporary researchers have suggested that the Wassermann test was so overly sensitive that it typically turned up as much as 25 percent false positives.[83] Many individuals during the 1930s suffered the consequences of the toxic syphilitic

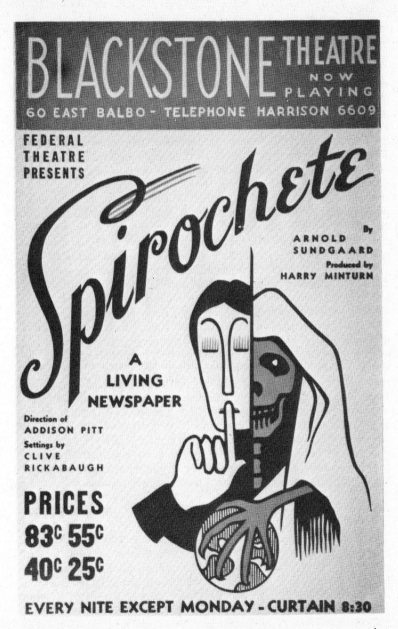

13. Arnold Sundgaard's *Spirochete*, produced by the Federal Theatre Project, was the centerpiece of the 1938 Chicago campaign against syphilis.

treatments although they were never infected; in some cases, these individuals were barred from marriage because of an incorrect Wassermann reading. They suffered the stigma associated with a disease they never had.

While massive testing for syphilis was undertaken in the 1930s, little interest in the other major venereal disease, gonorrhea, was expressed by public health officials. Although the federal legislation and public health efforts addressed the problems of all the venereal diseases, in reality they centered attention—as did Parran's publicity—on syphilis. Syphilis made headlines, while gonorrhea, four times more prevalent than syphilis, receded deeper in the public consciousness. Several factors explain why little effort was directed to gonorrhea. First, most physicians argued that the long-term pathology of the disease, though serious, was far less dangerous than syphilis. Second, diagnostic procedures for gonorrhea remained more complex and difficult to administer than the simple complement-fixation reactions that could identify syphilis through a blood test; microscopic smears were required to detect gonorrhea, a procedure few physicians could easily perform. Finally, medical science had little to offer an individual suffering from gonorrhea prior to the availability of the sulfonamides in the early 1940s. As Dr. William F. Snow pointed out: "Probably this disease will not be dramatized as syphilis has been in recent years unless some new and spectacular method of cure is devised."[84] Aware of the fact that gonorrhea was receiving short shrift in the anti-venereal campaign, however, doctors argued for the need to address the problem with equal force. N. A. Nelson cautioned Parran that his approach "seems to push gonorrhea another peg or two down the ladder." Accordingly, he suggested "it would not be out of place to carry the problem of gonorrhea into the public consciousness along with syphilis, since they have a common eipdemiological background." This critique, however, went largely unheeded during the 1930s. The *American Journal of Public Health* noted an alarming attitude toward gonorrhea : "Too many of our young men, for example, boast of having gonorrhea and regard it, if not as a matter of pride, as one showing that they know their way about and are men of the world." But to raise gonorrhea in the public mind, only to assert its untreatability, would have been a blow to the growing authority of science, medicine, and public health—the very authority behind the campaign against syphilis.

11

Thomas Parran's campaign against syphilis during the 1930s differed substantially from the reforms of the Progressive years and even the significant programs of World War I. Three essential themes characterized his effort. First, Parran rejected the traditional emphasis within the anti-venereal movement on sexual morality and ethics. Second, he hoped to place his crusade on the plane of science and medicine, to incorporate the battle against venereal disease within the tradition of efforts to combat infectious disease. And third, the surgeon general sought to force the State to accept certain fundamental responsibilities for the care of venereal sufferers. In each of these respects his program marked a watershed, a rejection of Progressive notions of voluntarism, charity, and morality.

Parran's campaign against venereal diseases represents the most positive elements of New Deal reform. Refusing to be limited by social conventions and political precedents, Parran clearly identified the problem and the available instrumentalities for its resolution. The struggle against venereal disease and the strong commitment of federal funds demonstrated the New Deal's resolve to expand the role and function of the federal government; to identify social problems of a magnitude that only a national government could effectively mitigate. The anti-venereal campaign is a neglected but important element in the history of New Deal social reform.

But just as the New Deal broke precedent, expanding the parameters of reform, so too, it met severe limitations and constraints. This, unfortunately, was also true in the case of the crusade against sexually transmitted diseases. Undercutting the dramatic success of Parran's battle were a number of subtle yet powerful views of the venereal diseases that continue to this day to limit our ability to deal with them effectively. These views, which were often at odds with the new sexual candor concerning the venereal diseases expressed during the 1930s, existed side-by-side with Parran's more dispassionate outlook, often undermining his goals.

The central problem that limited the potential of Parran's program to rid the nation of venereal infection was what became known as "syphilophobia"—the fear of syphilis, or for that matter, any venereal disease. In "The Next Great Plague To Go," Parran had actually advocated that "syphilis ignorance" be replaced by "syphilophobia." Though admitting that this might "create some neurotics" or aggravate some already strained family relationships, he suggested it would help to uncover unsuspected cases, bring new cases to treatment, and render many non-infectious. "Syphilophobia never killed anyone," declared Parran, "never brought a handicapped child into the world, never infected an innocent person." But the burden of syphilophobia, despite Parran's protestations, often generated unrealistic views of the disease, its impact and treatability—attitudes that ultimately made syphilis a more difficult problem to handle. *Hygeia*, a popular health periodical for laypeople, noted, for example: "As a menace to human health and happiness, cancer cannot begin to compare with [syphilis's] ravages."[85] Such views did not serve the attempt to make syphilis one of a number of infectious diseases that the techniques of medicine and public health could effectively control. Indeed, to the contrary, syphilophobia encouraged fear, stigma, and denial. This, of course, could ultimately lead to the bane of public health efforts: the hidden infection.

The fear campaign contradicted, in many respects, the very tenets of Parran's effort. Though education about the dangers of venereal diseases clearly was necessary, Parran often noted that the real emphasis should be placed on the medical profession's ability to treat syphilis effectively. Creating syphilophobia could only work against the goal of getting individuals in for treatment by heightening the stigma associated with the disease. Underlying the emphasis on fear, it seems, was a more traditional caution against promiscuous sexuality. The implicit message in repeated descriptions of the "ravages" of syphilis was the prescription: do not risk infection.

A number of contemporary writers noted the deleterious impact of syphilophobia on the anti-venereal movement. One critic observed in the *Survey*: "The public itself must recognize the irrationality of many of its fears of syphilis. It must stop being afraid." Dr. Thurman B. Rice of the Indianapolis Department of Health concurred, cautioning that the emphasis on syphilis might "frighten the population into a state of hysteria rather than to lead them into a constructive attitude toward the whole matter of sex." An iconoclastic venereal specialist from Chicago, Dr. Ben Reitman, proved to be one of the most steadfast critics of syphilophobia. Reitman, who closed his office to ride the rails in the summer with a group of hobos, dedicated his practice to taking care of the poor, prostitutes, and the down and out. Addressing the problem of fear and the venereal victim, he wrote:

> The social syphilophobia is more severe and dangerous today than any disease phobia that has ever been experienced in America. From time to time we have been panicy-stricken [sic] by smallpox, typhoid fever, and poliomyelitis, but usually there was some health officer or newspaper to put on the soft pedal. But in this syphilis propaganda the entire orchestra is striking a note of terror that is bound to produce a serious reaction.[86]

Parran's approach to the venereal problem, emphasizing its dangers, was thus fraught with a series of tensions. If raising the specter of fear of syphilis generated public attention and funding, so, too, it could create attitudes that could hinder the campaign as well.

Critics of syphilophobia often contended that the anti-venereal campaign played fast and loose with statistics, vastly overemphasizing the extent of the problem. Although most individuals active in the anti-syphilis campaign often cited the figure that one in ten Americans harbored an infection, actual tests for prevalence usually revealed a significantly lower number. The *New York State Journal of Medicine* remarked in an editorial: "No one will begrudge the money spent to combat venereal disease in recent years. Nevertheless we may question whether it is wise to base health measures on fear fostered by exaggerated morbidity figures."[87] Ben Reitman also argued that venereal statistics were greatly inflated to instill fear in the public. Perhaps overestimation of the number of infections did aid the campaign to generate funds, but the problem with inflating such statistics and increasing fears of epidemic contagion was that sexuality itself was under attack.

The persistence of certain beliefs about contagion long after they had been disproved contributed yet another aspect to syphilophobia. City and state health departments continued to pass ordinances requiring the examination for venereal disease of domestics and food handlers, although it was well-known that infections were rarely, if ever, transmitted without intimate sexual contact. Walter Clarke, executive director of the ASHA explained: "Health officers are practically unanimous in decrying the false impression upon which much of the public demand for the examination of food handlers is based, namely that syphilis and gonorrhea are spread by contact of infected people with articles of food or food utensils." Nevertheless, Clarke advocated the continued use of such ordinances as a case-finding method. "I have not felt it desirable personally to discourage communities where public opinion favors examination of domestics and food handlers," he concluded. But this view had the effect of endorsing the myth of non-genital infections. As one doctor testifying before the Senate explained: "I would suggest, if there is any doubt about this bill, that you have Dr. Parran see to it that the servants of all Members of Congress are given free tests. I think they will find it intimately enough connected with their lives to pass the bill very quickly."[88]

Ordinances such as those directed at domestics and foodhandlers stereotyped venereal victims, encouraging fears of social contact between social classes and ethnic groups. Although Parran's campaign had gone far towards making the point that venereal diseases reached all segments of society, the view persisted that these infections particularly affected the working class, the immoral, and certain racial and ethnic groups. "There may be from seven to ten out of every hundred persons in the United States who are infected, but among the criminal elements and the very dregs of human society from thirty to forty out of every hundred are found to be infected," observed Dr. Morris Fishbein without offering any substantiation for his statistics. Some individuals continued to argue that these infections could then reach into the upper classes. As one physician explained: "But even granted that syphilis were a reservoir of disease in the lowest social class of the population, scientists agree that such diseases always filter through and affect higher strata of society."[89] Again, the mode of such transmission remained a mystery.

Attitudes towards blacks and venereal diseases especially revealed the tension between the scientific-public health approach and the stereotyping moralism of syphilophobia. Since the early twentieth century, physicians, particularly those in the South, had suggested that blacks were unusually prone to venereal disease, a "syphilis-soaked race."[90] Typically, high rates of infection were attributed to the premise that blacks were promiscuous. Moreover, physicians argued that it was difficult to treat blacks because they could not be convinced of the danger that these diseases posed. Socioeconomic arguments for the prevalence of venereal infections among blacks were generally discounted. As surgeon genereal, Parran worked diligently to dispel these views, but he nevertheless fell under the weight of their tradition.

It is an ironic tragedy that, while the Public Health Service participated in a program that greatly benefited the black citizens of Chicago, it was at the same time conducting an experiment in Alabama that insured that some 400 black sharecroppers would never be treated for their syphilitic infections. In 1932 the PHS initiated an experiment known as the Tuskegee Syphilis Study that sought to determine the impact of syphilis if left untreated. The experiment was based upon two essentially racist precepts. First, the doctors who designed the study believed that virtually all southern blacks were infected. Second, they contended that the men involved would never be treated anyway. Over a forty-year period, the Public Health Service actively sought to prevent the men from receiving therapy, all the while telling the subjects that they *were* being treated by the government doctors. Many of the men—perhaps more than 100—died as a result of tertiary syphilis.[91]

The attitudes and opinions within the medical profession that made possible the Tuskegee Spyhilis Study and its continuation were strikingly persistent. In 1943 Dr. R. W. Williams of the Yazoo County Health Department wrote:

> I have one criticism to make about the treatment of the Negro in the South; he is babied too much. . . . It is my firm opinion that if the Negro right at this time was cast off from the white race, the majority would starve to death. His sense of responsibility is pratically nil.[92]

During the forty years that the Tuskegee Study continued, it was widely reported in medical journals without raising any significant objections on the part of the profession. Indeed, only reports of the study in the general press in 1972 finally brought it to an end.

Blacks justifiably took exception to the typical assessments of the venereal problem among their race. Many black physicians disputed the frequently cited statistics that blacks suffered from syphilis at rates five to six times that of whites. As Lester B. Granger, executive secretary of the National Urban League, commented:

> The National Urban League has constantly hammered on the point that it is not only unrealistic, but it is vicious to compare diseases and death rates among Negroes with those among whites, unless careful pains are taken to compare groups of similar income levels and living conditions. . . . In the meantime, constantly harping on a disproportionate rate of increase among Negroes merely intensifies a distorted picture that white society has of Negro family life, and makes it more difficult than ever for Negroes to find satisfactory adjustment in housing and employment situations.[93]

Moreover, black doctors raised objections to the notion that venereal disease had a fundamentally different pathological impact upon blacks because of biological differences between the races, a view held, for example, by Thomas Parran. These assumptions about race and venereal disease, like syphilophobia, had the effect of making these infections a problem of morals rather than medicine.

The final supposition underlying syphilophobia was that it was better to fear syphilis than to prevent infection. The campaign against venereal diseases during the 1930s consistently emphasized their dangers without ever giving serious attention to their prevention except through sexual abstinence. "Syphilis is always painted as a horrible, loathsome disease by medical men," declared Ben Reitman. "It is never explained that syphilis and gonorrhea are preventable."[94] Reitman repeatedly returned to this point in his critiques of the public health campaign. Despite the emphasis on science and medicine that Parran's efforts engendered, chemical prophylaxis was seldom advocated. Moreover, public health officials refused to encourage the use of condoms, also known to be effective preventives against disease. Even washing with soap and water after intercourse, shown at least to reduce the possibility of infection, never received the sanction of public health officials in their fight against venereal disease.

The response of the anti-venereal campaign to birth control is suggestive of the constraints upon the movement. The American Social Hygiene Association, concerned about the possibility of alienating their Catholic constituents, sought to avoid the issue of birth control altogether. This position, however, created concern among their primary sponsor, the Rockefeller-funded Bureau of Social Hygiene, which simultaneously sponsored some birth control research. The BSH believed that the ASHA was side-stepping an issue significantly related to their avowed interest in the American family. Though it was well-known that the condom served as both an effective preventive against pregnancy *and* venereal disease, the ASHA continued to refuse to endorse their use. As Ruth Topping of the BSH noted in a report: "Surely this is a strange position on the part of an organization with the avowed aim to reduce the menace of venereal disease."[95]

By 1940 the ASHA had still failed to promote, or indeed, even mention, the use of condoms in their educational literature. The Birth Control Federation of America bitterly noted this omission. Dr. Woodbridge Morris, general director of the Federation, wrote to the ASHA criticizing its defensive posture:

> In my strong conviction, as a citizen and as a physician, that venereal diseases must be controlled by every available means, I appeal to you to take a positive stand in this matter [condoms] before the public finds out that you are, in fact, permitting the spread of venereal disease because the most effective method to control it happens to be a method of contraception.

Walter Clarke of the ASHA sought to bury the issue, noting: "I believe that if we proceed cautiously we may continue to avoid battles on this touchy subject."[96] Thomas Parran also avoided the issue of condoms, although the advocacy of their use would have been consistent with his desire to approach the problem of venereal disease free of moral consideration. Indeed, Parran admitted fearing a decline in American morals:

> Whatever the causes for the double standard of morals . . . and its encouragement to commercial prostitution, it appears that our present trend is to a single standard unhappily in the direction of the old male standard of promiscuity rather than towards the woman's standard upon which was built the monogamous marriage.[97]

Parran, a Catholic, had perhaps already pushed his morality to the breaking point through his campaign against venereal disease; on the issue of prophylaxis, he simply could go no further.

In its response to birth control, the anti-venereal movement revealed its implicit outlook on American sexual ethics. Rather than accepting the fundamental changes that had occurred in American sexual life toward a more permissive premarital sexuality, many still hoped to turn back the clock. In this respect, prophylaxis was considered in much the same light as birth control; unwanted pregnancy and venereal disease had been used for some time as the principal means of controlling sexuality. To take the fear of these potential consequences out of sex was to many social critics to risk a breakdown of restraints on family and society. With the growing use of birth control in the 1920s and 1930s, the threat of venereal diseases became an even more potent injection against casual sex. Thus syphilophobia, rather than prophylaxis, became an elemental aspect of the campaign against the venereal diseases.

Thomas Parran and the New Deal's campaign nevertheless made dramatic strides against the venereal diseases. Parran had boldly defined the problem and acted to commit the federal government to its resolution. Before the 1930s, venereal disease had largely been viewed as a problem of personal willfulness and individual turpitude. Parran led the fight to see venereal disease as a social problem, worthy of government intervention. The times were attuned to such an effort, for the Great Depression had called into question—as few events could—Progressive notions of individual responsibility. The traditional view of the venereal victim as undeserving of aid was significantly weakened during the 1930s. Moreover, the social and economic costs of not dealing with the problem were, at last, made explicit. Parran's campaign thus clearly fits into the larger corpus of New Deal reform.

During the Progressive years the definition of venereal disease had changed from carnal scourge to family poison. During the 1930s the representatives of modern science and public health attempted to redefine venereal disease as a curable disease, but met with only partial success. Parran's goal of a nation freed from the burden of sexually transmitted diseases was never reached, despite the subsequent advent of more effective medical treatment. Venereal disease remained—in spite of Parran's efforts—a symptom of social decay and sexual evil. The discourse about the diseases reinforced this view, making venereal disease that much more difficult to deal with effectively. Even Thomas Parran failed to discern the close alliance of fear, stigma, and taboo: an alliance whose power continues to hold sway.

V

Dr. Ehrlich's Magic Bullet:
Venereal Disease in the Age of Antibiotics

1

At the height of Thomas Parran's campaign against syphilis in 1940, Warner Bros. produced a feature film celebrating Paul Ehrlich's chemotherapeutic breakthrough of 1910—the discovery of Salvarsan. *Dr. Ehrlich's Magic Bullet* starred Edward G. Robinson in the lead role, toiling against the hypocrisy of his time to advance medical progress. Ehrlich's prediction of the discovery of specific chemotherapeutic agents for specific diseases—"magic bullets" to root out and destroy infecting organisms—was the promise of modern medicine. Indeed, the so-called biomedical model of disease and treatment, upon which most twentieth-century therapeutics are based, stems from Ehrlich's initial discovery. Penicillin, discovered to be effective in treating syphilis and gonorrhea in 1943, seemed to be the answer to the search for a magic bullet. Unfortunately, however, the promise of the magic bullet has never been fulfilled. The control of many infectious diseases through antibiotics revealed a whole new set of systemic, chronic diseases, unresponsive to these drugs. Moreover, many infectious diseases, especially viral infections, still cannot be treated effectively.[1] And finally, even those infections that respond to antibiotics are still prevalent. Today, venereal diseases persist in epidemic proportions in spite of antibiotics. Effective against certain microorganisms, the magic bullets cannot combat the social and cultural determinants of these infections.

2

As World War II loomed on the horizon, the American military relied on traditional means of prevention and treatment for the venereal diseases. Penicillin was not to become widely available in the military until 1944. Instead of depending on therapeutics, anti-venereal programs developed during mobilization were closely modeled on those instituted during World War I. In early 1940 a joint meeting of the military medical services, the Public Health Service, and

161

the American Social Hygiene Association was held to develop plans for controlling venereal disease in the event of war. A resolution entitled the Eight Point Agreement resulted and was soon approved by the Conference of Territorial and State Health Officers.[2] This agreement endorsed an essentially conventional approach to venereal disease control: a combination of education, repression of prostitution, medical treatment of the infected, and rigorous casefinding and contact tracing.

Despite the agreement, the military failed to develop a comprehensive venereal disease program. In 1941 Parran and Raymond Vonderlehr published a stinging attack on military anti-venereal policy in a new book, *Plain Words About Venereal Disease*. They contended that the military was not taking sufficient precautions concerning the sexually transmitted diseases, risking the possibility of an all-out epidemic. "The framework for effective action against it is already in place," they explained. "The action as yet has not been taken."[3] In particular, Parran and Vonderlehr cited the growth of organized prostitution near army camps. The repression of prostitution had been the centerpiece of venereal control during World War I, and now, they argued, it was being overlooked by military officials. According to *Plain Words*, the machinery for dealing with the problem was growing rusty from disuse.

When local law enforcement proved inadequate in stemming a rising tide of prostitution in the vicinity of the military camps during mobilization, Congress took action. In January 1941 Representative Andrew J. May introduced legislation that made vice activities near military installations a federal offense.[4] The May Act, which became law in July 1941, was modeled on the World War I legislation that established "moral zones" free of alcohol and prostitution around the cantonments.

By the time *Plain Words* was published, however, no action had been undertaken to invoke the May Act despite a reportedly growing traffic in commercialized prostitution. "Unless vigorous Federal action is initiated, we may sink to the level of France in our tolerance of prostitution," cautioned the surgeon general. Again, as in World War I, the battle against venereal disease was pronounced a necessity of efficiency and morals. "Why subject these young men to the disease risks which 25 years ago were proved unnecessary?" Parran asked. "What would a Pershing and a Baker do now?" *Plain Words* demanded that the military invoke the May Act in a number of communities. "If it is stupid to waste money and materials at this juncture," Parran and Vonderlehr concluded, "it is treasonable to waste manpower."[5]

Parran's candid broadside did not find an appreciative audience in military and government circles among those eager to assure the nation of their concern for the troops' physical and moral welfare. Although the ASHA attempted to get Parran to soften his blows, their efforts were to no avail. William Snow, executive director of the ASHA, viewed the book as an unwarranted attack on Secretary of War Henry Stimson. Newspapers and magazines carried reports of Parran's views, noting the insufficiency of military programs to "protect" the troops. The political ramifications of this publicity soon became clear. Eventually President Roosevelt voiced concern, asking for a full report on venereal incidence in the Army and Navy. Roosevelt was particularly annoyed by the comments on the book's jacket, which castigated the federal government's apathetic policy. He angrily wrote to Paul McNutt, Parran's boss at the Federal Security Agency: "If the Surgeon General of the Army or the Surgeon General of the Navy had written this book before taking all prior steps called for, he would have been liable to immediate court martial." McNutt, in turn, reprimanded Parran: "There will be no repetition of such unethical and untactful procedure."[6]

Parran stood by his critique, despite the heat from his superiors, renewing his call for the vigorous repression of prostitution. To do otherwise, he explained, would result in higher incidence of disease and greater costs: "The indictment is against unnecessary disease: against a temporizing policy which requires increasingly large expenditures of public money for the treatment of disease without corresponding vigilance to reduce the cause of infection." Raymond Fosdick, who had directed the federal domestic campaign against venereal disease, during World War I, came to the surgeon general's defense, noting the need for a comprehensive program. The *American Journal of Public Health* also supported Parran's appraisal of the problem, commenting that "prostitution is an Axis partner."[7] With the invasion of Pearl Harbor, many such internal debates, including that about venereal policy, quieted, bringing together, in this case, the surgeon general with his military counterparts. The program that the military eventually developed during mobilization and the early years of the war, however, reflected few advances in policy from World War I.

3

Although the Commission on Training Camp Activities was not reconstituted during World War II, the military nevertheless sought to provide soldiers with education and amusements to divert their attentions and energies from "unwholesome" distractions. "Athletic activities, movies, and organized entertainment are provided on a scale never before attempted in order to dissuade soldiers from using their spare time looking for trouble in the form of alcoholic or sexual adventures," explained Major William Bisher. As in World War I, the Army developed a battery of educational materials on venereal disease prevention including pamphlets, lectures, and now-legendary films. Venereal education deliberately sought to create "syphilophobia" among the men, as two medical officers indicated:

> Fear is the dominant theme of many of the appeals that have been successfully used. We realize that much of pedagogical and medical opinion will differ with us on the value of fear as a motivation; yet we have found that it operates in the minds of the soldiers as one of the most potent reasons for the avoidance of venereal disease.[8]

Fear, they concluded, would serve to keep many men from straying from the path of continence.

But many did, in fact, disagree with this assessment. One medical officer noted somewhat ruefully, "The sex act cannot be made unpopular." Officials were forced to confront the limitations of the educational program. "There is little to indicate that we have been at all successful in converting to continence those individuals who were promiscuous before their entry into the service," admitted members of the Medical Corps evaluating venereal education. They found that "sexually stimulating motion pictures," "pin-up girls," and suggestive advertising all worked as countervailing forces to the military's campaign for sexual continence. Moreover, they suggested that, to men at war, the dangers of venereal infection might seem relatively inconsequential. "It may surprise you, indeed, to know what little importance the average enlisted man attaches to venereal infections," noted Lt. Commander Leo Shifrin. "Most of them think as little of a gonorrheal infection as they do of the ordinary common cold." After the introduction of antibiotics in late 1943, military physicians realized that the impact of scare tactics had been deeply undercut. The very nature and meaning of venereal infection had been transformed. "There is one important aspect of the use of fear as motivation that needs particular emphasis at this time," noted Drs. Larimore and Sternberg of the Medical Corps. "Namely, that fear of the venereal diseases themselves will be decreasingly effective from now on, as improved techniques of therapy render them less and less serious, and perhaps eventually relegate them to comparatively minor infections."[9]

Recognizing the limits of sex education to inculcate continence, the Army took measures to provide the troops with more effective preventive measures. As Joel T. Boone concluded: "We cannot stifle the instincts of man, we cannot legislate his appetite. We can only educate him to caution, watchfulness and the perpetual hazards of promiscuous intercourse; and furnish him with adequate preventive measures." The Army therefore devised a major program to ensure the provision of prophylaxis, both condoms and chemical treatments, to the troops. "If you can't say no, take a pro," was the oft-cited motto in the Army's campaign. "Realizing that angels rightfully belong only in heaven," as one medical officer explained, the Army established hundreds of stations in all theatres for chemical treatments after intercourse, as well as providing condoms *en masse*. For ten cents soldiers could obtain kits containing three condoms and a small tube of lubricating jelly; some units distributed these packets without charge. When women replaced men behind the sales counters at the Ships Service stores and Post Exchanges, sales of condoms reportedly fell. To overcome this problem, vending machines were installed "so that easy access is the rule at all hours." As many as fifty million condoms were sold or freely distributed each month during the war.[10] The provision of condoms, of course, marked an important reversal of World War I military policy. This policy constituted an implicit recognition of the inability of officials to control the troops' sexual drives.

The Army's emphasis on prevention and the liberal distribution of prophylactics nevertheless brought the program under fire from critics who suggested that the anti-venereal emphasis should be on sexual morals. "The bulk of military teaching," noted one dismayed physician, "is instruction in the use of pro-

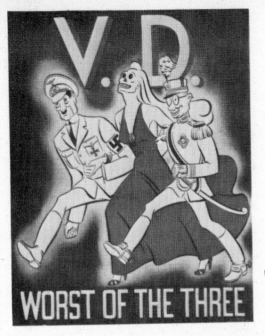

14. Venereal disease, typically portrayed as a woman.

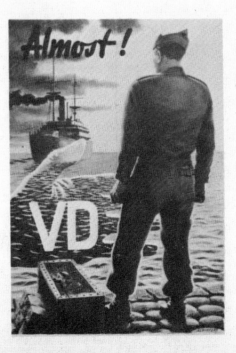

15. Venereal disease could keep a soldier from war.

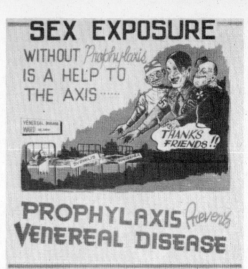

16. The Army Medical Corps vigorously promoted prophylaxis during World War II.

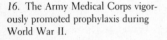

17. Despite the introduction of antibiotics, the military still sought to discourage sexual contacts.

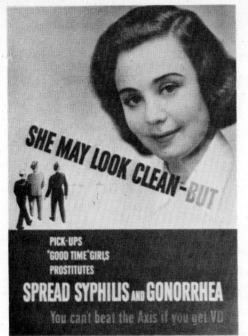

18. This popular poster asserted that even the woman who appeared "pure" could pose dangers for the soldier.

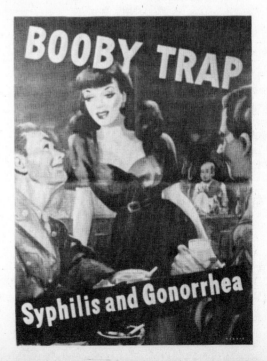

19. The dangers of loose women and pick-ups, a constant theme.

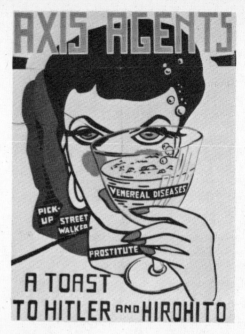

20. Venereal disease again attributed to the evil woman.

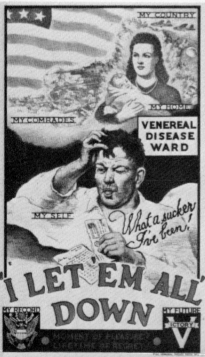

21. Regrets from the venereal ward.

phylaxis during sexual misbehavior." As in World War I, the easy availability of prophylaxis again drew criticism on this point. Dr. Morris Leider held that "the routine dissemination of prophylactic advice and material carries with it an inherent contradiction, in that it automatically suggests and sanctions promiscuity at the same time that it hopes to prevent disease danger of promiscuity."[11] Some physicians and social workers insisted that the only real way to contain the venereal problem was by controlling sexual behavior. "The horns of the dilemma cannot be evaded," explained Leider, "venereal disease control must be planned as behavior control." These individuals denied the validity of those traditional notions that held that continent men would not fight effectively and that extended sexual abstinence was against human nature. Organized Catholic groups protested; the Catholic War Veterans characterized the anti-venereal program as "indecent, repulsive, and un-American," suggesting that the military's campaign actually encouraged promiscuity. The Knights of Columbus deplored the "substitution of high-pressure publicity . . . and offensive frankness . . . for moral training."

Eventually these critics forced the withdrawal of several of the most graphic anti-venereal films in the military's repertoire. "The net effect," noted the New Republic, "is to leave the public with the impression that Catholics are strangely calm about the danger of venereal disease." This, of course, was not the case at all; they were deeply concerned about the problem, yet vehemently dissented from the military's efficiency-oriented approach. As the debate about the military programs illustrated, tensions between those whose primary concern was disease and those chiefly concerned with sexual morals had again been exacerbated. In Theodore Schroeder's view, there were still those who continued to assert the "spiritual value of syphilis" as a means of controlling sexuality.[12]

According to a military study, between 53 and 63 percent of all soldiers engaged in sexual intercourse during the war. This figure ranged approximately 10 percent higher among black soldiers. Among unmarried troops, more than 80 percent had sexual relations, while 50 percent of all married men engaged in extra-marital intercourse. The unreliable nature of these figures does not negate the fact that within the military it was recognized that most men would seek and find sex during their military tenures and that officials responded in an efficient and practical fashion. By the end of the war, the military reported difficulty in procuring sufficient quantities of condoms to meet the troops' demands.[13] As in World War I, the Medical Corps justified its pragmatic response on the basis of its effectiveness in controlling infections.

4

With the entry of the United States into the war, the anti-venereal program was reinvigorated with particular attention to the attack on prostitution. Although the ASHA had continued to express concern about the resurgence of vice after World War I, the campaign had receded during the 1920s and 1930s, and now the problem of prostitution in its relation to venereal diseases came again to the fore. Just as in World War I, the red-light district was equated to a swamp that bred malaria-carrying mosquitos. Moreover, social hygienists like Walter Clarke emphasized that military encampments tended to attract organized prostitution: "For wherever these men are gathered, those who seek to exploit them for gain will follow. And chief among the exploiters will be the procurer and prostitute, spreading disease and disorder among those upon whom our protection depends." The American Social Hygiene Association participated in the war program by sending its investigators to American cities to gather evidence of prostitution and vice—a virtual repeat performance of its World War I activities.[14] Secretary of War Stimson followed Newton Baker's lead, writing to all the state governors urging them to cooperate in ensuring that conditions free of commercial prostitution were maintained around the camps.

In late 1941 a new agency was created by Paul McNutt to enforce provisions to limit prostitution. The Social Protection Division (SPD), which operated within the Office of Community War Services, worked with the ASHA and the USPHS to investigate vice and aid the Department of Justice in May Act prosecutions. McNutt appointed the renowned Director of Public Safety of Cleveland, Eliot Ness, to direct the SPD. Ness, who had attracted a national reputation for cracking down on vice and organized crime in Cleveland, proved an effective leader, calling together police chiefs, mayors, and city managers to do their part in the campaign against prostitution. Ness even arranged through the National Cab Association to have taxi drivers' licenses revoked if they were found to be acting as go-betweens for prostitutes.[15]

The May Act provided the legal power necessary for the Department of Justice to assume the policing of areas deemed to be hazardous to the troops by the secretary of war or the secretary of the navy. In other words, if prostitution persisted in a given community, federal authorities could take action. The May Act was viewed as an indication of the seriousness of the government's commitment to repression of prostitution. As Federal Security Agency Administrator Paul McNutt noted, "Short of martial law there is hardly another field of local police power which can be forfeited to the Federal government." But invocation of the May Act, NcNutt explained, was to be avoided if possible; he sought to keep "local problems local," enlisting the assistance of city police. Although only invoked twice during the course of the war—in Tennessee and North Carolina—the May Act nevertheless served as a prod to local officials to "clean up" their communities or be deposed by federal officials.[16]

The war also elicited what was by then a classic debate concerning the regulation versus the suppression of prostitution. Although the Army opted to endorse complete repression, many doctors continued to argue that prostitution could best be handled by segregation and regular medical inspection. These physicians viewed prostitution as a lesser evil, an outlet for uncontrolled and uncontrollable sexual drives. Cited among the possible consequences of the repression of prostitution were homosexuality, seduction, and rape. "While the suppression of prostitution may greatly satisfy a puritanical mind, it will not answer the purpose for which it is taken," claimed Dr. Harry Benjamin. Some continued to express fear that the end of prostitution might force men to look elsewhere for sexual release. Dr. Sheldon Glueck explained to Ness's committee:

Here are the practical issues. In the first place you prevent prostitution; in the next place you allow boys to obtain contraceptives at army stations. Therefore where will they get their sexual gratification? Are you proposing that they shall invade the nonprofessional classes for this sort of thing? . . . I am just as concerned about the spread of illegitimate sex and disease among the better class of girls in the community as I am with the fighting efficiency of our forces.

In the vicinity of some camps medical officers arranged for medical inspection of prostitutes housed in brothels nearby. When knowledge of such action came to the attention of the surgeon general these physicians were reprimanded. "In an effort to correct the attitude of these officers and to forestall adverse public opinion," explained an official account of military policy, "a very strong Army-wide directive was published."[17]

The Army continued to contend that rates of venereal disease fell dramatically when communities closed down organized prostitution. Eliot Ness defended the government's anti-prostitution program:

Despite the alarums and dire prophecies of many critics of repression who were either honestly misinformed or whose financial interests were at stake, the more than 300 communities which clamped down on prostitution have not experienced great crime waves, or increases in rape cases.

Arrested women were subject to mandatory venereal exams and, if found infected, treatment under detention. Officials argued for vigorous measures to quarantine and detain women who were found to be carrying venereal infections. "We know that a person with small pox may so conduct himself that his infection will not be transmitted to others, but we do not hesitate at isolation, nevertheless," explained James D. Lade of the New York State Department of Health. "Why then are we chary of similar measures in venereal disease?" Nevertheless, thousands of women were institutionalized or detained. As a result, jails became overcrowded. Ness arranged for the creation of some thirty "civilian conservation camps" for young women as a means of relieving some of the pressure on existing facilities. In all, more than seven hundred cities and towns closed their red-light districts during the course of the war. Not since World War I had prostitution been so vigorously repressed in the United States.[18]

Despite the incarceration of thousands of prostitutes, it soon became clear that this could not in itself solve the venereal problem. Indeed, the impact of closing the red-light districts was sometimes disappointing to military officials. Increasingly army physicians reported that prostitutes constituted only a minority of the soldiers' sexual contacts. In the Third Service Command, for example, only 19 percent of the infections could be attributed to prostitutes; in other communities, even fewer infections could be so traced. As one journalist pointed out, "Fully 90 percent of the Army's cases in this country are traceable to amateur girls—teenagers and older women—popularly known as 'khaki-wackies,' 'victory girls,' and 'good-time Charlottes.' "[19]

The military soon turned its attention, therefore, to the "promiscuous" girl. Women of loose morals, eager to support the war effort, were determined by authorities to be the primary locus of infection. As venereal expert Dr. John Stokes explained:

The old time prostitute in a house or formal prostitute on the street is sinking into second place. The new type is the young girl in her late teens and early twenties, the young woman in every field of life who is determined to have one fling or better.

The harlot with the painted face had stepped aside for the girl-next-door. The Army now emphasized in its educational literature for soldiers that these "victory girls" could be just as infectious as the experienced prostitute. The most widely circulated World War II pamphlet was entitled, "She Looked Clean But. . . ." Again, such literature repeated the sorry association of "cleanliness" with chastity, impurity with disease. About these women a federal committee noted: "She is more dangerous to the community than a mad dog. Rabies can be recognized. Gonorrhea and syphilis ordinarily cannot."[20]

The attention centered upon promiscuous girls as the major foci of venereal infection reflected a ubiquitous double standard of sexual morality. Indeed, the word "promiscuous" was firmly anchored to "girl"—a promiscuous man was, by definition, an oxymoron. Women in this view, were the keepers of sexual mores—their indiscretions led to a deterioration of morals. "They" infected the soldiers; in this view, venereal disease could only be transmitted in one direction. Therefore, as sexual mores did in fact change, the burden of this transformation came to be placed upon women. The fact that controlling prostitution did not control sexuality forced many to confront the change in American sexual mores.

The anxiety about the increase of promiscuity reflected more than a simple concern regarding incidence of venereal disease. Some physicians suggested that the increase indicated a breakdown in traditional social restraints, especially in the family. They advocated the need for reinvigorated parental authority. "It is very disturbing to see misguided young girls, often bedraggled and undernourished without family or friends, caught up in the prostitution-repression program—jails and courts—when the whole situation might be handled by a stern father and a good doctor," explained Dr. Thomas Turner. Again, the concern about prostitution and promiscuity signaled the expansion of the doctor's role. Indeed, promiscuity often became the focus of medical attention instead of disease. John Stokes explained: "It is not the patient under treatment who spreads disease, but the promiscuous individual before and after treatment. In other words, we must move against promiscuity rather than, or in addition to, disease." The persistent tension in the anti-venereal campaign between morals and medicine once again became explicit. After reading a new pamphlet, Bascom Johnson wrote to a member of the Social Protection Division to inquire about the objectives of the program: "Is it to cut down venereal disease or is the reduction of VD a by-product of the real objective which is the prevention and reduction of sexual promiscuity?"[21] Johnson's question went unanswered.

Though military policy concerning the venereal diseases essentially mirrored the program of World War I, there was one significant difference. Although it had been Army policy since 1912 to withhold pay from soldiers for injury or disease incurred "not in the line of duty," Congress had actually passed a statute in 1926 making this injunction uniform. In January 1943 the surgeon general of the Army recommended that the law requiring the loss of pay for servicemen infected with a venereal disease be repealed. The surgeon general's request touched off a bitter debate, demonstrating both an important shift in attitudes regarding venereal diseases as well as the recalcitrance of positions held since the early twentieth century and before that emphasized personal responsibility for infection. Many continued to view the law as an important deterrent to exposure; nevertheless, a number of medical officers now argued that it did not effectively serve this purpose. According to a member of the Army Air Force medical staff, for example, the law had led to the concealment of infection, and clandestine treatment. Pilots were found to be continuing to fly while taking treatment, a considerable risk.[22] Others, prominent in the venereal disease control movement, joined the campaign against the law. J. E. Moore, chairman of the Subcommittee on Venereal Diseases of the National Research Council, argued vigorously for repeal, suggesting that concealment of infection merely led to additional infections. Moreover, the biological inequity implied—that some men became infected while others escaped despite exposure—was also offered as an argument against the no-pay provision.

Members of the medical corps had fundamentally revised certain notions of individual responsibility for health promulgated during World War I. They recognized that the risk of infection should not be borne by the individual soldier alone. As Thomas Sternberg explained: "When men are taken from the relative safety of their home environment and placed in situations where the risk of infection is many times as great, the Government should be ready to assume some share of the responsibility, just as it has always done in the care of other diseases." But a number of critics suggested that revising this provision would only lead to greater promiscuity among the troops, and thus to higher rates of infection.[23] The debate over the no-pay provision thus went right to the heart of the evaluation of the meaning of venereal disease and its causality. Was venereal disease merely the result of an individual's willful exposure, or should external, environmental, and social factors that might contribute to a tendency to exposure be considered? Moreover, did punishment for incurring an infection serve the military's purpose? Congress settled the debate in September 1944 by repealing the provisions calling for loss of pay. Soldiers infected during the war would not suffer punishment by the federal government as one of the consequences of the disease.

This change was among the factors credited by military officials for their ability to keep venereal disease under control. Parran's national campaign during the late 1930s had already lowered incidence before conscription. Among the first two million men drafted, 48 in every 1,000 were found to be infected with syphilis. Rates among blacks ran particularly high, with 272 per 1000 infected. The rate of infection in the South was found to be four times the rate in the North. During the early years of mobilization individuals discovered to be infected with a venereal disease during draft physicals were rejected for service. According to military officials, the induction of these men would have created an impossible burden for the medical service. Early in 1942, however, the Army reversed this policy, which many critics had found objectionable, and began inducting individuals with uncomplicated cases of gonorrhea, syphilis, and chancroid. As one military physician explained: "The Army benefitted by obtaining a large number of individuals suitable for military service at a time when the manpower situation was acute."[24] By December 1945, some 200,000 individuals had been treated at thirty-four barrack-hospitals upon joining the military; 170,000 of these had syphilis. Even before the advent of antibiotics, new treatment procedures had shortened the length of stay in these hospitals to a mere ten days before reassignment to a training camp. With penicillin, days lost to venereal disease were again significantly decreased.

Although in 1940 the venereal disease rate in the Army had risen to 42.5 per 1000, by 1943 it had fallen to 25. This, it should be remembered, occurred before the provision of penicillin. In fact, Army data for rates of infection within the military were essentially equivalent to civilian rates. For the entire duration of the war the average incidence of venereal disease was 37 per 1000. Perhaps even more significant from the standpoint of military efficiency, days lost to service because of venereal disease dramatically decreased as treatment regimes were refined. In 1940, for each 1000 men, 1,278 days a year were lost from duty because of venereal infections. By 1943 this level had been reduced to 368 days.[25]

5

The discovery of the effectiveness of penicillin had a remarkable impact on the ability to control venereal diseases, both during the war and the years which followed. In early 1943 Dr. John Mahoney of the U.S. Public Health Service was provided with strains of penicillin by a group of investigators at Oxford, England. Injecting the penicillin into syphilitic rabbits, Mahoney found that their symptoms dramatically disappeared, as did miscroscopic evidence of the spirochete. Realizing the potential implications of his discovery, Mahoney moved directly to repeat the experiment with a human subject. By September, he had announced his findings, and the massive production of penicillin was under way. The Office of Scientific Research and Development financed much of the research of production and costs of testing penicillin, allocating more than $2 million to this effort. The Northern Regional Research Laboratory of the Department of Agriculture made two significant discoveries that yielded greater quantities of penicillin: they found that growth in corn steep liquor increased the yield, and they identified a strain of penicillin more productive than the original Oxford variety. By 1949, some 650 billion units per month were produced; prices dropped from $20 per vial of 100,000 units to less than a dollar in 1945, and 30 cents in 1947. The exigencies of war had dramatically collapsed the normal time for testing, research, production, and distribution. Such rapid medical innovation was virtually unprecedented. The medical department concluded that without penicillin a major epidemic might have been possible, particularly as discipline broke down during demobilization.[26]

Within a year of Mahoney's September 1943 announcement, more than

10,000 patients had received penicillin for treatment of early syphilis. Rates of cure were an unprecedented 90 to 97 percent. Researchers soon demonstrated equally impressive results with penicillin against gonorrhea. Penicillin also proved to be of benefit for patients with late syphilis and paresis; though improvement was often slower, it was, nevertheless, significant in most cases. Although rates of infection had been falling since the provisions of the National Venereal Disease Control Act brought many new cases under treatment in the late 1930s, as penicillin became widely available rates began to fall dramatically. In the postwar years incidence of syphilis continued to drop. In 1940 the death rate for syphilis had stood at 10.7 per 100,000; a decade later, after the widespread availability of antibiotics, it was 5 per 100,000. By 1955, the rate had again been cut in half. In 1970, it was only 0.2 per 100,000. Deaths among infants from congenital syphilis fell even more precipitously: 5.3 per 10,000 births in 1940; 0.57 in 1950; 0.04 in 1968. Early cases of syphilis in New York City, for example, declined some 90 percent from 1946 to 1955. During these same years admissions to New York State mental hospitals for syphilis dropped by more than 50 percent, from 384 to 167.[27] Without question, antibiotics had transformed the nature of venereal disease. Though they were still important and prevalent public health problems gonorrhea and, in particular, syphilis, no longer held the danger that they had in the pre-penicillin years.

By the middle of the 1950s it seemed that venereal infections could no longer be considered a major public health threat. In 1949 Mahoney had written, "As a result of antibiotic therapy, gonorrhea has almost passed from the scene as an important clinical and public entity." An article in the *American Journal of Syphilis* in 1951 asked, "Are Venereal Diseases Disappearing?" Although the article concluded that it was too soon to tell, by 1955, at the height of optimism, the *Journal* itself had disappeared. *The Journal of Social Hygiene*, for half a century the leading publication on social dimensions of the problem, also ceased publication. And in 1956, the Joint Commission of Accreditation of Hospitals scotched the blood-test requirement for hospital admissions it had maintained in the past. In 1957 the number of cases of primary and secondary syphilis reached an all time low of 3.9 per 100,000; gonorrhea, always more prevalent than syphilis, had fallen to 127.4 per 100,000. In 1947 these rates had stood at 66.4 and 270.0 respectively. As the incidence fell, John Mahoney reflected upon the implications for venereal disease and public health policy:

> Hence, because of antibiotic therapy, the two important venereal diseases have undergone major changes in character. Their importance as public health entities, based upon their ability to produce human suffering, definitely has changed. It should not be inferred that there are not remaining problems which require solution. However, the practical health administrator must weigh the relative importance of what is left of the venereal disease field, against the demands of such potent factors as heart disease, cancer, arthritis, and mental health. In this comparison, the venereal group loses much of its importance.[28]

In the last years of the 1950s it appeared that the venereal diseases would join a host of other infectious diseases from polio to tuberculosis, now under the command of modern medicine.

6

The quick cure that penicillin offered for syphilis and gonorrhea raised considerable concern about its impact on sexual mores. After the war, the military significantly revised policies concerning the venereal diseases, once again emphasizing a moral approach rather than prophylaxis. The so-called "score techniques," emphasizing the use of condoms and prophylaxis, were replaced by what the Army called "character guidance;" companies were directed to spend at least one hour each week "building character." In phraseology reminiscent of the World War I educational campaign, soldiers were told to "work hard and play hard. . . . Some day a healthy little youngster will be glad to call you father." The Army recalled shock films and replaced graphic posters with family pictures titled, "Remember They Are Waiting, Avoid Venereal Disease." Programmatic statements stressed "self-control, self-discipline, and the worth of right conduct, clean living and its rewards." Moreover, the previous centrality of prophylaxis was now questioned: "Prophylaxis will be mentioned and discussed in a scientific manner, bringing out its limitations," explained the Medical Corps. "No more than ten percent of the time of one lecture should be expended on the subject of prophylaxis." In addition, it was now recommended that venereal patients be restricted from leaves and not recommended for promotion; this marked a return to the policy of punishment for venereal infection.[29] Without the exigencies of war, it seemed, the military could afford to revert to this approach.

This dramatic shift in military policy reflected a growing concern about venereal disease control in the age of antibiotics. Now that the venereal diseases were no longer the health menace that they once were, fear surfaced that a moral debacle might be the ultimate result. This is most clearly seen in the reactions of some physicians to the widespread use of penicillin. Dr. John Stokes, for example, soon reached the conclusion that effective treatment would make the problem worse. He commented in 1944: "Quick and easy cure is turning out . . . to be less of a device for the control of infection than an incentive to epidemicity through incitement to exposure. . . . Our boys and girls need help and knowledge to face this promiscuity that is rotting the family at its roots. There is no family immunity to these diseases." Several years later, Stokes's alarm had increased: "Mere treatment of venereal disease is certainly not the answer. And were it the answer, and were venereal diseases wiped out, it is now clear that the accomplishment would have heavy costs in the social, moral, and material life of man. A world of accepted, universalized, safeguarded promiscuity is something to look at searchingly before it is accepted." It is important to remember just who Stokes was. An original member of the Clinical Cooperative Group, he had been fundamental in establishing effective treatment regimens in the 1920s and 1930s. Indeed, as Director of the Institute for Venereal Disease Control at the University of Pennsylvania he was one of the leading clinical syphilographers in the nation, as well as author of one of the two most important textbooks concerning the treatment of venereal disease. Yet penicillin forced Stokes to have second thoughts. His view was not unlike that expressed by the military physician, Dr. Glantz, in William Styron's play about venereal disease during World War II, *In the Clap Shack*:

> Won't [penicillin] open up the floodgates of vice? For if a libertine knows he can indulge himself with impunity, he will throw all caution to the winds. What universal debauchery this might portend for our nation![30]

Antibiotics prompted those whose primary concern had always been sexual mores rather than disease to rethink their priorities. Stokes commented that antibiotics might have the impact of "subsidizing venery" and "may inaugurate a world of accepted, universalized, safeguarded promiscuity." In the view of Philip Mather of the ASHA, sexuality itself had become the problem: "When you get into venereal diseases you get into sex and when you get into sex you get into the most fundamental thing in the human race. We can't *cure* it." In this turn of phrase, Mather transformed sexuality itself into disease. Solving the venereal disease problem, in this view, made the problem of sexuality that much more difficult. William Snow, for almost half a century the leader of the American Social Hygiene Association, directly confronted this issue at a conference held at the end of the war:

> It is obvious . . . that sexual morality should not be taught to young people primarily because it serves as a method of avoiding venereal disease infection. Sex promiscuity is only one of many 'symptoms' of departure from the moral and ethical principles upon which our culture is based, and venereal disease is one of the many damaging results of misuse of the reproductive instinct.

With venereal disease no longer a threat, the rationale for public health involvement in public mores became increasingly tenuous. Public health officials noted that the increase in promiscuity threatened the basic family structure: "Sexual promiscuity is sexual irresponsibility. The place of the family as the indisputable unit of society cannot be secure so long as sexual irresponsibility is the order of the day." This was a task which many health officers now saw as beyond their scope. "It is not the responsibility of the health officer, alone, to teach people how to behave or why they should behave," noted an editorial in the *American Journal of Public Health*.[31]

Penicillin posed, fundamentally, the problem of medicine's role in sexual prescription. As Stokes made clear, implicit in the physician's response to venereal disease was the question of the doctor's function as social and sexual arbiter—a role which Stokes considered particularly important:

> It is a reasonable question, whether by eliminating disease, without commensurate attention to the development of human idealsim, self-control, and responsibility in the sexual life, we are not bringing mankind to its fall instead of fulfillment. When as he sometimes does, the physician takes the stand that his business is the extinction of disease by any and every method, regardless of its moral repercussions, and lets the chaplain look after the rest, he is on dangerous ground. First of all, he is

a leader and secondly, a servant of bodily health. If he debases the spirit of man by the methods he employs to save his body, he is indeed the Devil's servant. . . . If he is to measure up to his humanistic tradition he must concern himself constructively with the conservation of family living, and with education for it.

Indeed, Stokes's response to penicillin's efficacy is fully analogous to Prince Morrow's reaction to Salvarsan a generation earlier. These doctors, deeply committed to solving the problem of venereal disease, nevertheless harbored fears concerning the medical treatment of these ailments because they anticipated a sort of "Frankenstein effect" in which the cure could be worse than the disease. To solve the problem of venereal disease without directing sufficient attention to the ancillary "problem" of sexual morality would, to these physicians, be an abdication of their social responsibilities. This reflects a more fundamental medicalization of sexuality—a significant theme in twentieth-century medicine. All this, of course, is not to suggest that these physicians sought in any way to restrict the use of effective treatments, but that they voiced anxieties about the social implications of their own prescriptions. Deputy Surgeon General William F. Draper effectively exposed the fallacy underlying Stokes's argument:

> The doubt on the part of those concerned about the possibility that effective treatment may remove inhibitions against exposure to venereal disease is based on the assumption that fear of infection in the past has served as an effective brake. Considering the wide prevalence of syphilis and gonorrhea before the new treatment methods were introduced, the effectiveness of fear as a preventive of venereal disease is questionable.
>
> Carrying to their ultimate conclusion the implication of the idea that effective treatment encourages the spread of venereal disease do we not arrive at the amazing position that in order to prevent venereal disease we should stop treating it, or search for treatment methods of only partial effectiveness?[32]

By 1946, when Draper wrote this, there was considerable evidence that "syphilophobia" had failed as an effective preventive measure. There were some, however, who refused to relinquish the metaphor of venereal disease to therapy.

7

Unfortunately, the decline of venereal disease as a significant public health problem proved short-lived. By the last years of the 1950s and the first years of the 1960s, venereal rates had begun to climb once again. In the decade from 1965 to 1975, cases of gonorrhea more than tripled, rising to over 1 million per year. By 1980 most projections suggested that more than 2.5 million cases were communicated, with a small but growing number resistant to standard antibiotic therapy. Gonorrhea, according to reports of the federally operated Centers for Disease Control, constitutes the nation's most common and costly communicable disease. Although rates of syphilis rose at a somewhat slower rate, and its long range hazards were often mitigated by antibiotic treatments, it, too, remained a significant problem. From a low point in 1958, cases had more than quadrupled by 1975, which made syphilis the third most prevalent communicable disease behind gonorrhea and chicken pox.[33] As the extent of the new epidemic became clear, the optimism of the 1950s gave way.

Many public health officials and physicians attributed this increase to what they called the three "p's": permissiveness, promiscuity, and the Pill. In this view the so-called "sexual revolution" of the 1960s led to increased premarital sexual activity and more infections. There is little doubt that a fundamental shift in American sexual mores did indeed take place in that decade, but it is important to note that premarital sexual relations had been occurring with greater frequency throughout the century. Alfred Kinsey reported in his renowned 1948 study of male sexuality that 44 percent of college men had engaged in premarital sex by the age of 20. This percentage rose gradually, depending upon the locale and sample population; a 1968 study found that 58 percent reported having had prematiral intercourse. Data from women indicate a more fundamental shift. In 1953 Kinsey reported that 20 percent of college women had engaged in premarital coitus; a 1967 study found this percentage had climbed to 44 percent. Many attributed a relatively sudden rise in female premarital relations to the widespread availability of oral contraceptives after 1965. Unquestionably, another element of this "sexual revolution" or new permissiveness, as many of its critics chose to call it, was the upsurge of the gay rights movement and increased sexual activity within the gay community. As a new emphasis on individual consent has increasingly supplanted societally imposed moral strictures, tolerance of varied sexual practices grew.[34] By the late 1960s an undeniable sexualization of many facets of American life had occurred. Notably, advertising, mass media, and other elements of consumer culture self-consciously promulgated sexual images and encouraged attention to sexual aspects of everyday life. The rise in venereal rates was increasingly attributed to these changes, and venereal disease incidence was calculated by some critics of the new mores as a statistical index of immorality.

Changes in sexual practices cannot alone account for the sudden increase in venereal rates. It is overly simplistic, for instance, to cite the Pill as a "cause" of this rise in rates of infection. Studies have shown that women who rely on the Pill for contraception are at no greater risk to contract a venereal disease than those who use any form of birth control and, indeed, those who use no form of birth control at all. In fact, some recent studies have demonstrated that the Pill may actually act to prevent the development of pelvic inflammatory disease. Barrier forms of contraception—especially condoms and diaphragms—are also known to decrease the possibility of some infections. Some contraceptive foams and spermicides apparently have bacteriocidal properties, particularly for gonococcus. The relationship of contraceptive technique to the prevention of venereal disease has too often been overlooked in clinical practice; further research seems clearly indicated. Ironically, birth control, frequently cited as the principal cause of the new epidemic, may provide a means of combatting the problem. Moreover, according to several recent studies, individuals with venereal infections report the same number of sexual partners as does a similar population free of infection.[35] There is no clear correlation between promiscuity, birth control, and disease.

Additional factors therefore need to be assessed to understand the rise in venereal rates. Even as sexual mores were liberalized in the 1960s, attitudes towards the venereal diseases proved more resistant to change. The introduction of sex education into secondary school curricula, for example, was bitterly opposed in many communities. In 1964 NBC cancelled plans to air a two-part drama on two popular television series, "Mr. Novak" and "Dr. Kildare," in which a high school student contracted venereal disease. An NBC official explained: "If the drama were to be valid, it would have to contain passages and dialogue, including a discussion of sexual intercourse, that the network considered inappropriate for television." NBC refused to relent despite the protests of the American Public Health Association and the U.S. Public Health Service. Dr. Kildare would have to restrict his practice to diagnosing and treating rarer and more respectable diseases. Even the American Medical Association, which instituted a publicity campaign for the control of syphilis and gonorrhea in the 1960s, deleted these words from its advertisements. Moreover, the AMA refused to discuss preventive techniques such as the use of condoms, seeking not to appear to sanction promiscuity. "The consequences of this prudery," noted the *Nation*, "are far more damaging than the immorality which its adherents fear to encourage." In 1982 the staff of the State Commission of Education in Texas recommended the deletion of all references to venereal disease in all textbooks. The deputy commissioner explained, "The bottom-line issue is, when you're talking about sexually transmitted diseases you're relating it to 'How do you get it.' "[36] Despite significant shifts in sexual mores, attitudes that associate venereal disease with sin persist, inhibiting physicians from reporting their cases and making contact tracing and control more difficult.

Although many attributed the resurgence in venereal rates to the sexual revolution of the 1960s and 1970s, the failure of public health institutions to meet changing needs in the area of sexually transmitted diseases seems at least equally important. The effectiveness of penicillin, a shift in priorities within the public health establishment, and a desire to reduce federal expenditures all led to substantial reductions in appropriations for venereal disease control during the 1950s. In 1949 during a period of rising venereal rates in the immediate post-war years, Congress had made the largest commitment of federal funds for the venereal disease program ever: nearly $18 million. The following year, however, as rates decreased, this sum was cut by $7 million. In 1953 funding had been reduced to under $10 million; a year later the appropriation had been halved again. By 1955 venereal disease control received only $3 million from the federal budget. "The partial success in treatment and control, while justifying a feeling of satisfaction," Dr. Thomas Sternberg explained in 1952, "hardly warrants the flagging interest so evident today."[37]

Given the fact that effective treatment had preceded the introduction of the antimicrobials, it should have been clear that antibiotics alone could not solve the venereal problem. But the remarkable successes achieved with penicillin did appear to make the venereal diseases a problem which merited considerably less attention. James K. Shafer explained: "The heart of the matter today is whether, with venereal disease under partial control, we shall dismantle our control machinery instead of reorienting it to changing needs." As appropriations fell during the 1950s many public health workers and the ASHA began to express alarm:

Five years ago, the forces of V.D. Control were on the offensive, in state after state aggressive control programs were gaining the advantage. Before an intergrated system of information, case-finding, referral, and rapid treatment, the venereal diseases were melting away. The resulting optimism proved disastrous. Forgotten, even by some health officials, was the carefully perfected epidemiological apparatus that brought the patient and the penicillin together. The infectious syphilis rate was pitched so sharply downward (and gonorrhea rates had also started down) that it was inconceivable they would stop, even if all programming ceased. Anybody could get and take penicillin.

The intervening years and the painful review of some carefully documented hindsight have established the fact that drugs alone do not stop venereal disease.[38]

By the late 1950s much of the machinery, especially procedures for case-finding, tracing, and diagnostics, had been cut back. In addition, continued reliance on earlier public health techniques despite changing conditions limited the impact of some progams. Premarital testing, for example, revealed few infections, often only reaching a population at a relatively lower risk for venereal infection. In 1976 in New York City, for instance, only 39 cases of previously undetected syphilis were found in approximately 116,000 premarital venereal examinations. The total costs of these tests was $2.3 million; therefore, the cost of uncovering these cases was almost $60,000 per case. National figures for the costs of case-finding from premarital exams were equally striking. More than $80 million was spent by prospective brides and grooms to reveal but 456 cases. Meanwhile, screening programs for higher-risk populations such as homosexuals, college students, and sexually active teenagers were rarely, if ever, instituted. Programs for the distribution of condoms—known to prevent effectively the transmission of most infections—remained severely limited. As recently as 1977, eleven states still had statutes prohibiting stores from publicly displaying prophylactics.[39]

After the introduction of penicillin, the tracing of contacts—a key aspect of control efforts—became much more difficult. Many physicians no longer saw the importance of identifying contacts when treatment could be applied with such great effect so quickly, and patients often no longer saw the need to identify partners, if the diseases held so little danger. Moreover, the moralistic tenor of some venereal disease workers discouraged patients from revealing contacts. In the early 1950s, the Public Health Service had established a class on interviewing techniques. Contact epidemiologists were advised to show "no outward concern" during the interviews with patients. Robert R. Swank, who conducted these courses, explained why, in his view, it was difficult to get patients to cooperate in revealing their sexual contacts:

> Because of egocentricism, the patient's prestige, or his social status. Someone has said that 97 out of 100 people are liars and that liars lie most often when their prestige is involved. A person with VD is caught in an immoral and illegal act . . . acts which lower his prestige.[40]

With this persistent set of assumptions, it is small wonder that many individuals withheld the names of their contacts, or attempted to circumvent such interviews altogether. Despite his admonition to "judge not," Swank told his classes, "Discount 99½ percent of all rape stories."

Most significantly, federal expenditures for controlling the sexually transmitted diseases remained at low levels while the social and economic costs of the new epidemic continued to rise. Pelvic inflammatory disease, for example, frequently a complication of untreated gonorrhea, led to the hospitalization of some 22 million women in 1976 alone, at a cost of $229 million; in the same year the total congressional appropriation for venereal disease control was $18 million. Although a federal commission recommended that $43.3 million would be needed by 1977 to establish an adequate venereal disease control program, Congress allocated only $23 million; this, despite the fact that cases of gonorrhea had risen by more than 250 percent in the preceding decade. Although the incidence of gonorrhea had begun to climb rapidly as early as 1961, it was not until 1972 that the Public Health Service established a specific program designed to control the epidemic. Commenting on the dramatic increases in all types of venereal infections, one federal health official noted, "No one would have allowed this to happen with measles or polio." Funding for research concerning the venereal diseases has also remained extremely limited. In 1976 venereal diseases received only one-fifth of one percent of the National Institutes of Health's $2.5 billion budget, a total of approximately $8 million. By 1980 this figure, adjusted for inflation, had actually fallen.[41] With such limited funding, hopes for the development of vaccinations to prevent infection have dimmed.

It thus seems clear that it is not possible to attribute the new epidemic of venereal disease to a change in sexual mores alone. There has been a fairly direct correlation to government spending in the area of venereal disease control and rates of infection; shortly after federal funding peaked in the early 1950s, rates reached all time low points. After funding was severely cut back in the late 1950s, incidence of infection again began to climb. Public health institutions and practice, too, are subject to social and economic forces which may limit their application. Leading the fight for venereal disease appropriations has rarely been viewed as a springboard to a wider constituency, as many other health care issues now are. In this sense, one could argue that the new epidemic, rather than being merely the result of the new mores, is also the result of a more traditional ethic that has emphasized behavioral and moral means as the best way of combatting venereal disease, rather than medical and public health approaches. In this view, the answer to the venereal epidemic is relatively simple: reduce promiscuity.

8

The current epidemic of venereal diseases has eaten away the last vestiges of reticence. It seems almost impossible, given the power of the contemporary media, not to be aware of the venereal problem. Advertisements for clinics and hot lines announcing opportunities for diagnosis and treatment are aired frequently, especially for late-night television viewers, and articles can be found in newspapers and national publications outlining the extent of the problem. In 1980 alone more than two million cases of gonorrhea were reported in the United States. Syphilis and gonorrhea have been joined by a myriad of other sexually transmitted infections with less familiar names: non-gonococcal urethritis, chlamydias, and antibiotic resistant strains. Widely publicized because of its prevalence and incurability is herpes simplex virus II (HSV-2), or genital herpes. Estimates of the incidence of genital herpes in the United States vary from 5 million to the more frequently cited figure of 20 million, with 600,000 new infections now occurring annually.[42] The response to herpes indicates several of the most important themes in the social history of venereal disease.

Herpes, named for the Greek word "herpein" meaning "to creep," is a virus that crawls along the nerve pathways. There are some seventy varieties of herpes viruses, ranging from chicken pox and shingles to the common cold sores that three-quarters of the population experience at one time or another. Outbreaks of genital herpes are usually marked by clusters of small red lumps that soon turn into painful blisters on the genitalia, buttocks, and thighs. Rates of infection are high because genital herpes is incurable. Once infected, a herpes victim carries the virus—though it may often be in a dormant phase—in the nerve endings near the base of the spine. Although some individuals never experience symptoms after the initial outbreak, in most cases the virus will periodically travel back down the nerve and erupt in new skin lesions. There is no way of predicting when or how frequently this process may occur. Researchers have found that factors ranging from diet to stress may trigger the dormant virus to enter its active phase. When the virus does erupt it is highly contagious and herpes patients are advised to abstain from all sexual relations.[43]

A number of recent articles in the popular press have raised the specter of genital herpes in a forbidding and foreboding tone. *Time* called the infection the "new sexual leprosy"; in a later cover story, it chose to label herpes "today's scarlet letter." The heavy emphasis in these and other assessments is on sexual behavior; herpes and other venereal infections are portrayed as the seamy underside of the sexual liberation of the 1960s and 1970s. "It is beginning to seem that the new mores may be every bit as physically dangerous as the old mores were psychologically repressive," concluded New York's *Soho Weekly News*.[44]

In these assessments of the current herpes epidemic, three major themes characteristic of the history of venereal disease in the twentieth century are generally expressed, themes that illuminate the particular social and cultural values associated with venereal disease. First, venereal disease is considered a disease of behavior, a punishment (be it just or unjust) for those who take risks. Second, the danger of venereal disease is raised to argue (at least implicitly, but often explicitly) for a more restricted sexuality. And finally, venereal infection is viewed as not just a disease but as a symptom of a more profound sociosexual maladjustment, a failure of control. As the *Soho Weekly News* explained: "Perhaps it's current sexual practice that is the real epidemic and the rash of sexually transmitted diseases raging through the city simply a symptom."[45] This statement bears scrutiny, for the author has transformed venereal disease, the biomedical entity, into a symptom of social decay.

Increasingly, venereal disease is seen as a revenge against the sexual revolution and the modern medical technology that helped to make it possible. Attitudes have been expressed that are not unlike those that characterized the nineteenth century view of disease as the logical and deserved result of immorality. Herpes is now cited as proof that you cannot fool Mother Nature. Evangelist Billy Graham recently argued: "We have the Pill. We have conquered VD with penicillin. But then along comes Herpes Simplex II. Nature itself lashes back when we go against God."[46] In this view, science itself becomes a culprit; modern medicine, through contraception, abortion, and the antibiotic treatment of syphilis and gonorrhea, has spurred a shift in mores that is seen as violating basic religious and moral precepts.

In a number of other ways, the herpes epidemic forces a return to the first decades of the twentieth century, before the advent of Salvarsan. Today, for example, herpes is frequently cited—as were syphilis and gonorrhea in 1900— as the tell-tale sign of philandering. "Wives now give their husbands smiling lectures on the ravages of disease to keep them faithful," noted *Time*. Phyllis Schlafly, the nemesis of contemporary feminism, has counseled—as did her Victorian ancestors—"marry only a virgin." As it was in the early decades of the century, the possibility of extra-genital infections has been raised: two UCLA researchers reported that the herpes virus can live on towels and toilet seats. This finding, which, significantly, other researchers failed to confirm, serves to generate fears of contamination.[47]

Herpes seems to be feared among the public beyond its real dangers to health. Although, in reality, the long-term dangers of herpes are minor compared to those of syphilis, in a recent poll 47 percent of those questioned believed that genital herpes is a more dangerous disease than syphilis; only 23 percent responded that syphilis presented greater danger. Herpes does raise some significant health problems, especially for women. If a pregnant woman has active herpes during delivery, her child may become infected leading to retardation or death; this possibility, however, can be avoided by caesarean section. Some studies have indicated that women with herpes have a higher incidence of cervical cancer, and should receive more frequent Pap smears; on the other hand, no causal connection has been established between herpes and cervical cancer. Generally, the dangers of herpes have been exaggerated. As one physician at the National Institutes of Health notes: "If you total up the more serious complications from herpes there are only a couple of thousand or so cases a year."[48]

From a strictly scientific standpoint genital herpes is more of an annoyance than a danger; but for many who become infected it is a serious problem. As many physicians have made clear, the most dangerous sequelae of herpes, if treated and carefully watched, are psychological. Guilt, anger, and remorse are all widely reported among herpes sufferers. A frequent response of those infected, according to many reports, is to feel contaminated or "poisoned." "You never think you're clean enough," explained one herpes victim. Many come to reject sex altogether. As one medical assistant remarked: "We hear it over and over: 'I won't have sex again.' "[49] Stress builds for herpes victims with the possibility of each new relationship or potential sexual encounter. These attitudes, however, are not merely a consequence of the disease; rather, they are the result of the historical assumptions and values which have shaped the definition and response to venereal disease in this century. In this sense, victims suffer not just from the virus, but from the burden of history as well.

Clearly, for many individuals who become infected, herpes is a tragedy. It is a tragedy, however, not because of its physiological implications, but because of the stigma and psychological ramifications the disease carries with it. Here is a case where the disease—the biological entity—is of far less consequence than the illness—the individual's subjective response to disease. This response is refracted through the weighty stigma that is associated with infection.

The image of the herpes victim portrayed in most accounts is stereotyped and stigmatized: the mindless narcissist, the hedonistic orgiast, the promiscuous young professional. Individuals with herpes are viewed as lepers, lurking in the sexual community: "With visions of herpes sores clouding each new encounter, would-be lovers who used to gaze romantically into each other's eyes now look for the telltale blink or averted glance of the dissembling herpetic." According to *Time*, herpes sufferers are unusually angry, unusually dishonest, and unusually promiscuous. Indeed, the stereotypical view of the individual infected with herpes, applied by *Time* and a host of other recent commentaries, is not unlike the views of venereal victims ascribed throughout the century. The moral judgment is explicit; these diseases are received only through choice—a willful choice of questionable morals and mores. Moreover, the implication that herpes victims have got what they ultimately deserve runs beneath the surface of all these discussions. "Like many women who grew up during the sexual revolution, Susan was determined to take control of her life—to be free, whatever that meant," noted one journalist. "But now she is out of control in the worst way possible—out of control of her own body."[50]

These stereotypes, unfortunately, are even tacitly endorsed by those seeking to aid victims. When the American Social Health Association set up a hot line and organization for assisting individuals with herpes, they called the group HELP, an acronym for Herpetics Engaged in Living Productively. The contradiction between the medium and the message is explicit. First, the whole notion of a noun which identifies the infected individual by the disease itself—herpetic—contributes to the stigma the infection carries. Few other diseases have generated such words and almost all of those which have are stigmatized in particular ways: diabetic, epileptic, syphilitic, schizophrenic; the patient *is* the disease. Second, the notion of "Living Productively" reinforces the stigma; why would there be any assumption to the contrary, if not for prevailing views of these individuals and their morality? The irony of a group so named, organized to aid individuals with the psychological adjustment to the disease, is remarkable.[51]

The persistent tension between a rational, scientific program and a behavioral, moralistic approach continues to characterize current efforts to deal with venereal diseases, as it has throughout the twentieth century. In its consideration of herpes, for instance, *Time* emphasized the behavioral aspects of the problem, concluding that the current epidemic was already having a salutary impact on American sexual practice. According to *Time*, the proliferation of herpes was fundamentally altering behavior: "Those remarkable numbers [of infections] are altering sexual rites in America, changing courtship patterns, sending thousands of sufferers spinning in months of depression and self-exile and delivering a numbing blow to the one night stand." "The herpes counter-revolution," declared *Time*, in curiously celebratory fashion, "may be ushering a reluctant, grudging chastity back into fashion." There is scant, if any, evidence to indicate that the herpes epidemic is bringing about such a change. Heightened fears of infection, generated in part by sensational coverage, do not necessarily lead to behavioral change. *Time* chose to conclude by seeing positive implications in the herpes epidemic:

> Perhaps not so unhappily, it may be a prime mover in helping to bring to a close an era of mindless promiscuity. . . . For all the distress it has brought the troublesome little bug may inadvertently be ushering in a period in which sex is linked more firmly to commitment and trust.[52]

This seems an unusually optimistic and unwarranted assumption. Even if herpes was to lead to less promiscuity, would it necessarily lead to healthier and more fulfilling sexual relationships?

Herpes became a social symbol for a corrupt sexuality; it was *used* by social critics to argue for restraint. But heightened stigma and fear do not necessarily lead to less sexually transmitted disease. Herpes did make clear that even in the age of antibiotics, infections might prove intransigent to treatment. Soon the herpes epidemic, shaped and defined by the media, would be overshadowed by a far more serious and threatening disease, AIDS.

VI

"Plagues and Peoples": The AIDS Epidemic

1

As we have seen in the course of chronicling responses to sexually transmitted diseases in the twentieth century, the process by which a disease is defined has a fundamental impact on the character of policies devised to eliminate it. In the unfolding of the AIDS epidemic, we see this process at work.[1]

In light of the history of sexually transmitted diseases in the last century, it is almost impossible to watch the AIDS epidemic without experiencing a sense of *déjà vu*. AIDS raises a host of concerns traditional to the debates about venereal infection, from morality to medicine, sexuality and deviancy, prevention and intervention. In many instances the situation today with AIDS is similar to that with syphilis in the early twentieth century. Like syphilis, AIDS can cause death; presently has no effective treatment; education and social engineering characterize efforts to halt the epidemic—given that no magic bullet is on the horizon; fears, reflecting deeper social and cultural anxieties about the disease, its victims, and transmissibility, abound.

And yet AIDS is different.

2

In June 1981 in a weekly report surveying disease patterns in the United States, the federally operated Centers for Disease Control announced an unusual outbreak of disease in Los Angeles. Five homosexual men were reported to have a rare form of pneumonia caused by *Pneumocystis carinii*, a protozoan infection usually seen only in individuals whose immune systems have been compromised. The report suggested the possibility of "an association between some aspect of homosexual lifestyle or disease acquired from sexual contact."[2] By the following month, CDC revealed that Kaposi's sarcoma, a rare cancer, had been diagnosed in 26 gay men during the previous two and a half years. Kaposi's sarcoma is also associated with damage to the immune system. Physicians, recognizing a growing pattern of gay men with an assortment of infections in San Francisco, New York, and Los Angeles, soon defined a new syndrome, known initially as Gay Related Immune Disease or GRID. Because of the obviously stigmatizing nature of this label the name was changed to AIDS, for Acquired Immunodeficiency Syndrome. This change was also appropriate in light of the recognition that the disease did not affect gay men only. Cases were reported among intravenous drug users, Haitians, as well as a few who fit no specific group. By 1982, AIDS had been diagnosed in hemophiliacs, patients who had received blood transfusions, heterosexual women, and young children.[3]

AIDS is usually characterized at its beginning by a series of symptoms: fevers, night sweats, chronic diarrhea, and enlarged lymph nodes. In addition, some patients present with oral "thrush," a yeast infection of the mouth, or Kaposi's sarcoma, which is characterized by purplish skin lesions. The diseases seen in AIDS patients had been known to occur only among those whose immune systems had been severely impaired either by drugs used to combat malignant disease or by those used to facilitate transplants by warding off rejection. Because the virus attacks the immune system, AIDS patients are subject to infection by microorganisms that are usually harmless to healthy individuals. Such "opportunistic infections" as pneumocystis pneumonia and cytomegalovirus are difficult to treat because of the compromised state of the patient's immune system; they are often the cause of death for AIDS patients. Later it was found that the infection could affect the central nervous system and lead to chronic meningitis, encephalopathy, and dementia. AIDS can thus cause an agonizing death, leading up to which the victim may become confused and demented; patients usually die within three years of the onset of symptoms. To date (late 1986) there are no effective treatments for the disease.[4]

By 1983 most researchers had come to believe that AIDS resulted from a transmissible virus. This expectation was confirmed in early 1984 when candidate viruses were isolated in both French and American laboratories. The day before Secretary of Health and Human Services Margaret Heckler's news conference to announce that Robert Gallo, a NIH scientist, had discovered a virus that is a principal cause of AIDS, it was learned that a team of researchers at the prestigious Pasteur Institute in Paris had also made such a discovery. Gallo named the virus HTLV-III, short for human T-cell leukemia virus, type III, while the French team under Luc Montagnier called it LAV for lymphadenopathy-associated-virus. Later research would confirm that they had found the same organism, a human retrovirus that destroys T4 helper cells, the white blood cells that detect invading viruses and activate the immune system.[5] Shortly after the discovery of HTLV-III/LAV, a test for antibodies to the virus was developed in Gallo's laboratory. The test, known as ELISA for Enzyme Linked Immunosorbent Assay, can reveal with relatively high accuracy whether or not an individual has been exposed to the virus.[6]

A bitter priority battle over the discovery of the virus ensued, eventually leading to litigation, when the French challenged the U.S. government's patent for the ELISA test. Although there have been outstanding examples of cooperation in AIDS research, the HTLV-III/LAV controversy and subsequent patent suit made clear that power, status, and money are also at stake. The dispute reveals some aspects of the culture of elite bioscience and its system of reward and prestige. Within scientific circles it is recognized that a Nobel Prize may well be the ultimate reward for AIDS research. AIDS, not surprisingly, has not been immune to scientific politics.[7] In an attempt to develop a neutral descriptive nomenclature, an international committee recently decided to call the AIDS virus HIV (Human Immunodeficiency Virus).

Much of the early research on the AIDS virus (HIV) has focused on producing a vaccine. The problem of developing a vaccine for AIDS indicates the complex interrelationship between technical biomedical questions and social, political, and economic issues. The scientific obstacles to developing a safe and effective vaccine for HIV are formidable. The virus mutates frequently—up to 1000 times as fast as a typical influenza virus. According to Dr. William Haseltine, "Trying to develop a vaccine for AIDS is like trying to hit a moving target."[8]

The discovery of an effective vaccine in the laboratory may in the end be less difficult than the process of negotiating its actual testing, production, and distribution. It will be difficult to identify an appropriate group of test subjects for any experimental application of the vaccine. Moreover, the extended incubation period of the disease—perhaps longer than five years—will complicate assessment of the vaccine's safety and efficacy. Even when these hurdles are cleared, the liability problems may turn out to be insurmountable without federal legislation.[9] As AIDS has exposed so many problems in contemporary biomedicine, the question of liability in vaccine manufacturing is yet another.

Even if all these difficulties could be overcome, an effective vaccine would not solve the AIDS problem. For the more than one million individuals already infected with the virus, a vaccine would be of no use. The only hope for these individuals is the development of effective treatments. Although there are now a few promising possibilities, none has yet been demonstrated. A major cooperative trial using anti-viral agents such as HPA-23, Foscarnet, ribavarin, and azidothymidine is currently being initiated at centers around the United States.[10] But these drugs are known to have serious, sometimes debilitating side effects, which is particularly worrisome in that they may have to be taken for life in order to prevent the virus from multiplying.

Despite the lethal virulence of the AIDS virus, it is not easily transmitted. There are only two demonstrated sources of infection: blood and semen. The virus has been most often spread through sexual intercourse, the most efficient mode of sexual transmission being anal receptive intercourse. By 1986, gay males accounted for almost 75 percent of all cases in the United States. The second source is through blood and blood products. Communication via infected blood accounts for the high rates of disease among intravenous drug users who share needles; addicts account for about 20 percent of all cases. In addition, there is a small percentage of cases of individuals who have received transfusions of infected blood or blood clotting factors that were contaminated. Children have been infected perinatally when their mothers carried the virus; others because they received infected blood transfusions or blood products.[11]

Although the relative number of transfusion-related cases remained low (approximately 1 percent), they raised alarm that the blood supply was contaminated. In March 1983 the U.S. Public Health Service formally requested that members of high-risk groups not donate blood. By early 1985 the ELISA test made it possible to screen all blood donations. Any blood found to be positive would then be destroyed. If the first ELISA test is positive it is usually repeated and supplemented by another test (the Western blot) to avoid the possibility of a false result. Since the establishment of screening procedures for all blood banks, the blood supply is no longer a serious risk for the transmission of the disease. Concerns about transmission through transfusion have nevertheless persisted, and a National Institutes of Health consensus panel recommended in 1986 that individuals facing elective surgery should donate their own blood in advance where possible. Storage of blood for unanticipated future use, however, was considered logistically impractical.[12]

Although most cases of AIDS have been associated with the two principal high-risk groups, homosexual males and intravenous drug users, the virus can be transmitted through vaginal intercourse. Infected men can transmit the virus sexually to a female partner. Though probably a less efficient mode of transmission, it is also possible for an infected woman to pass the infection to a male during sexual contact. In Central Africa and Haiti, rates of infection are divided evenly between men and women, suggesting that the virus may be passed in either direction. The effectiveness of female to male transmission remains, however, an issue of considerable scientific and public debate.[13]

Although scientists have isolated the virus in saliva and tears, evidence seems persuasive that the virus is not transmitted in casual contact. Despite considerable concern early in the epidemic that health care workers might be at risk, there are no known cases of an individual getting the disease simply by caring for a patient, even though health care personnel have logged literally hundreds of thousands of hours doing so. The CDC concluded that if its basic procedures for taking specimens and handling blood and blood products were followed, safety would be assured. If AIDS is not transmitted to health care workers, any employees in other work settings would not be placed at risk. Researchers investigating the non-sexual household contacts of patients with AIDS and AIDS-Related Complex found that there was no risk of infection. Along with interviews, examinations and tests for the AIDS antibody were performed on family members and individuals who lived in the same household as an AIDS patient for three months or more. No family members became ill, nor had they developed antibody for the disease.[14]

3

Within fewer than five years, to the initial handful of cases thousands were added, with ominous predictions for the future. By mid-1986, some 21,000 cases of AIDS had been recorded. But diagnosed cases of AIDS are really only the tragic, lethal tip of an epidemiological iceberg. Many more individuals, perhaps five to ten times as many, are currently suffering some effects of HIV infection. Such individuals, who have not been diagnosed as having full-blown AIDS, which has a highly specific set of medical criteria, have what is known as ARC, AIDS-Related Complex. It is not known how many of these individuals will eventually develop AIDS itself. Individuals with ARC, many of whom are quite sick, have difficulty gaining social services, counseling, and disability benefits. Some critics suggest that AIDS has been defined too narrowly; that it is really a disease with a wide spectrum of clinical manifestations. For example, many patients with HIV infections who suffer neurological disturbances may nevertheless fail to be counted among those with AIDS. There are no requirements for reporting ARC cases, and therefore epidemiologic surveillance is inadequate. By counting and recording only cases diagnosed as AIDS, the scope of the epidemic has been underestimated. To calculate the current and future dimensions of the epidemic, cases of ARC, as well as the large numbers of healthy individuals already infected with HIV, must be assessed.[15]

Indeed, the numbers of individuals who have been infected with the virus but have no symptoms are particularly alarming. Epidemiologists project that between one and two million individuals have been "exposed" to the virus, meaning they carry the virus and can infect others despite the fact that they currently are healthy. Such individuals live under a dark cloud of medical uncertainty; how many of them will go on to develop AIDS or ARC is unknown. Although early reports suggested that the great majority would suffer no untoward results, recent studies have questioned this finding, concluding that most will eventually develop some symptoms, if not the full-blown disease. Among the theories to account for the development of AIDS after infection with HIV is the hypothesis that clinical disease occurs in those whose immune systems are weakened by other factors. This would account for the prevalence among gay men, intravenous drug users, Africans, and Haitians, many of whom have multiple other infections. Research into co-factors that promote (or inhibit) the development of AIDS after infection obviously needs to be pursued. Individuals found to be infected with HIV are currently advised of ways to avoid exposing others to the virus. But they are also told to eat well, get enough sleep, and practice general moderation of all behaviors which might make them prone to infection. Infected individuals are also counseled to avoid all further chances of being exposed to the virus, on the theory that multiple exposures promote the development of disease. Such other factors as the dose of the virus, the way it enters the body, frequency of exposure, and general environmental conditions may determine the course the infection takes in any particular person or groups.[16]

The latency period between infection and clinical manifestation of the disease, though still not precisely known, can be at least five years. Complicating matters from a public health standpoint is the ominous fact that this large group of healthy carriers will probably remain infectious for life, thereby increasing the likelihood that the number of infected individuals will continue to grow. In short, AIDS is a biologically complex medical problem with all the markings of a major medical disaster. No doubt the epidemic will worsen before it abates. Experts now estimate that by the early 1990s there will be more than 270,000 cumulative cases of AIDS in the United States; 179,000 individuals will have died as a result of the disease.[17] AIDS is already having an important epidemiological impact. In New York City, for example, it has become the leading killer of men aged 33 to 44. Given the large number of variables associated with the disease, it may be decades before a clear epidemiological picture of the disease emerges.

Although AIDS was first recognized as a clinical entity in the United States, soon cases were diagnosed throughout the world. Scientists have suggested that the virus first may have entered the human species in Central Africa, where AIDS is now epidemic. In fact, there is probably a higher rate of HIV infection there than in the United States or Western Europe, although the extent of the epidemic remains unclear. Researchers have reported, for example, that among prostitutes who come to clinics for treatment, 27 percent in Zaire, 56 percent in Kenya, and 88 percent in Rwanda are infected with the AIDS virus. Individuals in cities tend to have higher rates of positivity than do those who live in the country. According to one recent report, between 1 and 2 percent of the entire African population now carries the AIDS virus. This has led to speculation that perhaps some environmental factor has led to such high rates of infection. Most striking is the differing epidemiological pattern in Africa, where the disease is equally divided between men and women, suggesting that heterosexual transmission is far more prevalent there than in the United States.[18] In this age of world travel there are no clear epidemiologic boundaries. AIDS is already a health problem of international dimensions.

Dr. Donald McDonald, Acting Assistant Secretary of the Department of Health and Human Services, described the epidemic as "staggering" and "devastating." Not only is it expected that the number of cases will increase dramatically, the disease is also expected to spread geographically. Although currently New York and San Francisco account for more than 40 percent of all cases in the United States, by 1990 it is projected that these cities will account for only 20 percent. This epidemiological shift could have an important impact on social responses to the disease. The problem, McDonald said, "is bigger than the Public Health Service."[19]

4

Given the absence of effective treatments and the inability to render non-infectious those who carry the virus, the only current means of controlling the epidemic are preventive measures. Approaches to prevention have therefore centered on altering behavior patterns that are most closely associated with the transmission of the virus. Because many gays have multiple sexual partners, and anal intercourse is an efficient means of spreading AIDS, the disease spread rapidly within the gay population. Estimates of seropositivity in San Francisco among the gay male population were over 50 percent by mid-1986. AIDS forced the gay community to rethink the sexual mores which had become a symbol of their movement for wider social and political liberation.[20]

Although it is difficult to generalize about sexual practices, the advocacy of sexual freedom had been a hallmark of the gay rights movement. Casual, anonymous sex became a significant aspect of gay culture, especially in major cities like San Francisco and New York. Before AIDS, sexually transmitted diseases were epidemic in these communities, especially in the so-called fast track gay culture. With the beginning of the AIDS epidemic, many physicians counseled caution; as Dr. Daniel C. William explained:

> We had taught people that being sexually active was an acceptable sex risk. We were wrong. AIDS changed the rules. I'm very regretful that this recognition has been slow in coming.

"I don't consider it morality," William concluded, "I consider it survival."[21]

In the early years of the epidemic some leaders in the gay community saw in the disease an attempt to exert control over gay sexual culture. Given the limited public policies available for controlling the epidemic, the bathhouses in San Francisco and New York, frequented by gay males, became the focus of discussion. Both cities, after considerable debate, took action to close baths and clubs where, officials determined, sexual activities which might spread AIDS were openly practiced. Closing the baths touched off a bitter debate within the gay community about civil liberties, public health, and gay sexual identity. Some saw the necessity of public interventions; others viewed the closings as an attack on gay culture. As the writer Frances FitzGerald noted, "for most gay leaders, [the baths] seemed to stand as a synecdoche for gay sexual freedom."[22] When several bathhouses in New York City were closed, Thomas B. Stoddard of the New York Civil Liberties Union noted, "The Governor and the Mayor have taken us down the slippery slope that may lead to criminalization of private sexual conduct."[23] But even gay leaders eventually came to believe that by closing bathhouses lives might be saved. Despite the publicity generated and the important educational function it may have served, however, the debate over the bathhouses was fundamentally symbolic; as an effective public health measure their closure offered little. And indeed, as the significance and extent of the epidemic became clear in the gay community, such businesses began to close due to the lack of clientele.

The gay community responded by mobilizing to attack AIDS. This, of course, required a change in sexual mores and practices. Developing "safe sex" guidelines and educational programs to encourage behavioral change became an issue of survival in the gay community. In 1982 the Gay Men's Health Crisis was established in New York City. Similar groups were created in other cities to serve the gay populations and to develop programs in response to the epidemic. Such groups have performed admirably to educate the gay community about the nature of the risk and how to avoid the disease; for those already infected, these groups have provided legal and social services, counseling, and access to health care.[24]

The gay press quickly informed the community that only by modification of high risk behaviors, in particular unprotected anal intercourse which risked the exchange of blood and semen, could infection with the deadly virus be prevented. An educational campaign led to dramatic changes in sexual behavior. Researchers concluded that there was a decline in numbers of partners, a rise in the use of condoms, and high levels of compliance with "safe sex" guidelines. One study demonstrated, for example, that the proportion of gay men in San Francisco following these guidelines increased from 69 percent to 81 percent between August 1984 and April 1985. The changes were reflected in the precipitous fall in rates of other sexually transmitted diseases among gay males, a population in which such infections had been prevalent.[25]

Although the AIDS epidemic has been typically associated in the public mind with homosexuality, infection also flourished among intravenous drug users. The sharing of needles, a common practice in "shooting galleries" where i.v. drugs are used, proved to be an effective mode of transmisssion of the virus. Although attempts have been made to discourage the use of unsterile needles, because of the criminal nature of drug use it has been difficult to provide appropriate and effective education. While there have been dramatic alterations of behavior in the gay community, changing at-risk behaviors among intravenous drug users is more problematic. Not only is the i.v. drug community less cohesive and less well-educated, the nature of drug addiction itself compromises compliance in avoiding the risk of infection.

Nevertheless, there have been reports of changing practices among addicts aware of the risk of AIDS. Many drug users reportedly have been seeking sterile needles at premium prices. In New York City, public health officials considered lifting some of the legal restrictions on the availability of sterile needles. Such proposals are controversial because they are seen as possibly encouraging the use of illegal drugs. David Sencer, the Health Commissioner for the city, responded persuasively to such critics, "People don't become addicted to needles. They become addicted to drugs."[26] In light of the overwhelming difficulties of controlling the infections among drug users, the provision of clean needles is one proposal which offers some hope. As the epidemic worsens such policies may well garner greater support.

Sterile needles, however, will be only a partial solution. As has so often been the case, AIDS has brought to light ingrained social problems: in this instance, the "epidemic" of drug abuse and the shortage of treatment programs for addicts. AIDS forces us to address social ills which for too long have been treated inadequately or ignored. Even addicts motivated to break their habits cannot immediately find places in programs. "If we persuade addicts how bad AIDS is, its like yelling fire in a crowded theater," explained Dr. June Osborn, Dean of the University of Michigan School of Public Health. "They call for help and get told we'll get back to you in three to six months."[27] In New York City, where drug use and AIDS has been most closely related, the proportion of drug-related cases has risen to more than one-third of all cases. Current projections suggest that more than 50 percent of an estimated 250,000 intravenous drug users in New York City have been exposed to HIV. This is particularly worrisome since it is likely that intravenous drug users may spread the disease to individuals who are not currently considered at "high-risk" for the disease and thus may be less aware of the dangers and means of avoiding infection.[28]

Behavioral means are the only current hope for preventing the further spread of the disease. And yet as the history of the sexually transmitted diseases makes clear, altering behavior is no simple matter. Sexuality is a powerful force, certainly subject to individual will, but not completely so. Such problems as intravenous drug use highlight the issue of addiction, the fact that behavior is not always subject to rational control. Behavioral practices, though clearly related to patterns of disease, are poorly understood in contemporary biomedicine. Indeed, the underlying assumption about behavior, and one deeply ingrained in our culture, is that it is entirely voluntary. According to this logic, once appropriately informed about risks, individuals "should" modify their behaviors. Moreover, we know too little about how to assist individuals who seek to make, and maintain, difficult behavioral alterations. This is as true for sexual behavior as it is for the problem of drug addiction, the two principal mechanisms for the transmission of the AIDS virus. Preventive medicine and health promotion have had inadequate attention in modern medicine, where the emphasis has been on treatment, cure, and technology—the search for magic bullets.

5

AIDS has threatened our sense of medical security. After all, the age of transmissible, lethal infections was deemed long past in the Western world. Ours was the age of chronic disease—heart diseases and cancers which principally strike late in life. Communicability—epidemics of infectious diseases—had receded in the public memory. Not since the polio epidemics of the 1950s has fear of infection reached such a high pitch as it has in the 1980s. Indeed, no epidemic since the swine flu pandemic of 1918 has had such a dramatic impact on patterns of mortality. And ironically, the concerns in 1976, about a new epidemic of swine flu that never materialized seemed to confirm that fear of epidemic infection was unfounded in this modern age of antibiotics. AIDS has fractured this false sense of confidence. Dealing effectively with such a problem is further complicated by its "social construction," those attitudes and values which shape the public view of the disease. The social construction of AIDS will in turn have a powerful impact on the choices made in responding to the disease.

Though AIDS is an enormous public health problem, public perceptions of the epidemic have not always been accurate; indeed, many of the fears about AIDS reveal underlying anxieties about contagion, contamination, and sexuality. In this light, the story of AIDS is consistent with the broader history of sexually transmitted diseases in the twentieth century.

Despite considerable evidence that AIDS is not easily communicated, there are widespread fears. Anxiety that AIDS can be casually transmitted is reminiscent of those earlier in the century when it was believed that syphilis could be communicated by shared use of drinking cups, toilet seats, and door knobs. What were late Victorian concerns are now cast in a contemporary light. In the fall of 1985 a *New York Times*/CBS poll found that 47 percent of Americans believed that AIDS could be transmitted via a shared drinking glass, while 28 percent believed that toilet seats could be the source of contamination.[29] Another survey found that 34 percent of those polled believed it unsafe to "associate" with an AIDS victim even when no physical contact was involved. The California Association of Realtors instructed its members to inform prospective buyers whether or not a house on the market had been owned by an AIDS patient.[30]

Because of the considerable fear engendered by the AIDS epidemic—and the fact that the disease has principally affected two already outcast social groups—patterns of stigmatization and discrimination have been directed at its victims. AIDS patients have lost jobs, housing, and social support. People with AIDS are at risk not just from a serious, terminal disease but from a series of social perceptions and attitudes that encourage discrimination and isolation. Even the medical profession has not been free from the fear of AIDS. Early in the epidemic there were physicians who refused to treat AIDS patients, despite assurances that the virus was not easily transmitted.[31]

The hysteria has led to attempts to segregate victims. The first major skirmish in this battle arose over whether children with AIDS should be permitted to attend school. Ryan White, a thirteen-year-old AIDS victim, was banned from his Indiana school. This issue has attracted a vehement debate, but most jurisdictions have permitted children with the disease to attend when no risk was posed to other students. In Queens, New York, angry parents kept their children home in two school districts because a child with AIDS was permitted to go to school. The school boycott reflected a pervasive distrust of scientific authority, as well as a lack of understanding about uncertainty in science. Could officials assure—absolutely—that the disease could *not* be passed in the classroom? Medical science, which deals in probabilities, could not offer the definitive guarantees that many demanded.[32]

Stigma goes beyond AIDS patients to anyone considered at risk of carrying the infection. Indeed, not only have AIDS patients been subject to discrimination but the public response to the disease has been accompanied by a rise in attacks on homosexuals. Fire officials have refused to resuscitate men they suspected might be homosexuals. Police have worn gloves when apprehending suspects in some municipalities.[33]

Our understanding of AIDS and its meaning has been powerfully shaped by the media. This has been a complex process. AIDS has generated outstanding science writing as well as scurrilous reports bent on raising irrational fear and public hysteria. The death of movie idol Rock Hudson in October 1985 reflects the paradoxical relationship of AIDS and the media. Hudson's death became the occasion for the recognition that AIDS was a vast problem that merited more attention; his death put a human face on the epidemic for many Americans. It also became the occasion for speculation about Hudson's sexuality and a prurient interest in the gay subculture. Hudson's plight was heavy with irony. This macho screen star, the press now speculated, had lived a secret life. AIDS brought a pale, thin, dying Hudson out of the closet. President Ronald Reagan finally uttered the dangerous monosyllable "AIDS." But Hudson's death also led to heightened fears of hidden disease. Who knew who was gay? Who knew who might have the disease? Hudson's death created alarm in Hollywood that the disease might be contracted in the course of making movies and television shows. Some critics suggested that Hudson had acted irresponsibly by not informing his fellow cast members of the TV serial *Dynasty* and kissing his co-star Linda Evans in one episode. In this respect, Hudson's death again raised concerns about AIDS victims and those who carry the virus placing others at risk. Shortly after his death, Hudson's estate was sued by his lover, who claimed that Hudson had never informed him that he had AIDS.[34]

The fact that the two principal high risk groups are already highly stigmatized in American culture has had a powerful impact on responses to the epidemic. Some have seen the AIDS epidemic in a purely "moral" light: AIDS is a disease that occurs among those who violate the moral order. As one journalist concluded: "Suddenly a lot of people fear that they and their families might suddenly catch some mysterious, fatal illness which until now has been confined to society's social outcasts." AIDS, like other sexually transmitted diseases in the past, has been viewed as a fateful link between social deviance and the morally correct. Such fears have been exacerbated by an expectant media. "NO ONE IS SAFE FROM AIDS," announced *Life* in bold red letters on its cover.[35] Implicit was the notion that "no one is safe" from gays and intravenous drug users. The disease had come to be equated with those who are at highest risk of suffering its terrible consequences.

Underlying the fears of transmission were deeper concerns about homosexuality. Just as "innocent syphilis" in the first decades of the twentieth century was thought to bring the "respectable middle class" in contact with a deviant ethnic, working-class "sexual underworld," now AIDS threatened the heterosexual culture with homosexual contamination. In this context, homosexuality—not a virus—*causes* AIDS. Therefore, homosexuality itself is feared as if it were a communicable, lethal disease. After a generation of work to have homosexuality removed as a disease from the psychiatric diagnostic manuals, it had suddenly reappeared as an infectious, terminal disease.[36]

The AIDS epidemic thus offered new opportunities for the expression of moral opprobrium for homosexuality. Patrick Buchanan, conservative columnist and Reagan speech writer, explained, "The poor homosexuals—they have declared war upon Nature, and now Nature is exacting an awful retribution."[37] Criticizing government expenditures on research to produce a vaccine, the editor

Norman Podhoretz wrote, "Are they aware that in the name of compassion they are giving social sanction to what can only be described as brutish degradation?" Podhoretz's position—that gays get what they deserve, that to investigate treatments would merely encourage unhealthy behaviors—though a characteristic position in the history of sexually transmitted diseases, indicated a remarkably uninformed view of the epidemic, as well as a complete disregard for the public health.[38]

In a now classic work, sociologist Erving Goffman defined what he considered to be three distinct types of stigma. The first is an abomination of the body; clearly AIDS and all venereal diseases could be so categorized. The second is a blemish of individual character; again victims of sexually transmitted diseases have traditionally been seen as lacking control, as immoral and promiscuous. And third, Goffman identified the tribal stigmas of race, nation, or religion. This, too, has been a recurring theme in considerations of venereal disease—the notion that particular groups were especially prone to infection. Perhaps the sexually transmitted diseases carry a particularly weighty stigma because they cut through each of these categories; an undesired *difference*—of a sexual nature—that sets its victims apart. Victims of AIDS thus suffer the biological consequences of a terrifying disease as well as the deep social stigma.[39]

Fear of disease and the homophobia that it has generated have forced the gay rights movement into defensive action to fight a rising tide of discrimination. The AIDS epidemic threatens to undo a generation of progress toward gay rights. Not only does AIDS threaten the lives of many members of the gay community, it has unleashed a considerable political and legal threat. In June 1986 the Justice Department issued a decision which held that it is permissible for employers to bar AIDS patients or those infected with the virus from work. The ruling held that federal law did not protect the civil rights of those who *might* be considered dangerous to others; moreover, the ruling left the evaluation of such "real or perceived" risks to the employer. The decision was issued despite the fact that government scientists had repeatedly stated on the basis of considerable epidemiologic and biological evidence that the disease was not casually transmitted.[40] Public health officials openly expressed their dismay with the ruling, which threatened to encourage the irrational fears of the disease they had worked diligently to alleviate. An editorial in the *New York Times* called the ruling a "license to hound AIDS victims":

> No one should want to curb the powers of public health officials to control a disease as deadly as AIDS. But to throw AIDS victims out of their jobs is a capitulation to unwarranted fear that protects no one.[41]

As journalist Charles Krauthammer noted, the ruling undercut all antidiscrimination legislation:

> The whole point of such laws is to say this: it may indeed cause you psychological distress to mix with others whom you irrationally dislike or fear. Too bad. The state has decided that these particular prejudices are destructive and irrational. Therefore the state will prohibit you . . . from acting upon your groundless prejudices.

As Krauthammer concluded, "It should not matter if people think you can get AIDS in the Xerox room. You can't. Ignorance is a cause of discrimination. It is not a justification for it."[42]

Such a ruling may not be upheld in court. But the courts have not supported recent attempts to provide basic civil liberties for the homosexual population. Several days after the Justice Department ruling, the Supreme Court upheld in a 5 to 4 decision the constitutionality of a state's sodomy law in a case that was considered a major setback to the gay rights movement.[43] This ruling, which conflicted with the Court's recent affirmations of the right to privacy, can be fully understood only in the context of the AIDS epidemic.

Given the fact that AIDS cannot be casually transmitted, it is worth assessing why public concern has remained so high. Indeed, these fears are reminiscent of those that surrounded syphilis at the turn of the century. In one sense the fear of AIDS is not surprising; it is, after all, a terrifying disease. But the hysteria has reflected other forces as well: fears of homosexuality, irrational concerns about sexual contamination, and a failure of scientific authority.

6

While scientific knowledge of AIDS has grown at an exponential rate, much remains unknown. Nevertheless, AIDS presents a series of highly problematic social policy questions that must be addressed even in this context of incomplete medical knowledge of the disease and of widespread fear. AIDS makes explicit a central tension in our polity: the premium we place on the rights of the individual to fundamental civil liberties versus the notion of the public good and the role of the state in assuring public welfare. Both sets of values, highly prized in our culture, have been brought into conflict by the AIDS crisis. In the course of the twentieth century, the notion of civil liberties was expanded and strengthened in the courts. But this makes the conflicts posed by AIDS even more contentious.

Nowhere is this more clearly seen than in the current debate about testing and screening for HIV antibody. The discovery of the ELISA test not only made possible the screening of blood to preserve the quality of the blood supply, it also made it technically possible to identify individuals who have come in contact with HIV. While many, especially in the gay community, have viewed the test with grave concern for the potential to identify and segregate or even quarantine individuals found to be positive for HIV antibody, others have viewed the test as the critical element in a successful campaign to stem the epidemic. The debate currently rages about the appropriate use of this test.

In late 1985 the Department of Defense announced that all new recruits for military service would be screened for HIV antibody and rejected if found to be positive. One justification of the screening program was that military personnel receive a wide variety of live-virus vaccinations which might cause serious disease in individuals who were immune compromised. Military officials also contended that combat would provide a high risk for transmission of HIV, where soldiers might be asked to serve as blood donors in the field. Although the military suggested that the screening program would maintain absolute confidentiality, in practice this may be difficult to achieve. Rejected candidates may suffer the stigma of HIV infection. Critics of the military screening program argued that the test was being used to identify and remove gays from service.[44]

The military screening program was merely the first; many others have been proposed from the mandatory screening of high-risk groups, premarital testing, testing in prisons, and universal screening. While some have called for mandatory testing of high-risk individuals, such proposals fail to recognize the implicit impossibility of identifying such groups and requiring them to be tested.[45] How would officials go about implementing legislation mandating testing for only certain ill-defined social groups? Because such proposals are impossible to enforce, only universal screening programs could be mandated. But such programs would have obvious problems.

Conservative columnist William F. Buckley, Jr., has recommended mandatory universal screening, with all individuals found positive to be tatooed on their forearms and buttocks. This, he suggested, would serve to stem the epidemic by warning those who might share needles or have sex with such individuals. Buckley's sorry logic, however, is more than apparent. First, throughout his tortured argument, he failed to differentiate those with AIDS and those positive for the antibody. Second, he failed to note the possibility of false positives in the test, which with mandatory testing will become much more likely. "We face a utilitarian imperative," wrote Buckley.[46] But there is no evidence whatsoever that such an invasive and stigmatizing program would slow the spread of this epidemic. His proposal is all the more remarkable in light of his consistent attacks on intrusive government. Only thinly veiled in such proposals is a powerfully moralistic homophobia.

When the epidemic worsens, as it most certainly will, the social desire to segregate those individuals who are infected will probably become more intense, even though massive compulsory screening would offer little in the interest of public health. Such policies will be resisted only if the full costs and negligible benefits are clearly understood. Otherwise the irrational desire to segregate may be persuasive.

Finally, it is worth questioning the purpose of testing, especially in light of the current reality that there is no effective treatment for the disease. In the 1930s, when states began to mandate premarital blood testing for syphilis, individuals found to be infected could seek treatment, become non-infectious, and go on with their lives. Contacts of individuals with syphilis could be found, tested, and, if infected, treated. Such programs served the interests of the individuals who were infected as well as the public interest in assuring that disease was not spread further. Such a program is not possible in the case of AIDS, where there is presently no effective treatment and no means of rendering non-infectious those individuals who carry HIV.

Some have argued that testing is advisable because knowing one's antibody status will encourage individuals to act responsibly, avoid spreading the infection, and perhaps avoid further risks which could contribute to the development of disease. This may be true for some, but it has yet to be determined; individuals may have quite variable psychological and behavioral responses to finding out whether or not they are infected. Many individuals, especially in the gay community, have altered their behaviors without knowledge of their antibody status. The test has risks in that it is difficult, even in the best of circumstances, to guarantee that the results will be held strictly confidential. Fears that a positive test could lead to discrimination seem realistic in light of the highly stigmatized view of the disease and such rulings as that by the Justice Department.[47]

All this, of course, is not to argue that testing is useless. Many individuals, especially those likely to have come in contact with the virus, may want to be tested to learn their antibody status. Obviously, such individuals should be able to do so under the strictest confidentiality. Moreover, as treatments become available in the future, it is likely that they will be most effective if initiated before the development of symptoms; therefore, it would become important for infected individuals to find out while they are still asymptomatic—so they may be made aware of the need to seek treatment.

It is crucial to maintain the distinction between voluntary use of the test and mandatory screening. Mandatory screening could have the effect of creating an "underground" epidemic in which infected individuals, fearing discrimination, isolation, or quarantine, refuse to cooperate with public health officials. Hidden infection is the nemesis of any effective campaign to halt an epidemic disease. The test could be used as a "marker" to license discrimination in employment, housing, and the availability of health and life insurance.

Among those asserting their right to require individuals to take the ELISA test are insurance companies. These companies have argued that individuals who have been exposed to HIV are likely to have higher health care costs than the population in general; therefore, they contend, such individuals should pay higher premiums. "If America's private voluntary-insurance system is to remain workable, AIDS tests must be allowed so the disease can be underwritten in the same manner as heart disease, cancer, or alcohol and drug abuse," explained Claire Wolkoff of the American Academy of Actuaries. "The alternative is to spread the risk factor over the whole population, thus raising the price of insurance for everyone."[48] Several states have taken legislative action to bar insurers from requiring the test, or to assure its absolute confidentiality. When the District of Columbia passed such a resolution, Senator Jesse Helms, the conservative Republican from North Carolina, said, "The truth is the so-called homosexual rights crowd has snookered the entire District of Columbia into footing the bill to provide special treatment for those who are at health risk because of AIDS." At least four life and health insurance companies announced a decision to stop doing business in the District rather than comply with the legislation.[49]

At the heart of the debate about insurance testing is the question of who will bear the cost of AIDS. Should the costs of the epidemic be spread over the whole society, or should they be borne by those who have been and will be infected by HIV? Early studies estimated that the average health care costs for

AIDS patients were about $150,000. Later investigations soon determined that this figure might be overestimated by as much as 100 percent. Total direct and indirect costs—the losses from medical care and income—rose to $3.3 billion by mid-1986. An added problem was that hospitals often had to pick up the tab on unpaid bills for AIDS patients. This has been particularly true in New York City, where close to 30 percent of all cases are among intravenous drug users, whose health care costs tend to be higher, and who are less likely to be insured.[50] In this respect, AIDS again reveals deep and persistent social problems, in this instance, the problem of financing of health care. How should the risks of catastrophic disease be spread? Shall we apply an individualist ethic? Or look to social programs to allocate the costs of disease more equitably? These questions have been on the national agenda for more than a generation. AIDS forces them out of the shadows. At issue on who should bear the costs of the epidemic is the critical question: who is responsible? This has been an especially significant question in the history of sexually transmitted diseases, which have traditionally been seen as diseases of individual moral failing.

The debate over screening for HIV antibody is ultimately part and parcel of a larger debate in American society over testing in general. New biotechnologies make it possible for tests to reveal a great deal about any individual, his or her health status, behaviors, medical risks, and genetic make-up. This is information that not only insurers but employers and the state might want to have. The right to require tests, and in whose interests such tests are conducted, promises to be a bitter and controversial issue in the years ahead. Indeed, testing raises the question of whose interest medical science will serve. Compulsory testing raises the most fundamental tensions between civil liberties and social control.

7

Although Edward Brandt, the government's top health official, called AIDS the nation's "number one priority" in public health in mid-1983, the federal government's response has been poorly coordinated and haphazard. In 1985 the Office of Technology Assessment (OTA) issued a report analyzing the effectiveness of the federal government's response to AIDS. The report revealed a number of significant shortcomings. First, the government had been slow to respond. Although CDC had identified AIDS in 1981, research at the NIH did not begin in earnest until 1983. Bureaucratic procedures prevented a more timely response to this public health emergency. Second, when NIH did take up the problem of AIDS, research funding was inadequate. In 1982 and 1983 the administration did not budget any money for AIDS research; nevertheless Congress allocated $33 million. The following year, the administration asked for $39 million—Congress appropriated $61 million. In 1986, Congress allocated $234 million, but the Reagan administration proposed cutting this to $213.2 million; this, despite the fact that cases have been doubling every year.[51] Underlying this debate over funding was the controversial nature of AIDS itself and its close association with homosexuality. Funding for sexually transmitted diseases has always been suspect in the federal health budget.

The OTA report also pointed out the lack of attention to social and psychological factors associated with the disease. This was especially noteworthy in that preventive measures offered the only immediate hope of slowing the epidemic. Nevertheless, funds for education have been meager. In 1986 the CDC had $25 million available for education, although a full program would have required three times that amount. As Harvey V. Fineberg, Dean of the Harvard School of Public Health, noted, "We understand enough about the cause and spread of the AIDS virus to give people the knowledge they need to protect themselves."[52] And yet, outside the gay community, this is not being done. Sex education has traditionally been an area of significant controversy. How to present the AIDS epidemic to school children of various ages has been the subject of considerable debate. As Dr. Walter Dowdle explained: "The sense of urgency is somewhat different here. It's not a matter of philosophy and religious taboos. We are talking about prevention in life and death situations."[53] AIDS has again raised the historic debate of addressing the problem of sexually transmitted diseases from a relatively dispassionate, instrumental standpoint versus the notion that only a proper moral standard will prevent their spread. The federal government refused to issue educational materials explicitly advising "safe sex" practices. Apparently, it was feared that this would be construed as an "endorsement" of homosexuality.

8

AIDS makes explicit, as few diseases could, the complex interaction of social, cultural, and biological forces. Given the social history of venereal disease in the United States, this is hardly surprising. But, as disease is shaped by its particular social and historical context, the response to AIDS will be informed by the forces of our time. Nevertheless, the analogues which AIDS poses to the broader history of sexually transmitted diseases in the United States are striking: the pervasive fear of contagion; concerns about casual transmission; the stigmatization of victims; the conflicts between protecting public health and assuring civil liberties; the search for magic bullets. How these issues will be resolved as the AIDS epidemic continues to unfold in the years ahead is far from certain.

History is not a predictive science. AIDS is not syphilis, and the historical moment has shifted. But one thing is certain: the response to AIDS, as already can be seen, will not be determined strictly by its biological character; rather, it will be deeply influenced by our social and cultural understanding of disease and its victims. And, indeed, even our scientific understanding of the disease will be refracted through our cultural values and attitudes. It is an understanding of this process which gives the historical record relevance and meaning. How will the response to AIDS be shaped by prevailing social and cultural mores? History does provide us with a way of understanding and approaching the present. The recognition of this process by which disease is defined provides us with an opportunity to guide and influence the response to AIDS in ways which may be more constructive, effective, and humane.

A series of difficult dilemmas are just off stage. How can the impact of this disease be mitigated? Can we protect the rights of victims of the disease while avoiding the victimization of the public? What types of public policies should be employed? And how will these policies reflect our understanding of the disease? How will the conflict between individual liberties and public welfare be resolved? [54]

In the months and years ahead the problem of constructing cost-benefit ratios for various policies will be confronted. Who will bear the burdens of any particular intervention? What will the motives be? How will information be used? Ideally? In practice? What are the potential unintended consequences of any particular policy? Already there has been a tendency to invoke traditional public health policies: screening, testing, reporting, contact tracing, isolation, and quarantine. Will these measures be effective in the case of AIDS, which is complicated by the large number of healthy carriers perhaps infectious for life? Does the fact that no effective treatments for the disease currently exist change the nature of potential public health interventions?

There are two criteria upon which any proposal must be evaluated. The first should be: will it work? There must be considerable evidence that any particular policy offers substantial benefit. The second criteria for public interventions should be: is it the least restrictive of all possible positive measures? Are there any better alternatives consistent with a desire to guard civil liberties as well as protect the public welfare? In short, how do we construct a just and effective policy? How do we protect civil liberties while protecting the public good?

But the answers to these difficult questions will be shaped by our scientific, social, and cultural understanding of the disease. This, of course, has been further complicated by the substantial fear surrounding the epidemic. Although there is much that we know about AIDS, there is much that lies outside current scientific understanding. Scientists and physicians have experience in tolerating such ambiguities, such a level of uncertainty, however, is often hidden from or denied by the larger society. Policies relating to AIDS will, of course, be created in this atmosphere of uncertainty. Moreover, the decline of the authority of experts—from Three Mile Island, to Love Canal, to the Space Shuttle, to Chernobyl—has had the effect of creating significant distrust in the public. [55] The fact that as a society we have been fortunate not to have had to address any major infectious disease on an epidemic level since polio accounts for our relative lack of social and political experience in dealing with such problems. And, indeed, we would probably have to go back to the influenza pandemic of 1918 to identify a pathogen as dangerous as the AIDS virus. In this light, we have few models for dealing with public health issues of this magnitude and complexity.

Our notions of cost-benefit analysis and social policy are characterized by a belief in policies without costs. All social policies carry certain costs, but in our political culture we tend to reject policies when the costs become explicit, even if they promise significant potential benefits. This has been seen in two proposals to slow the spread of the infection. As in the early twentieth century, education has been put forward as one of the few positive activities which might slow the further spread of the disease. But discussions must assess the meaning and content of such education. Explicit sexual education has been rejected by some officials because it is viewed as encouraging homosexuality; the costs are thus evaluated as being too high. Another recent proposal has met a similar fate—the idea of providing sterile needles to intravenous drug abusers to slow down the rapid spread of the disease which has already taken place in that community. This idea has been rejected because it is seen as contributing to the drug problem. Underlying such assessments, of course, is the idea that AIDS is a "self-inflicted" disease.

As was the case in the early twentieth century, public health measures that require dramatic infringements of civil liberties are again being proposed. All too often such measures have had no positive impact on the public health. For example, rates of venereal disease climbed rapidly during the First World War, despite radical government measures for the incarceration of prostitutes. This is not to suggest the purely pragmatic notion that if an intervention works it is right. But rather, that if it does not produce results, and yet it is supported by officials and the public, one must look for secondary reasons to explain the intervention. The issue thus becomes not the desire to protect the public from hazard—an idea so basic to modern governments that few would question it in principle; indeed, our most fundamental notions of social welfare are based upon it. Rather, these activities indicate a transformation from protection to punishment; a clear signal that the disease and those who get it are socially disvalued.

In the context of fear that surrounds AIDS, there is a clear potential for policies which despite having little or no potential for slowing the epidemic could have considerable legal, social, and cultural appeal. What can be done to separate realistic concerns from irrational fears? How can victim-blaming and stigmatization of high risk groups, already socially outcast, be avoided? In many respects the process of dividing victims between the blameless and blameful—analogous to early twentieth-century notions of venereal disease *insontium*—has been activated once again. This can be seen, for example, in assessments such as the following offered by a journalist in the *New York Times Magazine* in 1983:

> The groups most recently found to be at risk for AIDS present a particularly poignant problem. Innocent bystanders caught in the path of a new disease, they can make no behavioral decisions to minimize their risk: hemophiliacs cannot stop taking bloodclotting medication; surgery patients cannot stop getting transfusions; women cannot control the drug habits of their mates; babies cannot choose their mothers. [56]

This passage raises a number of problems. First, it suggests that the disease is somehow more "poignant" when it attacks non-homosexuals rather than homosexuals. Second, if these groups are "innocent bystanders," then those at highest risk of contracting AIDS may be assumed to be "guilty." Implicit in this discussion is the view that the entire community is at risk from the sexual practices of homosexuals. In some quarters the misapprehension persists: AIDS is caused by homosexuality rather than a retrovirus. In this confused logic, the answer to the problem is simple: repress these behaviors. Implicit in this approach to the problem are powerful notions of culpability and guilt.

Indeed, assessments of AIDS—as of most sexually transmitted diseases in the twentieth century—rest on the essentially simplistic view that the problem can be solved if individuals act more responsibly in their sexual conduct. The assumption that an individual's behavior is free from external forces—that life style is strictly voluntary—is explicit. These assumptions with which we still live regarding health-related behavior rest upon an essentially naive, simplistic view of human nature. If anything has become clear in the course of the twentieth century it is that behavior is subject to complex forces, internal psychologies, and external pressures, all not subject to immediate modification, or, arguably, to modification at all. Sexuality is subject to a number of powerful influences, social and economic, conscious and unconscious, many more powerful than even the fear of disease. In this view, sexuality is equated with other risk-taking behaviors—smoking, drinking, poor diet, driving too fast. These are behaviors for which, of course, individuals can in part be held accountable, but the question of to what extent, and whether they should be is not as simple.

The persistence of such values and attitudes calls into question the received view of the sexual revolution in the midst of which we live. No doubt there have been serious and important changes in sexual mores and practices, the gay liberation movement is but one example. But this makes certain continuities all the more striking. Social values continue to define the sexually transmitted diseases as uniquely sinful—indeed, to transform disease into an indication of moral decay. There remain those who believe fear of disease will lead to a higher morality. It thus seems naive and wishful to assert that we have conquered the Victorians within ourselves, for underlying tensions in American sexual values persist, tensions that are brought forward in our approach to AIDS as well as other venereal diseases. To those who subscribe to this belief, the message is clear: the way to control sexually transmitted disease is not through medical means but rather through moral rectitude. A disease such as AIDS is controlled by controlling individual conduct.

The current trend in health care policy is to accept this model of disease and to apply it to a myriad of other illnesses, to reduce the emphasis on social or external determinants of disease and health, and to stress individual responsibility.[57] This model, however, has failed venereal disease, and the historical record renders it a dubious precedent. The presumption nevertheless remains. Behavior—bad behavior at that—is seen as the cause of disease. These assumptions may be powerful psychologically, and in some cases they may influence behavior, but so long as they are dominant—so long as disease is equated with sin—there can be no magic bullet.

In this sense the old scare-tactics have failed; denial and repression of sexuality have failed; victim-blaming and moralizing all have failed as effective public health mechanisms. While biomedical solutions offer much hope, they too have failed to free us of infectious disease. More creative and sophisticated approaches to this set of diseases are necessary. Now that we recognize that behavioral changes may be a significant factor in disease, we know that new techniques to assist those who seek to change are required. Moreover, we must recognize that behavioral change does not mean encouraging celibacy, heterosexuality, or morality; rather, it means developing means to avoid coming into contact with a pathogen.

AIDS makes painfully explicit the limits of our ability to intervene against the course of the biological world. Sexual contact is one of a number of ways in which microorganisms are transmitted from human to human. New or altered infectious agents are passed this way; no single medical treatment has proven effective for these infectious organisms. This, then, makes evident a fundamental flaw in the biomedical model: the search for magic bullets. Venereal diseases, and indeed all infectious diseases, constitute complex bio-ecological problems in which host, parasite, and a number of social and environmental forces interact. No *single* medical or social intervention can thus adequately address the problem. Just as social mores and practices change, so too the biological system is in flux. New infections such as AIDS may appear, or older infectious diseases, once controlled, such as gonorrhea, may become intransigent in the face of agents whose effectiveness is attenuated as the organism itself changes. As one observer recently remarked, the battle against infectious disease is an ongoing "leap-frog war."[58]

Caught in the complex web of social and scientific questions surrounding AIDS, we easily forget the dimensions of the tragedy. While disease tells us much about the nature of our society, it also reveals the nature of illness, suffering, and death and dying. The high mortality associated with AIDS and the growing number of cases could become the justification for drastic measures. "Better safe than sorry" could well become a catch phrase to justify dramatic abuses of basic human rights in the context of an uncertain science. Moreover, the social construction of this disease, its close association in much of the public's eye with violations of the moral code could contribute to spiralling hysteria and anger which has already led to further victimization of victims, the double jeopardy of lethal disease and social oppression.

The social costs of ineffective draconian public health measures would only augment the crisis we know as AIDS. But such measures will be avoided only if we are adept in both our medical and cultural understanding of this disease; if we are sophisticated in our ability to create an atmosphere of social tolerance. For we need to perform a difficult task; that of separating deeply irrational fears from scientific understanding. Only when we recognize the ways in which social and cultural values shape this disease will we be able to begin to deal effectively and humanely with a problem as serious and complex as AIDS.

AIDS is an unfinished chapter in our medical and social history. It reveals the contemporary nature of biomedical science and research; our beliefs about health, disease, and contagion; our ideas about sexuality and social responsibility. AIDS demonstrates how economics and politics cannot be separated from disease; indeed, these forces shape our response in powerful ways. In the years ahead we will, no doubt, learn a great deal more about AIDS and how to control it. We will also learn a great deal about the nature of our society from the manner in which we address the disease. AIDS will be a measure upon which we may calibrate not only our medical and scientific skill but our capacity for justice and compassion.

Appendix

CASES OF VENEREAL DISEASE REPORTED BY STATE HEALTH DEPARTMENTS, AND RATES PER 100,000 POPULATION
(Known Military Cases Excluded) United States Total: Calendar* Years 1941-1979

| Year | All Stages** | | Syphilis | | | | | | | | Gonorrhea | | Chancroid | | Granuloma*** Inguinale | | Lympho-granuloma Venereum | |
| | | | Primary and Secondary | | Early Latent | | Late and Late Latent | | Congenital | | | | | | | | | |
	Cases	Rates	Cases	Rates	Cases	Rates	Cases	Rates	Cases	Rates	Cases	Rates	Cases	Rates	Cases	Rates	Cases	Rates
FISCAL YEARS 1941-1947																		
1941	485,560	368.2	68,231	51.7	109,018	82.6	202,984	153.9	17,600	13.4	193,468	146.7	3,384	2.5	639	0.4	1,381	1.0
1942	479,601	363.4	75,312	57.0	116,245	88.0	202,064	153.1	16,918	12.8	212,403	160.9	5,477	4.1	1,278	0.9	1,888	1.4
1943	575,593	447.0	82,204	63.8	149,390	116.0	251,958	195.7	16,164	12.6	275,070	213.6	8,354	6.4	1,748	1.3	2,593	2.0
1944	467,755	367.9	78,443	61.6	123,038	96.7	202,848	159.6	13,578	10.7	300,676	236.5	7,878	6.1	1,759	1.3	2,858	2.2
1945	359,114	282.3	77,007	60.5	101,719	79.9	142,187	111.8	12,339	9.7	287,181	155.8	5,515	4.3	1,857	1.4	2,631	2.0
1946	363,647	271.7	94,957	70.9	107,924	80.6	125,248	93.6	12,106	9.0	368,020	275.0	7,091	5.2	2,232	1.6	2,603	1.9
1947	372,963	264.6	106,539	75.6	107,767	76.4	121,980	86.5	12,271	8.7	400,639	284.2	9,039	6.4	2,403	1.7	2,688	1.9
CALENDAR YEARS 1947-1979																		
1947	355,592	252.3	93,545	66.4	104,124	73.9	122,089	86.6	12,200	8.7	380,666	270.0	9,515	6.7	2,330	1.7	2,526	1.8
1948	314,313	218.2	68,174	47.3	90,598	62.9	123,312	85.6	13,931	9.7	345,501	239.8	7,661	5.3	2,469	1.7	2,429	1.7
1949	256,463	175.3	41,942	28.7	75,045	51.3	116,397	79.5	13,952	9.5	317,950	217.3	6,707	4.6	2,402	1.6	1,925	1.3
1950	217,558	146.0	23,939	16.7	59,256	39.7	113,569	76.2	13,377	9.0	286,746	192.5	4,977	3.3	1,783	1.2	1,427	1.0
1951	174,924	116.1	14,485	9.6	43,316	28.7	98,311	65.2	11,094	7.4	254,470	168.9	4,233	2.8	1,352	0.9	1,300	0.9
1952	167,762	110.2	10,449	6.9	36,454	24.0	105,238	69.1	8,553	5.6	244,957	160.8	3,738	2.5	951	0.6	1,200	0.8
1953	148,573	95.9	8,637	5.6	28,295	18.3	98,870	63.8	7,675	5.0	238,340	153.9	3,338	2.2	667	0.4	983	0.6
1954	130,697	82.9	7,147	4.5	23,861	15.1	89,123	56.5	6,676	4.2	242,050	153.5	3,003	1.9	618	0.4	875	0.6
1955	122,392	76.2	6,454	4.0	20,054	12.5	86,526	53.8	5,354	3.3	236,197	147.0	2,649	1.7	490	0.3	762	0.5
1956	130,201	78.7	6,392	3.9	19,783	12.0	95,097	57.5	5,491	3.3	224,346	135.7	2,135	1.3	357	0.2	500	0.3
1957	123,758	73.5	6,576	3.9	17,796	10.6	91,309	54.2	5,288	3.1	214,496	127.4	1,637	1.0	348	0.2	448	0.3
1958	113,884	66.4	7,176	4.2	16,556	9.7	83,027	48.4	4,866	2.8	232,386	135.6	1,595	0.9	314	0.2	434	0.3
1959	120,824	69.2	9,799	5.6	17,025	9.8	86,740	49.7	5,130	2.9	240,254	137.6	1,537	0.9	265	0.2	604	0.3
1960	122,538	68.8	16,145	9.1	18,017	10.1	81,798	45.9	4,416	2.5	258,933	145.3	1,680	0.9	296	0.2	835	0.5

Year																		
1961	124,658	68.8	19,851	11.0	19,486	10.8	79,304	43.8	4,163	2.3	264,158	145.8	1,438	0.8	241	0.1	787	0.4
1962	126,245	68.7	21,067	11.5	19,585	10.7	79,533	43.3	4,070	2.2	263,714	143.5	1,344	0.7	207	0.1	590	0.3
1963	124,137	66.5	22,251	11.9	18,235	9.8	78,076	41.9	4,031	2.2	278,289	149.2	1,220	0.7	173	0.1	586	0.3
1964	114,325	60.4	22,969	12.1	17,781	9.4	68,629	36.2	3,516	1.9	300,666	158.8	1,247	0.7	135	0.1	732	0.4
1965	112,842	58.8	23,338	12.2	17,458	9.1	67,317	35.1	3,564	1.9	324,925	169.4	982	0.5	155	0.1	878	0.5
1966	105,159	54.3	21,414	11.1	15,950	8.2	63,541	32.8	3,170	1.6	351,738	181.6	838	0.4	148	0.1	308	0.2
1967	102,581	52.4	21,053	10.8	15,554	8.0	61,975	31.7	2,894	1.5	404,836	207.0	784	0.4	154	0.1	371	0.2
1968	96,271	48.7	19,019	9.6	15,150	7.7	58,564	29.6	2,381	1.2	464,543	235.1	845	0.4	156	0.1	485	0.2
1969	92,162	46.2	19,130	9.6	15,402	7.7	54,587	27.3	2,074	1.0	534,872	267.9	1,104	0.6	154	0.1	520	0.3
1970	91,382	45.5	21,982	10.9	16,311	8.1	50,348	25.0	1,953	1.0	600,072	298.5	1,416	0.7	124	0.1	612	0.3
1971	95,997	47.0	23,783	11.6	19,417	9.5	49,993	24.5	2,052	1.0	670,268	328.1	1,320	0.6	89	0.0	692	0.3
1972	91,149	44.2	24,429	11.8	20,784	10.1	43,456	21.0	1,758	0.9	767,215	371.6	1,414	0.7	81	0.0	756	0.4
1973	87,469	42.0	24,825	11.9	23,584	11.3	37,054	17.8	1,527	0.7	842,621	404.9	1,165	0.6	62	0.0	408	0.2
1974	83,771	39.9	25,385	12.1	25,124	12.0	31,854	15.2	1,138	0.5	906,121	432.1	945	0.5	47	0.0	394	0.2
1975	80,356	38.0	25,561	12.1	26,569	12.6	27,096	12.8	916	0.4	999,937	472.9	700	0.3	60	0.0	353	0.2
1976	71,761	33.7	23,731	11.1	25,363	11.9	21,905	10.3	626	0.3	1,001,994	470.5	628	0.3	71	0.0	365	0.2
1977	64,621	30.1	20,399	9.5	21,329	9.9	22,313	10.4	463	0.2	1,002,219	466.8	455	0.2	75	0.0	348	0.2
1978	64,875	30.0	21,656	10.0	19,628	9.1	23,038	10.6	434	0.2	1,013,436	468.3	521	0.2	72	0.0	284	0.1
1979	67,049	30.7	24,874	11.4	20,459	9.4	21,302	9.7	331	0.2	1,003,958	459.4	840	0.4	76	0.0	250	0.1

*Fiscal years 1941-1947, Fiscal Year – Twelve-month period ending June 30 of year indicated. Calendar years 1947-1979.

**Includes stage of syphilis not stated.

***Rates less than .05 are shown as .0. NOTE: Rates per 100,000 population.

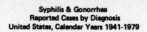

Syphilis & Gonorrhea
Reported Cases by Diagnosis
United States, Calendar Years 1941-1979

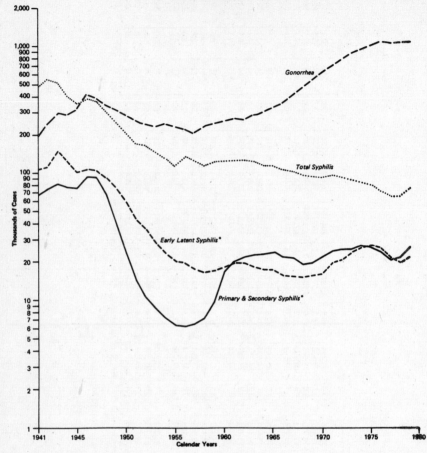

*1941-1946 Fiscal Years: Twelve month period ending June 30 of years specified. 1947-1979 Calendar Years.

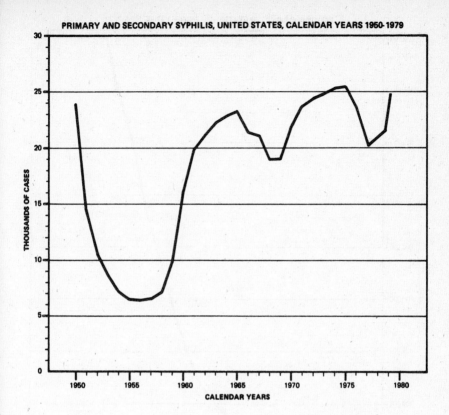

PRIMARY AND SECONDARY SYPHILIS, UNITED STATES, CALENDAR YEARS 1950-1979

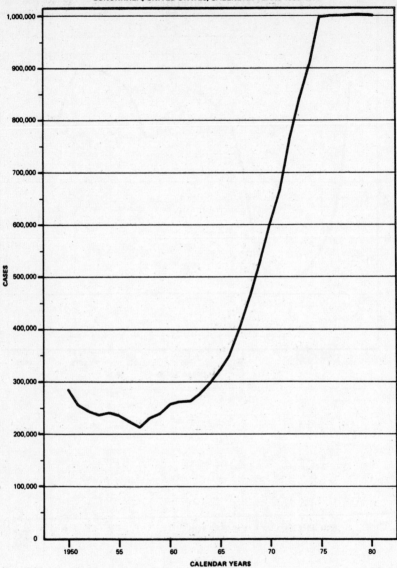

GONORRHEA, UNITED STATES, CALENDAR YEARS 1950-1979

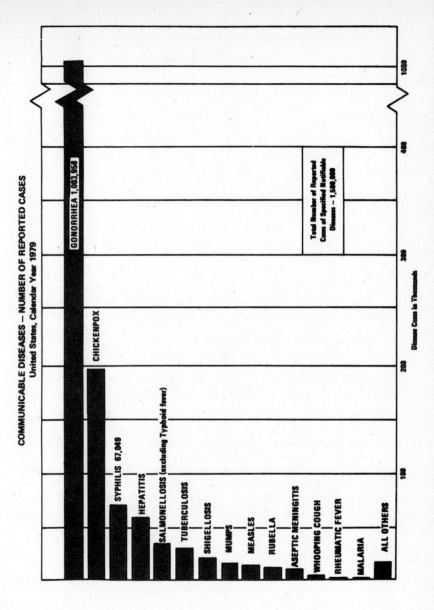

COMMUNICABLE DISEASES — NUMBER OF REPORTED CASES
United States, Calendar Year 1979

GONORRHEA 1,003,958

CHICKENPOX

SYPHILIS 67,049

HEPATITIS

SALMONELLOSIS (excluding Typhoid fever)

TUBERCULOSIS

SHIGELLOSIS

MUMPS

MEASLES

RUBELLA

ASEPTIC MENINGITIS

WHOOPING COUGH

RHEUMATIC FEVER

MALARIA

ALL OTHERS

Total Number of Reported
Cases of Specified Notifiable
Diseases — 1,560,000

Disease Cases in Thousands

100   200   300   400   1000

Note on Sources

In tracing the history of venereal disease since the late nineteenth century, I consulted a wide variety of published and unpublished source materials. Venereal disease was frequently analyzed, debated, and researched in the pages of the American medical press, and I have relied heavily on this published material. The *Index-Catalogue of the Library of the Surgeon-General's Office, United States Army* [1st ser.], 16 vols. (Washington, 1880–95) and *Index Medicus* which began publishing in 1879 provide an excellent guide into this documentary corpus. This voluminous medical literature is an unusually rich resource for social historians. Additionally, I have utilized a range of popular journals, newspapers, and published pamphlets directed to the question of venereal disease control.

This work relies in great measure on the repositories of unpublished materials—letters, reports, memoranda, research notes—devoted to addressing the problem of venereal disease. In particular, the National Archives literally holds thousands of feet of public health and military records documenting governmental efforts regarding the control of venereal disease. Foundations, voluntary agencies, and welfare organizations also have records which I have consulted in this study. Finally, collections of personal papers of individuals active in the campaigns against veneral disease proved indispensable.

A list of manuscript sources and abbreviations used in the endnotes follows.

Manuscript Sources

National Archives, Washington, D.C.

Record Group 62, Records of the Council of National Defense, (Washington-National Records Center, Suitland, Maryland (WNRC)).

Record Group 69, Records of the Works Projects Administration.

Record Group 90, Records of the U.S. Public Health Service.

Record Group 112, Records of the Office of the Surgeon General (Army).

Record Group 120, Records of the American Expeditionary Forces, 1917–1923.

Record Group 165, Records of the War Deparmtent General and Special Staffs.

Record Group 200, National Archives Gift Collection, Records of the American National Red Cross.

Record Group 215, Records of the Office of Community War Services, Social Protection Division.

Collected Papers

American Social Hygiene Association Papers, Social Welfare History Archives Center, University of Minnesota, Minneapolis, Minnesota. (ASHA Papers).

Newton D. Baker Papers, Library of Congress, Washington, D.C.

Bureau of Social Hygiene Papers, Rockefeller Archives Center, Hillcrest, Pocantico Hills, North Tarrytown, New York (BSH Papers).

Committee of Fifteen Papers, New York Public Library, Annex, New York, New York.

Committee of Fourteen Papers, New York Public Library, Annex, New York, New York.

Josephus Daniels Papers, Library of Congress, Washington, D.C.

Ethel Sturges Dummer Papers, Schlesinger Library, Radcliffe College, Harvard University, Cambridge, Massachusetts.

Raymond Fosdick Papers, Seeley G. Mudd Manuscript Library, Princeton University, Princeton, New Jersey.

Library of Congress Federal Theatre Project Collection, George Mason University Libraries, Fairfax, Virginia.

Massachusetts Society for Social Health Papers, Schlesinger Library, Radcliffe College, Harvard University, Cambridge, Massachusetts.

National Young Men's Christian Association Papers, National YMCA Library, New York, New York.

Thomas Parran Papers, Library of the School of Public Health, University of Pittsburgh, Pittsburgh, Pennsylvania (TP MSS).

Ben L. Reitman Papers, Special Collections, University Library, University of Illinois at Chicago, Chicago, Illinois.

Oral Histories

Columbia Oral History Collection, Columbia University. (COHC)
"The Reminiscences of Haven Emerson. (1950)
"The Reminiscences of Thomas Parran." (1965)

Abbreviations

AJClinMed	*American Journal of Clinical Medicine*
AJObst	*American Journal of Obstetrics*
AJPH	*American Journal of Public Health*
AJSyph	*American Journal of Syphilis*
AJUr	*American Journal of Urology*
ASHA Bull	*American Social Hygiene Association Bulletin*
AmQ	*American Quarterly*
BHM	*Bulletin of the History of Medicine*
BMS	*Boston Medical and Surgical Journal*
JAH	*Journal of American History*
JAMA	*Journal of the American Medical Association*
JHI	*Journal of the History of Ideas*
JHMAS	*Journal of the History of Medicine and Allied Sciences*
JSocHy	*Journal of Social Hygiene*
JSSMP	*Journal of the Society for Sanitary and Moral Prophylaxis*
LHJ	*Ladies' Home Journal*
MedRec	*Medical Record*
MilSurg	*Military Surgeon*
MRR	*Medical Review of Reviews*
NEJM	*New England Journal of Medicine*
NYMJ	*New York Medical Journal*
NYStJM	*New York State Journal of Medicine*
SocHy	*Social Hygiene*
SocDis	*Social Diseases*
TASSMP	*Transactions of the American Society for Sanitary and Moral Prophylaxis*
TNR	*The New Republic*
VDI	*Venereal Disease Information*
WMJ	*Women's Medical Journal*

Notes

Introduction

1. Alfred Crosby, *Epidemic and Peace* (Westport, Connecticut, 1976). On the devastating impact of infectious disease see also, William H. McNeill, *Plagues and Peoples* (New York, 1976).

2. The fullest exposition of the now considerable debate on the cause of the decline of mortality and the rise of population is Thomas McKeown, *The Role of Medicine* (Princeton, 1980). McKeown argues, quite convincingly, that mortality had fallen substantially before modern medicine could effectively address most infectious diseases. See also Thomas McKeown, "A Historical Appraisal of the Medical Task," in McKeown and Gordon McLachlan, eds., *Medical History and Medical Care*, (London, 1971), 29–50; T. McKeown and R. G. Record, "Reasons for the Decline of Mortality in England and Wales During the Nineteenth Century," in M. W. Flinn and T. C. Smout, *Essays in Social History* (Oxford, 1974), 218–50; Edward Meeker, "The Improving Health of the United States, 1850–1915," *Explorations in Entrepreneurial History* 9 (Summer 1972): 353–73; and Peter Mathias, "Disease, Medicine, and Demography in Britain During the Industrial Revolution," *Annales Cisalpines d'Histoire Sociale* 2 (1973): 1045–84.

On the impact of modern therapuetics see Harry F. Dowling, *Fighting Infection: Conquests of the Twentieth Century* (Cambridge, 1977); and Paul B. Beeson "Changes in Medical Therapy During the Past Half Century," *Medicine* 59 (1980): 79–85.

3. "STD Fact Sheet—1980" (Washington: DHHS, 1981); and *New York Times*, January 23, 1977.

4. In the last two decades, studies of cholera, pellagra, and hookworm have deepened our understanding of disease in its social context. See Charles E. Rosenberg, *The Cholera Years* (Chicago, 1962); Elizabeth W. Etheridge, *The Butterfly Caste* (Westport, Connecticut, 1972); and John Ettling, *The Germ of Laziness*, (Cambridge, 1981).

5. On the history of the American medical profession and issues of professionalization see Paul Starr, *The Social Transformation of American Medicine* (New York, 1982); Burton Bledstein, *The Culture of Professionalism* (New York, 1976); Jeffrey Berlant, *Profession and Monopoly: A Study of Medicine in the United States and Great Britain* (Berkeley, 1975); Bernard Barber, "Some Problems in the Sociology of the Professions," in Kenneth Lynn, ed., *The Professions in America* (Boston, 1965), 15–34; Rosemary Stevens, *American Medicine and the Public Interest* (New Haven, 1971); and Martin S.

Pernick, "A Calculus of Suffering: Pain, Anesthesia and Utilitarian Professionalism in Nineteenth Century American Medicine," Ph.D. dissertation, Columbia University, 1979.

6. For critiques of the biomedical model see, for example, René Dubos, *The Mirage of Health* (New York, 1959); and Elliot G. Mishler, *Social Contexts of Health, Illness, and Patient Care* (New York, 1981).

7. See Susan Sontag, *Illness as Metaphor* (New York, 1978). Sontag demonstrates in this brilliant polemic that disease has throughout history attracted metaphors and symbolic language that reveal implict beliefs about the disease and its victims. Sontag believes, however, that science can free medicine from the metaphors of disease. In this essentially positivist framework, she assumes that once a disease is understood and treatable, the metaphors will wither away. This, of course, denies the notion that science, too, is subject to the power of cultural values and beliefs.

8. The notion of dirt and contamination is most clearly developed by cultural anthropologist Mary Douglas. Douglas has examined the nature of dirt, disorder, and contamination in a number of cultures. See her *Purity and Danger: An Analysis of the Concepts of Pollution and Taboo* (London, 1966).

9. Among the recent important discussions on the historiography of sexuality see Martha Vicinus, "Sexuality and Power," *Feminist Studies* 8 (Spring 1982): 133–156; also Jeffrey Weeks, *Sex, Politics and Society since 1800* (London, 1981), 1–18; also, Robert Padgug, "Sexual Matters: On Conceptualizing Sexuality in History," *Radical History Review* 20 (Spring/Summer 1979): 1–22; John C. Burnham, "American Historians and the Subject of Sex," *Societas* 2 (Autumn 1972): 307–16; and Ronald G. Walters, "Sexual Matters and Historical Problems: A Framework for Analysis," *Societas* 6 (Summer 1976): 157–75.

Chapter I

1. In his history of the American family, *At Odds: Women and the Family in America From the Revolution to the Present* (New York, 1980), Carl Degler provides a survey of recent scholarship; see also Michael Gordon, ed., *The American Family in Social and Historical Perspective* (New York, 1974, 1979).

2. On the changing composition of families see Ansley J. Coale and Melvin Zelnik, *New Estimates of Fertility and Population in the United States* (Princeton, 1963), 36; also Xarifa Sallume and Frank W. Notestein, "Trends in the Size of Families Completed Prior to 1910 in Various Social Classes," *American Journal of Sociology* 38 (November 1932): 398–408; Frank W. Notestein, "The Decreasing Size of Families from 1890 to 1910," *Quarterly Bulletin of the Milbank Memorial Fund* 9 (October 1931): 181–88; and Daniel Scott Smith, "Family Limitation, Sexual Control and Domestic Feminism in Victorian America," *Feminist Studies* 1 (Winter-Spring 1973): 40–57.

3. See William L. O'Neill, *Divorce in the Progressive Era* (New Haven, 1967); also G. V. Hamilton and Kenneth MacGowan, *What is Wrong with Marriage* (New York, 1929); and Elaine Tyler May, *Great Expectations: Marriage and Divorce in Post-Victorian America* (Chicago, 1980).

4. Theodore Roosevelt, "Race Decadence," *Outlook* 97 (April 8, 1911); 765; see also Roosevelt, "A Premium on Race Suicide," *Outlook* 105 (September 20, 1911): 163–64; Roosevelt, "The Greatest American Problem," *Delineator* (June 1907), 966–67; Linda Gordon, *Woman's Body, Woman's Right: A Social History of Birth Control in America* (New York, 1976), 136–42.

5. "Marriage and Marital Customs," *American Medicine*, n.s. 6 (August 1911): 395.

6. Because of its heterogeneous nature, Progressivism remains a central problem in American historiography. The two classic works on the history of progressive reform are Richard Hofstadter, *The Age of Reform* (New York, 1955); and Robert H. Wiebe, *The Search For Order* (New York, 1967). On the complexity of reform and its constituents, see Peter G. Filene, "An Obituary for the Progressive Movement," *AmQ* 20 (1968), 20–34; and Daniel T. Rodgers, "In Search of Progressivism," *Reviews in American History* 10 (December 1982): 113–132.

7. See Alfred Fournier, *Syphilis and Marriage*, trans. Prince A. Morrow (New York, 1880); and L. Duncan Bulkey, *Syphilis in the Innocent* (New York, 1894).

8. William Allen Pusey, *The History and Epidemiology of Syphilis* (Baltimore, 1933), 53–61; John T. Crissey and Lawrence C. Parrish, *The Dermatology and Syphilology of the Nineteenth Century* (New York, 1981), 80–94.

9. Rudolf Virchow, *Ueber die Natur der Constitutionell Syphilitischen Affectionen* (Berlin, 1859); Pusey, *The History and Epidemiology of Syphilis*, 59–61.

10. See Fancis Welch, "On Aortic Aneurism in the Army and Conditions Associated with It," *Med-Chirurgery* 41 (1876): 41; also William Osler, "Syphilis and Aneurysm," *British Medical Journal*, (November 27, 1909): 1509–14; and Lewis A. Connor, "Development of Knowledge Concerning the Role of Syphilis in Cardio-Vascular Disease," *JAMA* 102 (February 24, 1934): 575–81; P. S. Conner, "The Late Manifestations of Syphilis," *Transactions of the American Congress of Physicians and Surgeons* 2 (1891): 78–93; also Homer F. Swift and Arthur W. M. Ellis, "The Direct Treatment of Syphilitic Diseases of the Central Nervous System," *NYMJ* 96 (July 13, 1912): 53; Hideyo Noguchi and J. W. Moore, "A Demonstration of Treponema Pallidum in the Brain in Cases of General Paralysis," *Journal of Experimental Medicine* 17 (February 1913): 232.

11. Prince A. Morrow, "The Relations of Social Diseases to the Family," *American Journal of Sociology* 14 (March 1909): 629; also Allan J. McLaughlin, "Syphilis as a Public Health Problem," *SocHy* 2 (January 1916): 63; Philip S. Goodhart, "Syphilis and the Nervous System with Especial Reference to its Sociological Aspect," *SocDis* 4 (October 1913): 144–53.

12. William Osler, "Internal Medicine as a Vocation," in *Aequanimitas: With Other Addresses to Medical Students, Nurses and Practitioners of Medicine*, 3rd ed. (Philadelphia, 1932), 131–46; Osler, "Syphilis and Aneurysm," *British Medical Journal* (November 27, 1909): 1509.

13. Prince A. Morrow, "Publicity as a Factor in Venereal Prophylaxis," *JAMA* 47 (October 20, 1906): 1244; William Osler, "The Campaign Against Syphilis," *Lancet* (May 26, 1917): 789.

14. Ricord had explained, "A woman frequently gives gonorrhea without having it." Quoted in Prince A. Morrow, *Social Diseases and Marriage* (New York, 1904), 84; see also Harry F. Dowling, *Fighting Infection*, (Cambridge, 1977), 86–87.

15. Owsei Temkin, *The Double Face of Janus* (Baltimore, 1977), 473; Arthur Bloomfield, *A Bibliography of Internal Medicine: Communicable Diseases* (Chicago, 1958), 185–92; also Dowling, *Fighting Infection*, 86–87; P. S. Pelouze, *Gonorrhea in the Male and Female*, 3rd ed. (Philadelphia, 1939).

16. Diday argued that an apparently healthy child born of syphilitic parents should be treated. P. Diday, *Traite de la Syphilis des Nouveau-nes et des Enfants a la Mamelle* (Paris, 1854).

17. Symptoms developed at least three years, or even later, after birth. Alfred Fournier, *La Syphilis Hereditaire Tardive* (Paris, 1886).

18. Emil Noeggerath, "Latent Gonorrhea, Especially with Regard to its Influence on Fertility in Women," *Transactions of the American Gynecological Association* 1 (1876):

292, 293. The other physicians gathered at this meeting took exception with Noegger-ath's findings; see also John G. Clark, "A Critical Summary of Recent Literature on Gonorrhea in Women," *American Journal of Medical Science* 119 (January 1900): 73–81.

19. On American medical education, see Donald Fleming, *William Welch and the Rise of Modern Medicine* (Boston, 1954), esp. 32–56; and Thomas N. Bonner, *American Doctors and German Universities* (Lincoln, Neb., 1963).

20. Morrow became the leader of American efforts to fight venereal disease. Unfor-tunately, biographical data are scant. A few scattered letters can be found in the ASHA Papers, Folders 1:4–5. Also, see "Morrow Memorial Number," *SocDis* 4 (July 1913); Edward L. Keyes, "Prince Albert Morrow," *VDI* 22 (February 1941): 39–43; and Charles Walter Clarke, *Taboo: The Story of the Pioneers of Social Hygiene* (Washington, D.C., 1961), 56–63; also John C. Burnham, "The Progressive Era Revolution in American Attitudes toward Sex," *JAH* 59 (March 1973): 885–908.

21. Alfred Fournier, *Syphilis and Marriage*, trans. Prince A. Morrow (New York, 1880); iii–iv.

22. Owsei Temkin, "Therapeutic Trends and the Treatment of Syphilis Before 1900," *BHM* 39 (July-August 1955): 309–16; also Jarold E. Kemp, "An Outline of the History of Syphilis," *American Journal of Syphilis* 24 (November 1940): 759–74.

23. Leonard J. Goldwater, *Mercury: A History of Quicksilver* (Baltimore, 1972), 215; quote in Dowling, *Fighting Infection*, 89.

24. See Charles E. Rosenberg, "The Therapeutic Revolution: Medicine, Meaning, and Social Change in Nineteenth Century America," in Rosenberg and Morris J. Vo-gel, eds., *The Therapeutic Revolution* (Philadelphia, 1979), 3–25.

25. Fessenden Otis, *Practical Clinical Lessons on Syphilis and the Genito-Urinary Diseases* (New York, 1883), 306–307; Frederick Hollick, *A Popular Treatise on Venereal Disease* (New York, 1852), 48–49; see also, Ann Douglas Wood, "The Fashionable Diseases: Women's Complaints and Their Treatment in Nineteenth Century America," *Journal of Interdisciplinary History* 4 (1973), 25–52; and Gail Pat Parsons, "Equal Treatment for All: American Medical Remedies for Sexual Problems, 1850–1900," *JHMAS* 32 (January 1977): 55–71.

26. Prince A. Morrow, "Report of the Committee of Seven of the Medical Society of the County of New York on the Prophylaxis of Venereal Disease in New York City," *NYMJ* 74 (December 21, 1901): 1146.

27. For military statistics, see *Report of the Surgeon General for the United States Army, 1910* (Washington, D.C., 1911); also "Venereal Diseases in American Army," *Survey* 29 (January 25, 1913): 539; Morrow quote in *New York Tribune*, April 7, 1912.

28. John S. Fulton, "The Medical Statistics of Sex Hygiene; Such as they Are," *AJPH* 3 (July 1913): 661; Richard C. Cabot, "Observations Regarding the Relative Frequency of the Different Diseases Prevalent in Boston and its Vicinity," *BMSJ* 165 (August 3, 1911): 155.

29. Prince A. Morrow, "The Frequency of Venereal Diseases: A Reply to Dr. Ca-bot," *BMSJ* 165 (October 5, 1911): 522, 524; Morrow, "Report of the Committee of Seven," 1192.

30. William Osler, "The Campaign Against Syphilis," *Lancet* (May 26, 1917): 787.

31. *Conference Internationale pour la Prophylaxie de la Syphilis et des Maladies Ve-nerienne*, 2 vols. (Brussels, 1899, 1902).

32. Morrow, *Social Diseases and Marriage* (New York, 1904); see also Morrow, "Sanitary and Moral Prophylaxis," *BMSJ* 154 (June 14, 1906): 674.

33. On nineteenth-century views of heredity, see Charles E. Rosenberg, "The Bitter

° Fruit: Heredity, Disease, and Social Thought," *Perspectives in American History* 8 (1974): 189–235.

During the late nineteenth century many physicians contended that syphilis could skip a generation and be traced in the third generation. See William Allen Pusey, *Syphilis as a Modern Problem* (Chicago, 1915), 61–65.

34. Morrow, *Social Diseases and Marriage*, 78–79; Abraham L. Wolbarst, "The Venereal Diseases: A Menace to the National Welfare," *American Journal of Dermatology* 14 (June 1910): 269.

35. Prince A. Morrow, "Blindness of the Newborn," *TASSMP* 2 (April 1908): 81; see also, Carolyn Conant Von Blarcum, "Blindness of the Newborn and its Causes," *JSSMP* 6 (January 1915): 23–32; and Charles Bull Stedman, "Opthalmia Neonatorum and Its Prophylaxis from the Standpoint of the Opthalmologist," *TASSMP* 3 (1910): 63–71.

36. K.S.F. Credé, *Die Verhutung der Augenentzundung der Neugeborenen* (Berlin, 1884).

37. P. C. Barsam, "Specific Prophylaxis of Gonorrheal Opthalmia Neonatorum," *NEJM* 274 (March 31, 1966): 731–33; also J. W. Kerr, "Opthalmia Neonatorum: An Analysis of the Laws and Regulations Relation Thereto in Force in the United States," *Public Health Service Bulletin* No. 49 (Washington, D.C., 1911).

The failure of midwives to use silver nitrate led to demands that they be more carefully supervised and licensed. See Frances E. Kobrin, "The American Midwife Controversy: A Crisis of Professionalization," *BHM* 40 (July-August 1966): 351; Abraham L. Wolbarst, "On the Occurrence of Syphilis and Gonorrhea in Children by Direct Infection," *American Medicine*, n.s. 7 (September 1912): 494; also Carolyn Von Blarcum, "The Harm Done in Ascribing All Babies' Sore Eyes to Gonorrhea," *AJPH* 6 (September 1916): 926–31; Edith Houghton Hooker, "The Scapegoat," *Survey* 35 (December 4, 1915): 254–55.

38. Morrow, *Social Diseases and Marriage*, 84; Morrow, "A Plea for the Organization of a 'Society of Sanitary and Moral Prophylaxis,' " *Medical News* 86 (June 4, 1906): 1075.

39. E. L. Keyes, *Syphilis* (New York 1908), 34.

40. Albert H. Burr, "The Guarantee of Safety in the Marriage Contract," *JAMA* 47 (December 8, 1906): 1887–88; Abraham L. Wolbarst, "The Venereal Diseases: A Menace to the National Welfare," 268; also "The Pity of It," *NYStJM* 13 (June 1913): 298.

41. Morrow, *Social Diseases and Marriage*, 109, 131; also Joseph Taber Johnson, "The Effects of Gonorrhea on the Female Generative Organs," *JAMA*, 44 (March 4, 1905), 757–59; and Abraham Jacobi, "Discussion," *SocDis* 2 (January 1911): 25.

42. Morrow, *Social Diseases and Marriage*, 269; also Henry D. Holton, "Birthrate and Decrease in Population as Affected by Syphilis and Gonorrhea," *JAMA* 44 (March 4, 1905): 761–62. On birth control practice see Linda Gordon, *Woman's Body, Woman's Right*, 95–115; Daniel Scott Smith, "Family Limitation, Sexual Control, and Domestic Feminism in Victorian America," 40–57; and James Reed, *From Private Vice to Public Virtue* (New York, 1978), 3–18.

43. See Carroll Smith-Rosenberg and Charles E. Rosenberg, "The Female Animal: Medical and Biological Views of Women," *JAH* 60 (September 1973): 332–56.

44. Morrow, *Social Diseases and Marriage*, 30, 31.

45. Prince A. Morrow, "The Society of Sanitary and Moral Prophylaxis: Its Objects and Aims," *American Medicine*, n.s. 9 (February 25, 1905): 318; also Morrow, "Education Within the Medical Profession," *TASSMP* 1 (1906): 47–57.

46. Rosenberg, "The Therapeutic Revolution," 3–26.

47. W. A. Purrington, "Professional Secrecy and the Obligatory Notification of Venereal Diseases," *NYMJ* 85 (June 29, 1907): 1207.

48. John A. Fordyce, "The Value of Education and Treatment as Safeguards in Venereal Infection Through Marriage," *TASSMP* 1 (1906): 150–51; see also William S. Gottheil, "Discussion," *TASSMP* 2 (1908): 111.

49. John H. Stokes, *The Third Great Plague* (Philadelphia, 1917), 129; Morrow, *Social Diseases and Marriage*, 51; Purrington, "Professional Secrecy," 1209.

50. Morrow, *Social Diseases and Marriage*, 61, 70; see also L. Stevenard, "The Professional Secret in Syphilis and Marriage," *AJUr* 12 (1916): 33–37.

51. Keyes, *Syphilis*, 64; Ann J. Lane, ed., *The Charlotte Perkins Gilman Reader* (New York, 1980), 118–19.

52. Morrow, "The Relations of Social Diseases to the Family," *American Journal of Sociology* 14 (March 1909): 635; Robert N. Willson, "The Relation of the Medical Profession to the Social Evil," *JAMA* 47 (July 7, 1906): 30.

53. Morrow, *Social Diseases and Marriage*, 30; William Lee Howard, "The Havoc of Prudery," *Pearson's Magazine* 24 (1910): 591. See also Charles Henry Huberich, "Venereal Disease in the Law of Marriage and Divorce," *American Law Review* 37 (1903): 226–36; also Christopher Lasch, "Divorce and the Family in America," *Atlantic Monthly* 218 (November 1966): 57–60.

54. See Mark H. Haller, *Eugenics: Hereditarian Attitudes in American Thought* (New Brunswick, N.J., 1963), esp. 50–57; also Richard Hofstadter, *Social Darwinism in American Thought* (1944; Boston, 1955), 161–67.

55. Prince A. Morrow, "Eugenics and Venereal Diseases," *Proceedings of the Child Conference for Research and Welfare* 2 (1910): 192; Morrow, *Eugenics and Racial Poisons* (New York, 1912), 11; See also Morrow, "Venereal Diseases and Their Relation to Infant Mortality and Race Determination," *NYMJ* 94 (December 30, 1911): 1315.

56. Morrow, *Eugenics and Racial Poisons*, 11; see also E. L. Keyes, "The Prenuptial Sanitary Guarantee," *NYMJ* 85 (June 29, 1907): 1202–1204.

57. J. W. Kerr and A. A. Moll, "Communicable Diseases: An Analysis of the Laws and Regulations," *Public Health Service Bulletin* No. 62 (Washington, D.C., 1913): 44–46; See also, "Should a Medical Certificate of Freedom from a Transmissable Disease be Required as a Condition of License to Marry?" *TASSMP* 3 (1910): 125–58; also Oscar Dowling, "The Marriage Health Certificate: A Deeply Rooted Problem," *AJPH* 5 (November 1915): 1145; Edward L. Keyes, "Can the Law Protect Matrimony from Disease," *SocHy*, 1 (December 1914): 9–14; and Evangeline Young, "The Conservation of Manhood and Womanhood," *WMJ* 29 (March 1910): 20.

58. E. L. Keyes, "Can the Law Protect Marriage from Disease?" 11.

59. See, for example, Paul Starr, *The Social Transformation of American Medicine* (New York, 1982), 79–144.

60. See John Higham, *Strangers in the Land: Patterns of American Nativism, 1860–1925* (New Brunswick, 1955; New York, 1963), 159; 100–112, 202–204.

61. Ralph Williams, *The United States Public Health Service, 1798–1950* (Washington, D.C. 1950), 525–27; U.S. Senate, *Reports of the U.S. Immigration Commission,* 61st Congress, 3rd session, Senate doc. 747 (Washington, D.C., 1911), 1: 34; Louise Eberle, "Where Immigration Medical Inspection Fails," *Colliers'* 50 (February 8, 1913): 27; also Frederick Whitin to William F. Snow, November 18, 1916, Papers of the Committee of Fourteen, New York Public Library.

62. W. Travis Gibb, "Criminal Aspect of Venereal Diseases in Children," *TASSMP*

2 (1908): 25; Howard Kelly, "The Best Way to Treat the Social Evil," *TASSMP* 1 (1906): 72; also Kelly, "What is the Right Attitude of the Medical Profession toward the Social Evil," *JAMA* 44 (March 4, 1905): 679–81; see also Abraham Wolbarst, "On the Occurrence of Syphilis and Gonorrhea in Children by Direct Infection," *American Medicine*, n.s. 7 (September 1912): 496.

63. L. Duncan Bulkey, *Syphilis in the Innocent*, 3–4.

64. See Egal Feldman, "Prostitution, The Alien Woman dnd the Progressive Imagination," *AmQ* 19 (Summer 1967): 192–206.

65. Bulkey, *Syphilis in the Innocent*, 21; Frederick Taussig, "The Contagion of Gonorrhea Among Little Girls," *SocHy* 1 (June 1915): 415–22.

66. "What One Woman Has Had to Bear," *Forum* 48 (October 1912): 451, 452–3, 454. See also, "New Laws About Drinking Cups," *Life* 58: (December 21, 1911): 1152.

67. "I will not come out and take care of venereal cases and put urology upon the basis of venereology. . . . That is where urology first got its black eye." Ernest G. Mark, *Transactions of the American Urological Association* 5 (1911): 14–15.

68. See, for example, Edward B. Vedder, *Syphilis and Public Health* (Philadelphia, 1918): 200–201.

69. Ellen Torelle, "Botany and Zoology as a Means of Teaching Sex-Hygiene," *TASSMP* 3 (1910): 167; Howard Kelly, "The Best Way to Treat the Social Evil," 75; also Kelly, "The Protection of the Innocent," *AJObst* 55 (April 1907): 477–81.

70. L. Duncan Bulkey, "Should Sex Instruction Be Given to Young Men of the Working Class?" *TASSMP* 1 (1906): 104; Howard Kelly, "Social Diseases and Their Prevention," *SocDis* 1 (July 1910): 17.

71. Robert N. Willson, "The Relation of the Medical Profession to the Social Evil," 32; Prince A. Morrow, "Publicity as a Factor in Venereal Prophylaxis," *JAMA* 47 (October 10, 1906): 1246; also W. J. Herdman, "The Duty of the Medical Profession to the Public in the Matter of Venereal Diseases, and How to Discharge It," *JAMA* 47 (October 20, 1906): 1247–48.

72. Morrow, "Sanitary and Moral Prophylaxis," *BMSJ* 154 (June 14, 1906): p. 676; Edward Bok, *The Americanization of Edward Bok* (New York, 1924), 345–51.

73. Margaret H. Sanger, *What Every Girl Should Know* (New York, 1912, 1920). The Post Office lifted the ban several weeks later. See Linda Gordon, *Woman's Body, Woman's Right*, 214. Morrow, "Publicity as a Factor in Venereal Prophylaxis," 1246.

74. Egbert Grandin, "Should the Great Body of the General Public Be Enlightened as to the Extent and Danger of the Venereal Diseases and Their Mode of Contagion, Direct or Indirect?" *Charities and Commons* (February 24, 1906), 4; D. E. Standard, "The Crime of Sexual Ignorance," *AJClinMed* 17 (November 1910): 1169; see also, Albert E. Carrier, "What Shall We Teach the Public Regarding Venereal Diseases?" *JAMA* 47 (October 10, 1906): 1250–52.

75. Grandin "Should the Public be Enlightened," 4; Ferdinand C. Valentine, "Educational Limitation of Venereal Diseases," *MedRec* 62 (November 8, 1902): 734–36; William A. Evans, "The Attack on Venereal Diseases Through Education and Publicity," *JSSMP* 5 (July 1915): 86.

76. Morrow, "A Plea for the Organization of a 'Society of Sanitary and Moral Prophylaxis,' " *Medical News* 86 (June 4, 1904): 1074; Morrow, "Sanitary and Moral Prophylaxis," *BMSJ* 154 (June 14, 1906): 674; Morrow, "The Society of Sanitary and Moral Prophylaxis: Its Aims and Objects," *TASSMP* 1 (1906): 32.

77. "The American Federation for Sex Hygiene," *SocDis* 1 (July 1910): 5; "The American Federation for Sex Hygiene: Its Objects and Proposed Method of Work," *SocDis* 3 (October 1912): 34–36; Morrow, "Report of Progress," *SocDis* 3 (April 1912): 1–17.

See Morrow, "The Society of Sanitary and Moral Prophylaxis: Its Objects and Aims," *TASSMP* 1 (1906): 26–36; Morrow, "Results Achieved by the Movement for Sanitary and Moral Prophylaxis—Outlook for the Future," *TASSMP* 3 (1910): 94–104.

See also, James Frank Gardner, "Microbes and Morality: The Social Hygiene Crusade in New York City, 1892–1917," Ph.D. dissertation, Indiana University, 1974, esp. 106–174.

78. Morrow, "Publicity as a Factor in Venereal Prophylaxis," 1245, 1246.

79. Prince A. Morrow, "The Teaching of Sex Hygiene," *Good Housekeeping* 54 (March 1912): 405; Robert N. Willson, "The Eradication of the Social Evil in Large Ctities," *JAMA* 69 (September 21, 1912): 925.

80. Morrow, "The Teaching of Sex Hygiene," 405; Willson, "The Relation of the Medical Profession to the Social Evil," 32.

81. Prince A. Morrow, *The Boy's Problem* (New York, 1906), 21–22; U.S. Public Health Service, *The Problem of Sex Education in the Schools* (Washington, D.C., 1919), 9; also, "Parents and Sex Hygiene," *MRR* 19 (June 1913): 352–53.

82. Frederic Henry Gerrish, "A Crusade Against Syphilis and Gonorrhea," unp. typescript, June 7, 1910, p. 15, ASHA Papers, Folder 1:4; Rose Woodallen Chapmen, "How Shall I Tell My Child?" *Ladies' Home Journal* (April 1, 1911), 66.

83. Bryan Strong, "Ideas of the Early Sex Education Movement in America, 1890–1920," *History of Education Quarterly* 12 (Summer 1972): 144–45.

84. Prince A. Morrow, *Health and the Hygiene of Sex*, ASSMP Educational Pamphlet No. 6 (New York 1914), 6.

85. Morrow, *Health and the Hygiene of Sex*, 31. On the history of masturbation, see H. Tristram Englehardt, Jr., "The Disease of Masturbation: Values and the Concept of Disease," *BHM* 48 (Summer 1974): 234–48; also E. H. Hare, "Masturbational Insanity: The History of an Idea," *Journal of Mental Science* 108 (1962): 2–25; and Robert H. MacDonald, "The Frightful Consequences of Onanism: Notes on the History of a Delusion," *JHI* 28 (July-September, 1967): 423–31.

86. Winfield Scott Hall, *Instead of Wild Oats* (New York, 1912), 25. On the history of the double standard see Keith Thomas, "The Double Standard," *JHI* 20 (April 1959): 195–216; and Ira L. Reiss, "The Double Standard in Premarital Sexual Intercourse," *Social Forces* 34 (March 1956): 224–30.

87. Morrow, *Social Diseases and Marriage*, 125; Frank D. Watson, "Discussion," *JSSMP* 5 (April 1915): 111; G. Stanley Hall, "The Needs and Methods of Educating Young People in the Hygiene of Sex," *TASSMP* 2 (1908): 196.

88. Prince A. Morrow to Mary Cobb, September 13, 1909, ASHA Papers, Folder 1:4; Morrow, "The Society of Sanitary and Moral Prophylaxis: Its Objects and Aims," *TASSMP* 1 (1906): 33; Abraham Wolbarst, "Discussion," *TASSMP* 3 (1910): 34; Margaret Cleaves, "Discussion," *TASSMP* 3 (1910): 31.

89. Max J. Exner, "Sex Education in the Colleges and Universities," *JSSMP* 6 (October, 1915): 131–33; Maurice A. Bigelow, "Discussion," *JSSMP* 5 (1915): 107; Bigelow, "The Selection and Training of Teachers for Sex Instruction," *JSSMP* 6 (October, 1915): 131–33.

90. B. S. Talmey, *Genesis: A Manual for the Instruction of Children in Matters Sexual* (New York, 1910), 135; Ferdinand C. Valentine, "Education in Sexual Subjects," *TASSMP* 1 (1906): 97; Woods Hutchinson, "What Not to Teach Our Children Upon Race Hygiene," *Good Housekeeping* 54 (April 1912): 530.

91. Morrow, "The Teaching of Sex Hygiene," 406; Maurice Bigelow, *Sex Education* (New York, 1916), 127.

92. See, for example, William Lee Howard, "The Havoc of Prudery," *Pearson's*

Magazine 24 (1910): 589–98; J. Riddle Goff, "Discussion," *TASSMP* 1 (1906): 118–19.

93. D. E. Standard, "The Crime of Sexual Ignorance," 1167.

94. Gerrish, "A Crusade Against Syphilis and Gonorrhea," 15. These medical views cannot, of course, be read as actual reflections of the sexual experience of women. See Carl N. Degler, "What Ought to Be and What Was: Women's Sexuality in the Nineteenth Century," *American Historical Review* 79 (December 1974): 1467–90; also Nancy F. Cott, "Passionlessness: An Interpretation of Victorian Sexual Ideology, 1790–1850," *Signs* 4 (1978): 219–36; and Charles E. Rosenberg, "Sexuality, Class, and Role," *AmQ* 25 (May 1973): 131–53.

95. Willson, "The Relation of the Medical Profession to the Social Evil," 32; Morrow quoted in New York *Tribune*, April 7, 1912; Charlotte Perkins Gilman, "Discussion," *TASSMP* 3 (1910): 28. See also, Emma Walker, "Protective Hygiene for Mothers and Girls," *TASSMP* 2 (1910): 8–16; Rosalie Slaughter Morton, "Lectures to Women of the Educated Classes," *TASSMP* 3 (1910): 17–25; Albert Vandeveer, "In the Relation We Bear to the Public What Use Shall We Make of Our Knowledge of the Evil Effects of Venereal Disease?" *AJObst* 64 (December 1911): 1033–42. For a vigorous feminist endorsement of social hygiene see Lavinia L. Dock's guide for nurses, *Hygiene and Morality* (New York, 1910).

96. "Circular No. 3," Massachusetts Association of Boards of Health, 1908 in ASHA Papers, Folder 4:2; Margaret A. Cleaves, "Education in Sexual Hygiene for Young Working Women," *Charities and Commons* (February 24, 1906), 9.

97. *Educational Review* 46 (October 1913): 318; George Whiteside, "What Should We Teach the Public Regarding Venereal Disease," *JAMA* 47 (October 20, 1906): 1253.

98. Mabel S. Ulrich, "Constructive Preventive Work Through Moral Education," *JSSMP* 6 (April 1915): 54; Miriam C. Gould, "The Psychological Influence Upon the Adolescent Girl of the Knowledge of Prostitution and Venereal Disease," *SocHy* 2 (April 1916): 195; Talcott Williams, "The Situation," *SocDis* 3 (October 1912): 3.

99. Prince A. Morrow, "Results of the Work Done by the Society of Sanitary and Moral Prophylaxis," *TASSMP* 2 (1908): 121; Grandin, "Should the Public Be Enlightened?" 5; Morrow, "Results of the Work Done," 127.

100. Newell Edson, "Status of Sex Education in High Schools," Bureau of Education, Department of the Interior, *Bulletin*, 1922, no. 14 (Washington, D.C., 1922): 3; James Pedersen, "The Social Evil," *NYStJM* 13 (February 1913): 101; George Meylan, "Discussion," *JSSMP* 5 (April 1914): 112. See also, Prince Morrow, "Report of Progress," *SocDis* 3 (April 1912): 17.

101. See Peter T. Cominos, "Late Victorian Respectability and the Social System," *International Review of Social History* 8 (1963): 18–48, 217–50; and Steven Marcus, *The Other Victorians: A Study of Sexuality and Pornography in Mid-Nineteenth Century England* (New York, 1966).

102. Ludwig Weiss, "The Prostitution Problem in its Relation to Law and Medicine," *JAMA* 47 (December 22, 1906): 2074. Katharine B. Davis, "The Department of Corrections and the Social Hygiene Movement," *JSSMP* 5 (October 1914): 165; also Edward B. Vedder, *Syphilis and Public Health*, 47–49.

103. On the nineteenth-century crusades against vice, see David J. Pivar, *Purity Crusade: Sexual Morality and Social Control, 1868–1900* (Westport, Conn. 1973); also Carroll Smith-Rosenberg, "Beauty, the Beast, and the Miltant Woman: A Case Study in Sex Roles and Social Stress in Jacksonian America," *AmQ* 23 (October 1971): 562–84.

104. The classic formulation of the social role of the prostitute was W. E. H. Lecky's:

"Herself the supreme type of vice, she is ultimately the most efficient guardian of virtue." See his *History of European Morals from Augustus to Charlemagne* (New York, 1955), 2:283; Morrow, *Social Diseases and Marriage*, vi; Morrow, "Eugenics and Venereal Diseases," 197.

105. Pivar, *Purity Crusade*, 24–43; Janes Addams, *A New Conscience and an Ancient Evil* (New York, 1912), 97.

106. Committee of Fifteen, *The Social Evil* (New York, 1902), 58, 69. Among the recent secondary studies of prostitution in the Progressive years and the vice crusades see Paul S. Boyer, *Urban Masses and Moral Order* (Cambridge, 1978) esp. 191–219; Jeremy P. Felt, "Vice Reform as a Political Technique: The Committee of Fifteen in New York, 1900–1901," *New York History* 54 (January 1973): 24–51; Eric Anderson, "Prostitution and Social Justice: Chicago, 1910–15, *Social Service Review* 48 (June 1974): 203–28; Roy Lubove, "The Progressives and the Prostitute," *Historian* 24 (May 1962): 308–30; Judith K. Walkowitz, "The Politics of Prostitution," *Signs* 6 (Autumn 1980): 123–35; Robert E. Reigel, "Changing American Ideas Toward Prostitution," *JHI* 29 (July-September 1968): 448–62; and especially Mark Thomas Connelly, *The Response to Prostitution in the Progressive Era* (Chapel Hill, 1980); and Ruth Rosen, *The Lost Sisterhood: Prostitution in America, 1900–1918* (Baltimore, 1982).

107. Vice Commission of Chicago, *The Social Evil in Chicago: A Study of Existing Conditions* (Chicago, 1911), 25–26; Between 1911 and 1916, twenty-seven American cities issued reports of vice investigations. The best account of these commissions is Connelly, *The Response to Prostitution in the Progressive Era*, esp. pp. 91–113.

108. Committee of Fifteen, *The Social Evil*, 8–9.

109. See, for example, Stokes, *The Third Great Plague*, 158–59; also Charles Chaissagnac, "Etiology of the Social Evil," *JAMA* 47 (December 22, 1906): 1075; and Vedder, *Syphilis and Public Health*, 214.

110. J. H. Landis, "The Social Evil in Relation to the Health Problem," *AJPH* 3 (October 1913): 1075; on the membership of the Committee of Fifteen see Felt, "Vice Reform as a Political Technique," 30; on the Chicago Vice Commission, see Anderson, "Prostitution and Social Justice," 208–211; also Boyer, *Urban Masses and Moral Order*, 211–17.

111. "National Merger to Fight White Slavery," *Survey* 27 (March 30, 1912): 1991–92; "New Methods for Grappling with the Social Evil," *Current Opinion* 54 (April 1913): 308–309; "The 'Vice Trust' in New York City," *Current Opinion* 54 (January 1913): 5–6; O. Edward Janney, *The White Slave Traffic in America* (New York, 1911), esp. 5–8, 22–23.

112. George Kibbe Turner, "The City of Chicago: A Study of the Great Immoralities," *McClure's Magazine* 28 (April 1907): 575–82; Peter Y. Sonnenthal, "The Origins and Early Enforcement of the White Slave Traffic Act, 1910–1917," M.A. thesis, Columbia University, 1977; see also Clifford G. Roe, *Horrors of the White Slave Trade: The Mighty Crusade to Protect the Purity of Our Homes* (New York, 1911).

113. George J. Kneeland, *Commercialized Prostitution in New York* (New York, 1913), 92; Maude E. Miner, *The Slavery of Prostitution* (New York, 1916), ix. see also, Willoughby C. Waterman, *Prostitution and Its Repression in New York City* (New York, 1932).

114. Addams, *A New Conscience and an Ancient Evil*, 89; Adolphus S. Knopf, "Some Thoughts on the Etiology, Prophylaxis and Treatment of the Social Evil," *TASSMP* 2 (1908): 218–35; Committee of Fifteen, *The Social Evil*, 10–11. Chicago Vice Commission, *The Social Evil in Chicago*, 43; also Margaret Dreier Robins, "One Aspect of the Menace of Low Wages," *SocHy* 1 (1915), 358–63; Weiss, "The Prostitution Prob-

lem in Relation to Law and Medicine," 2073. Department stores were singled out as particularly dangerous places to be employed. See, for example, Florence Kelly, "The Economic Causes of Prostitution," *SocDis* 3 (July 1912): 9–13.

115. See, for example, A. J. McLaughlin, "Pioneering in Venereal Disease Control," *AJObst* 80 (December 1919): 634, 642; also Ruth Rosen, ed., *The Maimie Papers* (New York 1977), 280, 287–90. Maimie Pinzer, a prostitute whose letters are collected here, lost an eye, apparently from a syphilitic infection.

116. See Estelle B. Freedman, *Their Sisters' Keepers: Women's Prison Reform in America* (Ann Arbor, 1981); and Richard Roland Wagner, "Virtue Against Vice: A Study of Moral Reformers and Prostitution in the Progressive Era," Ph.D. dissertation, University of Wisconsin, 1971.

117. On measures for regulating prostitution during the nineteenth century, see Pivar, *Purity Crusade*, esp. 32–34.

118. Henry P. DeForest, "Personal Observation of Police Methods of Dealing with Prostitution in Germany with Conclusions as to Their Sanitary Value," *TASSMP* 2 (1908), 141–70; Frederic Bierhoff, "The Problem of Prostitution and Venereal Diseases in New York City," *NYMJ* 93 (1911): 557–61; V. G. Vecki, "Can We Abolish, Shall We Ignore, or Must We Regulate Prostitution?" *American Journal of Dermatology* 11 (1910): 213–20; J. H. Landis, "The Social Evil in Relation to the Health Problem," *AJPH* 3 (October 1913), 1073–86; Denslow Lewis, "What Shall We Do with the Prostitute?" *American Journal of Dermatology* 11 (1907): 485–93; and George B. H. Swayze, "The Social Evil," *Medical Times* 34 (1906): 257. See also John C. Burnham, "Medical Inspection of Prostitutes in America in the Nineteenth Century: The St. Louis Experiment and its Sequel," *BHM* 45 (May-June 1971): 203–18.

119. See, for example, Prince A. Morrow, "The Sanitary and Moral Prophylaxis of Venereal Diseases," *JAMA* 44 (March 4, 1905): 675; also Howard Kelly, "The Regulation of Prostitution," *JAMA* 44 (February 10, 1906): 398; Abner Post, "What Should Be the Attitude of Boards of Health Toward Venereal Disease," *AJPH* 4 (January 1908): 47–48; and Abraham Flexner, "Legal and Administrative Phases of the Social Hygiene Problem," *JSSMP* 5 (October 1914): 215–23. On the rigorous debate regarding state regulation of prostitution in England, see Judith Walkowitz, *Prostitution and Victorian Society* (New York, 1980).

120. Committee of Fifteen, *The Social Evil*, 85; G. Frank Lydston, "The Social Evil and Its Remedies," *AJClinMed* 16 (March 1909): 281; Chicago Vice Commission, *The Social Evil in Chicago*, 25.

121. The law resulted from a commission chaired by State Senator Alfred Page to investigate the Magistrate's Court of New York City. See State of New York, *Proceedings of the Commission to Inquire Into Courts of Inferior Criminal Jurisdiction in Cities of the First Class*, 5 vols. (Albany, 1909); also *Final Report of the Commission* (Albany, 1910). See also "Hearings on the Page Bill," *Survey* 24 (May 1910), 923.

122. E. R. A. Seligman, "Sanitary Supervision of Prostitution," *SocDis* 2 (January 1911): 10.

123. See Julius Mayer, "Clause 79 of the Page Bill and the Sanitary Supervision of Prostitution," *SocDis* 1 (October 1910): 5; also Homer Folks, "Discussion," *SocDis* 1 (October 1910): 24–26; and Frederic Bierhoff, "Concerning the Protest by the Committee Representing Various Women's Clubs Against Paragraph 79," *NYMJ* 92 (December 3, 1910): 1108–12.

124. The Conference of All the Organizations of Women in Greater New York issued a statement in October 1910, declaring that the law endorsed the double standard of sexual morality. The New York City Federation of Women's Clubs passed a resolu-

tion demanding that section 79 also include the examination of men. See Gardner, "Microbes and Morality," 193–200. Alice Stone Blackwell wrote that the "law provides a heavier penalty for stealing a horse than for stealing a girl," *Survey* 25 (December 10, 1910): 437; Prince A. Morrow, "Sanitary Aspects of Clause 79 of the Page Law," *SocDis* 1 (October 1910): 8, 15.

125. Morrow, "Sanitary Aspects of Clause 79," 8.

126. "The End of Clause 79," *Survey* 26 (July 8, 1911): 552.

127. Prince A. Morrow to Mary Cobb, June 24, 1910, ASHA Papers, Folder 1:4.

128. John D. Rockefeller, Jr. to Edward L. Keyes, Jr., July 18, 1913, BSH Papers; American Social Hygiene Association, *First Annual Report, 1913–14* (New York, 1914); also Jerome Greene, "Memo on American Social Hygiene Association," unp. mss., July 18, 1916, BSH Papers. See also, "The Christening of the New Association," *ASHA Bull* 1 (April 1914); William F. Snow, "The American Social Hygiene Association: An Experiment in Preventive Medicine and 'Curative' Morals," *JSSMP* 5 (April 1914): 79–91.

129. For American Social Hygiene Association budgets see "Brief Historical Statement: Confidential Office Memorandum," unp. typescript, ca. 1948, ASHA Papers, Folder 1:1. On Rockefeller's interest in prostitution and social hygiene I have relied on Gardner, "Microbes and Morality."

130. John D. Rockefeller, Jr. to Frederick Gates, November 2, 1910; John D. Rockefeller, Jr., "The Origins, Work, and Plans of the Bureau of Social Hygiene," unp. typescript, January 27, 1913, BSH Papers; see also "The Bureau of Social Hygiene," *Outlook* 103 (February 8, 1913): 287–88; Jerome D. Greene, "The Bureau of Social Hygiene," *SocHy* 3 (January 1917): 1–9.

131. Unpublished memorandum, December 7, 1915, BSH Papers.

132. See George J. Kneeland, *Commercialized Prostitution in New York* (New York 1913); Abraham Flexner, *Prostitution in Europe* (New York, 1914); Raymond B. Fosdick, *European Police Systems* (New York, 1915); and Harold B. Woolston, *Prostitution in the United States* (New York, 1921). See also Fosdick, *Chronicle of a Generation: An Autobiography* (New York, 1958), 124–25.

133. John D. Rockefeller to Katharine B. Davis, November 13, 1911; Rockefeller to Davis, December 29, 1911; Davis to Bureau of Social Hygiene, January 13, 1915; "Minutes of Meeting of the Bureau of Social Hygiene," unp. typescript, April 28, 1917, BSH Papers.

134. See, for example, Edith R. Spaulding, *An Experimental Study of Psychopathic Delinquent Women* (New York, 1923); Charles B. Davenport, "Some Social Applications of Modern Principles of Heredity," *Transactions of the Fifteenth International Congress on Hygiene and Demography, 1912* (Washington, D.C., 1913), 4:661.

135. Dowling, *Fighting Infection*, 91; on the history of the Wassermann reaction see Ludwik Fleck, *Genesis and Development of a Scientific Fact*, trans. Trenn (1935; Chicago, 1979).

136. Homer F. Swift, "Dispensary Facilities of the Treatment of Syphilis," *NYMJ* 97 (May 17, 1913): 103; Dowling, *Fighting Infection*, 89; and Pelouze, *Gonorrhea in the Male and Female*, 3rd ed. (Philadelphia, 1939).

137. Quote in Martha Marquardt, *Paul Ehrlich* (New York, 1951), 91; M. P. Earles, "Salvarsan and the Concept of Chemotherapy," *Pharmaceutical Journal* 204 (April 18, 1970): 340–42; and Isador Rosen and Nathan Sobel, "Fifty Years' Progress in the Treatment of Syphilis," *NYStMJ* 50 (November 15, 1950): 2694–96.

138. Patricia Spain Ward, "The American Reception of Salvarsan," *JHMAS* 36 (January 1981): 59–60; also Harry F. Dowling, "Comparisons and Contrasts Between

the Early Arsphenamine and Early Antibiotic Periods," *BHM* 47 (May-June 1973): 236–49.

139. John Stokes, "Certain Technical Requirements in Methods of Intravenous Injections," *MedRec* 92 (September 29, 1917): 529.

140. See Barbara G. Rosenkrantz, *Public Health and the State: Changing Views in Massachusetts, 1842–1936* (Cambridge, 1972), esp. 97–127.

141. Robert N. Willson, "The Eradication of Social Disease in Large Cities," *Transactions of the Fifteenth International Congress of Hygiene and Demography, 1912* (Washington, D.C., 1913), 4:115; Gertrude Seymour, "A Summary of the New Public Health Measures for Combating Venereal Disease," *SocHy* 4 (July 1918): 380; Louis Chargin, "Recent Progress in the New York City Venereal Disease Campaign," *SocHy* 3 (October 1917); 477.

142. Allan J. McLaughlin, "Syphilis as a Public Health Problem," *SocHy* 2 (January 1916): 67; Hermann Biggs to New York City Board of Health, December 8, 1911, BSH Papers; Hermann Biggs, "Venereal Diseases: The Attitude of the Department of Health in Relation Thereto," *NYMJ* 97 (May 17, 1913): 1009.

143. William F. Snow, "The Status and Uses of Statistics on the Prevalence of Venereal Diseases," *JSSMP* 6 (July 1915): 70–83; also, Rosenkrantz, *Public Health and the State*, 110–12; and Gerald N. Grob, *Edward Jarvis and the Medical World of Nineteenth Century America* (Knoxville, Tenn., 1978), 83–107.

144. William F. Snow, "Public Health Measures in Relation to Venereal Diseases," *Proceedings of the Second Pan American Scientific Congress, 1915–16*, Section 8, Part I (Washington, D.C., 1917), 9:491; see also, George Goler, "The Municipality and the Venereal Disease Problem," *AJPH* 6 (April 1916): 355–59.

145. "Sanitary Control of Venereal Disease in New York City," *Monthly Bulletin of the Department of Health of the City of New York*, 3 (June 1913): 142–43; "Resolutions," *SocDis* 3 (April 1912): 50–51; Charles Bolduan, "Venereal Diseases: The Relation of the Public Health Authorities to Their Control," *AJPH* 3 (October 1913): 1089; Snow, "Public Health Measures in Relation to Venereal Diseases," 491; also Kerr and Moll, "Communicable Diseases: An Analysis of the Laws and Regulations," *Public Health Service Bulletin* No. 672 (Washington, D.C., 1913), 44.

146. Biggs quote in C.-E. A. Winslow, *The Life of Hermann Biggs* (Philadelphia, 1929), 235; see also "The Reminiscences of Haven Emerson," Columbia Oral History Collection (1950), 35; Jerome D. Greene to John D. Rockefeller, Jr., December 5, 1912, BSH papers; Biggs, "Venereal Diseases," 1011; *Weekly Bulletin of the Department of Health of the City of New York*, (May 20, 1916).

147. "Shall Venereal Diseases Be Reportable to the Board of Health?" *NYStJM* 11 (July 1911): 312; Quoted in W. A. Evans, "Municipal Health Officers and Venereal Disease," *AJPH* 5 (September 1915): 885; A. T. Bristow, "Discussion," *SocDis* 2 (July 1911): 23; also "The Professional Secret and the Reporting of Venereal Diseases," *MedRec* 81 (January 27, 1912): 170–71; and Hugh Cabot, "Syphilis and Society," *Transactions of the American Congress of Physicians and Surgeons* 10 (1916): 48. See also, S. L. Strong, "A Symposium on the Reportability and Control of Venereal Diseases," *BMSJ* 169 (December 18, 1913): 903–907.

148. "The Boston Dispensary and Venereal Diseases," *BMSJ* 97 (November 29, 1877): 630; Morris J. Vogel, *The Invention of the Modern Hospital* (Chicago, 1980), 69–72.

149. Bolduan, "Venereal Diseases," 1091; H. S. Newcomer, Russell Richardson, and Charlotte Ashbrook, "One Aspect of Syphilis as a Community Problem," *American Journal of Medical Science* 158 (August 1919): 145; Sigmund Pollitzer, "Syphilis in Relation to Some Social Problems," *AJObst* 73 (May 1916): 861; also A. D. Mewborn, "What Are

the Facilities for Treatment Open to the Venereal Patient in Dispensaries and Hospitals of New York?" *TASSMP* 2 (1908): 70–76.

150. Vogel, *The Invention of the Modern Hospital*: 72; J. Whitridge Williams, "The Significance of Syphilis in Prenatal Care in the Causation of Fœtal Death," *Bulletin of the Johns Hopkins Hospital* 31 (1920): 142.

151. Hermann Biggs, "Discussion," *SocDis* 2 (April 1911): 24; "Sanitary Control of the Venereal Diseases in New York City," *Monthly Bulletin of the Department of Health of the City of New York*, 3 (June 1913): 142–44; Ernest Lederle, "Health Department Control of Venereal Diseases," *SocDis* 3 (October 1912): 26; Bolduan, "Venereal Diseases," 1091.

152. See S. S. Goldwater, "Hospital Accommodations for the Treatment of Venereal Diseases," *NYMJ* 97 (May 17, 1913): 1016–18; E. H. Lewinski-Corwin, "The Medical and Social Importance of an Association of Dispensaries," *MRR* 19 (June 1913): 363; also Charles E. Rosenberg, "Social Class and Medical Care in 19th-century America: The Rise and Fall of the Dispensary," *JHMAS* 29(1974): 32–54.

153. Michael M. Davis, "Evening Clinics for Syphilis and Gonorrhea," *AJPH* 5 (April 1915): 310–11; See Michael M. Davis, "How Efficient Dispensary Clinics Can Help Solve the Medical-Social Problems of Venereal Diseases," *Proceedings of the National Conference on Charities and Correction*, 1915 (Baltimore, 1916), 273–81; Davis, "What the Campaign Against Venereal Disease Demands of Hospitals and Dispensaries," *AJPH* (April 1916), 346–54; Davis and Andrew R. Warner, "Pay Clinics," *Survey* 40 (June 22, 1918): 334–36. See also, Ralph E. Pumphrey, "Michael M. Davis and the Development of the Health Care Movement, 1900–1928," *Societas* 2 (Winter 1972): 27–41.

154. See Gardner, "Microbes and Morality," 308–12; Louis Chargin, "The Reporting and Control of Venereal Diseases," *AJPH* 5 (April 1915): 300; Archibald McNeil and B. S. Barringer, "Diagnosis and Advice in Venereal Diseases as Furnished by the Department of Health," *SocHy* 1 (December 1914): 53–60; *Weekly Bulletin of the Department of Health of the City of New York*, (April 7, 1917).

155. Gardner, "Microbes and Morality," 312–13; B. S. Barringer and Philip S. Platt, "A Survey of Venereal Clinics in New York City: A Statistical Efficiency Test," *SocHy* 1 (June 1915): 344–57; also Philip S. Platt, "The Efficiency of Venereal Clinics," *AJPH* 6 (February 1916): 136–37; "Venereal Disease Clinics," *SocHy* 6 (July 1920): 337–48.

156. Prince A. Morrow to Mary Cobb, April 10, 1912, ASHA Papers, Folder 1:4; Howard A. Kelly, "Status Praesens of the Prostitution Question," *Transactions of the Fifteenth International Congress on Hygiene and Demography, 1912* (Washington, D.C., 1913), 4:668; E. L. Keyes, Jr. "Morals and Venereal Disease," *SocHy* 2 (June 1916): 51.

157. Richard Cabot, "Are Sanitary and Moral Prophylaxis Natural Allies?" *JSSMP* 5 (January 1914): 23.

158. Eugene Brieux, *Damaged Goods*, trans. John Pollack (New York, 1913). Alfred Fournier, the noted syphilographer, assisted Brieux, insuring the accuracy of the medical details revealed on stage.

159. Edward L. Bernays, *Biography of an Idea: Memoirs of Public Relations Counsel Edward L. Bernays* (New York, 1965), 53–62; *New York Times*, April 6, 1913.

160. Brieux, *Damaged Goods*, 205; see also Barbara Gutmann Rosenkrantz, "Damaged Goods: Dilemmas of Responsibility for Risk," *Health and Society* 57 (1979): 1–37.

161. "Demoralizing Plays," *Outlook* 150 (September 20, 1913): 110; John D. Rockefeller, Jr., "The Awakening of a New Conscience," *MRR* 19 (May 1913): 281; also Cosmo Hamilton, "Syphilis and Education," *MRR* 19 (February 1913): 129; "Damaged Goods," *Hearst's Magazine* 23 (May 1913): 806; "Brieux's New Sociological Sermon in

Three Acts," *Current Opinion* 54 (April 1913): 296–97; *New York Times*, April 6, 1913.

162. H. L. Mencken, "The Flapper," *Smart Set* 45 (1915): 1–2.

163. Joyce Kilmer, "Drama as an Instrument of Sex Education," *JSSMP* 5 (April 1914): 50. William Dean Howells also expressed offense. See Howells, "The Plays of Eugene Brieux," *North Atlantic Review* 201 (March 1915): 403.

164. Agnes Repplier, "The Repeal of Reticence," *Atlantic Monthly*, 113 (March 1914), 297–304; "On Some Sex Books," *Medical Times* 45 (April 1917): 112; "Sex O'Clock in America," *Current Opinion* 55 (August 1913): 113.

165. William J. Robinson, "Venereal Disease as a Retribution for Illicit Intercourse," *AJUr* 12 (1916): 25; Robinson to Mary Cobb, December 7, 1910, ASHA Papers, Folder 1:4; Theodore Schroeder, "Our Prudish Censorship," *Forum* 53 (January 1915): 87.

166. E. L. Keyes, Jr., "Social Hygiene in 1914," *JSSMP* 5 (October 1914): 197; E. L. Keyes, *Syphilis* (New York, 1908): 6.

167. See Nathan G. Hale, Jr., *Freud and the Americans: The Beginnings of Psychoanalysis in the United States, 1876–1917* (New York, 1971), esp. 274–312.

168. Walter Lippmann, *A Preface to Politics* (New York, 1913), 135–36. See also Ronald Steel's *Walter Lippmann and the American Century* (Boston, 1980), esp. 46–49.

169. Quoted in E. L. Keyes, "Prince Albert Morrow, M.D.," *VDI* 22 (February 1941): 42.

Chapter II

1. On the relationship of Progressivism to World War I see Allen F. Davis, "Welfare, Reform and World War I," *AmQ* 29 (Fall 1967): 516–533; also Charles E. Forcey, *The Crossroads of Liberalism* (New York, 1961), esp. pp. 221–72.

Works which devote particular attention to Progressive attitudes towards science and technology are John D. Buenker, John C. Burnham, and Robert M. Crunden, *Progressivism* (Cambridge, 1977); Samuel Haber, *Efficiency and Uplift* (Chicago, 1964); and John C. Burnham, "Medical Specialists and Movements Toward Social Control in the Progressive Era: Three Examples," in Jerry Israel, ed., *Building the Organizational Society: Essays on Associational Activities in Modern America* (New York, 1972), 19–30.

2. George E. Harmon, "Venereal Diseases in the Navy and their Prophylaxis," *TASSMP* 1 (1906): 130. Colonel Valery Harvard told the group that "From the medical standpoint, venereal diseases are by far the most serious evil in our army, as well as all other armies." "Venereal Diseases in the Army and their Prophylaxis," *TASSMP* 1 (1906): 123.

3. For accounts of military activities on the Mexican border see Clarence C. Clendenen, *The United States and Pancho Villa* (Washington, 1961), and *Blood on the Border: The United States Army and the Mexican Irregulars* (New York, 1969); also Frank E. Vandiver, *Black Jack: The Life and Times of John J. Pershing* (College Station, Texas, 1977), 2: 660–65.

4. Jerome D. Greene to National Young Men's Christian Association, July 10, 1916, in National YMCA Archives, E213, New York, New York. Greene explained, "The conditions on the Mexican border present a peril of the gravest kind."

For an account of the meeting with Baker see Frederick Palmer, *Newton D. Baker: America at War* (New York, 1931), 1: 296–98.

5. Raymond B. Fosdick, *Chronicle of a Generation* (New York, 1958), 207. For a brief discussion of Fosdick's Progressive ideology, see Otis L. Graham, Jr., *An Encore*

for Reform: The Old Progressives and the New Deal (New York, 1967), 57, 112–13.

6. Raymond B. Fosdick, European Police Systems (New York, 1915) and Crime in America and the Police (New York, 1920).

7. Raymond B. Fosdick to Newton D. Baker, August 10, 1916, Fosdick Papers, Box 1, Princeton University. This memo is discussed in some detail in Palmer, Newton D. Baker: America at War, I: 298–302.

8. William Howard Taft, ed., Service With Fighting Men (New York, 1922), 1: 107, 108; M. J. Exner, "Prostitution in its Relation to the Army on the Mexican Border," SocHy 3 (April 1917): 208.

9. For rates of infection see U.S. Congress. House. Committee on Military Affairs. Hearings on Training Camp Activities. 65th Congress, 2nd session, March 14, 1918, p. 7; Fosdick to Baker, August 10, 1916. General John J. Pershing, who would later command the AEF, was among the officers who instituted such procedures on the border. See Vandiver, Black Jack, 2: 773–74.

Abraham Flexner's classic study of prostitution in Europe, written for the Bureau of Social Hygiene, argued forcefully against regulated prostitution. See Prostitution in Europe (New York, 1917), esp. pp. 130–36, 157–58, 216–18. Fosdick to Baker, August 10, 1916.

10. According to some officers, "Sissies were no use on the firing line. Soldiers must have women. They made poor soldiers if they did not have women." Quoted in Palmer, Newton D. Baker: America at War, 1:298. Exner, "Prostitution in its Relation to the Army on the Mexican Border," 218, 211; also, "The Militiaman's Morals," Literary Digest 53 (November 18, 1916): 121.

11. Exner, 202, 207, 211; New York Evening Post, July 14, 1917; see also Dorothy G. Ross, G. Stanley Hall (Chicago, 1972), 328, 383–85.

12. L. M. Maus, "A Sociological Study of the Enlisted Men of the Regular Army with Suggestions for the Protection of the Young National Soldier Against Moral Degeneracy and Diseases of Vice," unpublished typescript, n.d. (1917?), 5, ASHA Papers, Folder 131:2; see also, J. S. Taylor, "The Social Status of the Sailor," SocHy 4 (April 1918): 159–78. William Ernest Hocking, "Personal Problems of the Soldier," Yale Review 7 (July 1918): 715; see also his Morale and its Enemies (New Haven, 1918).

13. Exner, 206. Exner, 214.

14. Fosdick to Baker, August 10, 1916, Fosdick MSS; Fosdick, Chronicle of a Generation, 137–38; Palmer, Newton D. Baker: America at War, 1: 302–6.

15. Quotations in Palmer, Newton D. Baker 1:302, 303; Baker had been mayor of Cleveland, Ohio.

16. Typescript speech, November 16, 1918, Fosdick MSS, Box 3; Fosdick, Chronicle of a Generation, 141; Palmer, 1:307.

17. Baker frequently argued that a draft army—drawn from a cross section of American youth—would require the War Department to undertake greater precautions against immorality. See Palmer, 1:310–11.

18. M. J. Exner to Frank Ober, May 23, 1917, NARG 165, Box 574; Exner, "Prostitution in Relation to the Army on the Mexican Border," 205.

19. Mrs. R. G. Stone to Josephus Daniels, April 25, 1917, Daniels MSS, Box 459, Library of Congress, Washington, D.C; Mrs. E. L. Wunder to Woodrow Wilson, April 17, 1917, NA RG 165, Box 574; see also, Harrison S. Whitney to War Department, July 23, 1917, NA RG 165, Box 577; and Caroline Bunker to Woodrow Wilson, June 18, 1917, NA RG 165, Box 586.

20. See, for example, William F. Snow to Executive Committee, American Social Hygiene Association, August 31, 1917, NA RG 165, Box 572. On the work of the Na-

tional War Work Council see Luther Gulick, *Morals and Morale* (New York, 1919), esp. pp. 8–10; and Taft, ed., *Service With Fighting Men*, 1:103–107.

21. Quoted in Palmer, *Newton D. Baker*, 1:307; Fosdick, *Chronicle of a Generation*, 143.

22. Newton D. Baker, *Frontiers of Freedom*, (New York, 1918), 88; Baker, *Frontiers of Freedom*, 84–97; see also, Fred D. Baldwin, "The Invisible Armor," *AmQ* 16 (Fall 1964): 432–34.

23. Baker, *Frontiers of Freedom*, 231.

United States War Department, *Annual Report 1917* (Washington, 1918), 35; Baker quoted in Fosdick, *Chronicle of a Generation*, 143; For a discussion of the Progressive ideology underlying these programs see Paul S. Boyer, *Urban Masses and Moral Order in America, 1830–1920* (Cambridge, 1978).

24. Josephus Daniels, *Navy and the Nation* (New York, 1919), 58, 59; "Today as never before American manhood must be clean and fit," concluded Daniels. "America stands in need of every ounce of her strength. We must cut out the cancer of disease if we would live." See "Extracts from speech," unpublished typescript, November 15, 1918, Daniels MSS, Box 463.

25. Raymond B. Fosdick to Newton D. Baker, April 12, 1917, Baker MSS, Box 3, Library of Congress, Washington D.C.

26. Fosdick to Baker, April 12, 1917; on the Plattsburg camp see *New York Herald*, March 22, 1917; and Palmer, *Newton D. Baker* 1:310.

Baker conceived of the Commission as a means of organizing voluntary agencies: "The functions of the Commission will be largely advisory, but I will expect to consult it upon the whole question of police regulations outside the limits of the military camps." This idea was consistent with Progressive views of the limited role of government for social programs. Baker to Fosdick, April 18, 1917, Fosdick MSS, Box 1.

27. On the popular perception of the "Fosdick Commission," see Franklin Martin, *The Joy of Living* (New York, 1933), 1:121; and *New York Evening Post*, July 14, 1917. Other members of the Commission included Thomas J. Howells, Malcolm McBride, Charles P. Neil, Palmer E. Pierce, and Joseph Raycroft. See *Report of the Chairman of the Commission on Training Camp Activities* (Washington, 1918). In July 1917, at Josephus Daniels's request, a Navy Commission on Training Camp Activities was appointed with Fosdick as Chairman. The two Commissions actually functioned as one. See Raymond B. Fosdick to Josephus Daniels, June 21, 1945, Fosdick MSS, Box 28.

28. Raymond B. Fosdick, "The War and Navy Departments Commissions on Training Camp Activities," *Annals* 79 (September 1918): 131; see also Fred Davis Baldwin, "The American Enlisted Man in World War I," Ph.D. dissertation, Princeton University, 1964, pp. 31–64, 92–199.

29. Taft, ed., *Service With Fighting Men*, 1:110–13; John R. Mott, "The War Work of the Y.M.C.A.," *Annals* 79 (September 1918); Raymond B. Fosdick to E. C. Carter, August 22, 1919, Fosdick MSS, Box 1; also, Fosdick, *Chronicle of a Generation*, 148–50.

30. Fosdick, "The War and Navy Departments Commissions on Training Camp Activities," 136.

31. Joseph Lee, "The Training Camp Commissions," *Survey* 39 (October 6, 1917): 5; Edward Frank Allen, *Keeping Our Fighters Fit* (New York, 1918), 42, 47–48; United States War Department, *Annual Report 1918* (Washington 1918), 510, 658–59; Fosdick, "The War and Navy Departments Commissions on Training Camp Activities," 139.

32. William H. Zinsser, "Working With Men Outside the Camps," *Annals* 79 (Sep-

tember 1918): 195; Newton Baker often referred to the camps as "soldier-cities." See United States War Department, *Annual Report 1917* (Washington, 1918), 35. See also, Palmer, *Newton D. Baker: America at War*, 234–38; and Joseph Lee, "The Training Camp Commissions," 4; Fosdick, *Chronicle of a Generation*, 148–52; Allen F. Davis, "Welfare, Reform and World War I," *AmQ* 29 (Fall 1967): 516–33 and *Spearheads for Reform: The Social Settlements and the Progressive Movement* (New York, 1967), 225–26.

33. On the organization of the Social Hygiene Division see Raymond B. Fosdick to Commanding Officer, Fort Thomas, January 18, 1918, NA RG 165, Box 426; Walter Clarke, "Social Hygiene and the War," *SocHy* 4 (April 1918): 272.

34. Zinsser, "Working With Men Outside the Camps," 195–96. On Victorian sexual prescription see Ronald G. Walters, ed., *Primers for Prudery: Sexual Advice to Victorian America* (Englewood Cliffs, New Jersey, 1974). For discussions of the growing reliance on professionals see Burton Bledstein, *The Culture of Professionalism* (New York, 1976); Robert H. Wiebe, *The Search for Order* (New York, 1967); and Christopher Lasch, *Haven in a Heartless World* (New York, 1977).

35. H. E. Kleinschmidt, "Educational Prophylaxis of Venereal Diseases," *SocHy* 5 (January 1919): 27; Lee, "The Training Camp Commissions," 4; William C. Gorgas, "Venereal Diseases and the War," *AJPH* 8 (February 1918): 110.

36. Walter Clarke, "The Promotion of Social Hygiene in War Time," *Annals* 79 (September 1918): 189; Gorgas, "Venereal Diseases and the War," 108–10; see also, Gorgas, "The Credit Side of Our War Ledger," *Collier's Weekly* 61 (June 8, 1918): 11, 22–23 "Lecture to Troops," unpublished typescript, (December, 1917?), 5–6, NA RG 165, Box 418.

37. *Keeping Fit to Fight* (Washington, 1918), 1; "Syllabus Accredited for Use in Official Supplementary Lectures on Sex Hygiene and Venereal Diseases," unpublished typescript, (February 1918), NA RG 165, Box 433.

38. William Allen Pusey, "Handling of the Venereal Disease Problem in the United States Army in the Present Crisis," *JAMA* 71 (September 28, 1918): 1017; M. J. Exner to Frank Ober, May 23, 1917, NA RG 165, Box 574. The YMCA continued to assert that they could best handle the lecture program. See, for example, Norman F. Coleman to Walter Clarke, November 10, 1917, NA RG 165, Box 431. The CTCA suggested that the YMCA could give non-compulsory lectures on moral themes. Coleman replied: "I doubt if anything is to be gained by creating an artificial distinction between the so-called religious appeal in matters of sex and the so-called scientific appeal." Coleman to Thomas D. Eliot, January 22, 1918, NA RG 165, Box 431. See also M. J. Exner to Walter Clarke, December 24, 1917, NA RG 165, Box 420.

39. Pusey, "Handling of the Venereal Disease Problem in the United States Army in the Present Crisis," 1019; Lawrence quoted in Martin S. Pernick, "Progressives, Propaganda, and Public Health: Army Medicine and Venereal Disease Education Films," unpublished paper, 1974, 1; Charles P. Neil, a member of the CTCA explained that "since this was a matter in which science backed up a moral principle, it furnished a splendid opportunity for a big drive against immorality." "Minutes of the Commission on Training Camp Activities," unpublished notebooks, July 26, 1917, NA RG 165, Box 57.

40. Franklin H. Martin, ed., *Digest of the Proceedings of the Council of National Defense During the War* (Washington, 1934), 149. Though it is true that a group of purity crusaders had been calling for an end to the double-standard of sexual morality for some time, these reformers had never achieved such substantial backing for their claims. "Genteel morality" had been strictly the domain of the genteel middle class. See

Nathan Hale, Jr., *Freud and the Americans: The Beginnings of Psychoanalysis in America* (New York, 1917); also John S. Haller and Robin M. Haller, *The Physician and Sexuality in Victorian America* (Urbana, 1974), esp. pp. 191–234; and David J. Pivar, *Purity Crusade* (Westport, Connecticut, 1973).

41. Martin, ed., *Digest of Proceedings of the Council of National Defense*, 149–50. The resolution was endorsed by the American Medical Association. See *New York Evening Post*, July 14, 1917, and *New York Times*, October 18, 1917.

42. *Keeping Fit to Fight* (Washington, 1918), 5–6; F. G. Barr, "Talk to Soldiers," unpublished typescript, March 1918, NA RG 165, Box 246; "Lecture to Troops," unpublished typescript, (December 1917?), 11, NA RG 165, Box 418.

43. See, for example, Prince A. Morrow, *Social Diseases and Marriage* (New York, 1904), esp. pp. 345–64; "Lecture to Troops," 12, 21–22; *Don't Take a Chance* (New York, 1918), a pamphlet distributed by the YMCA and the National Committee for Trench Comfort Packets. Masturbation was also considered to be wasteful sexual energy. See G. J. Barker-Benfield, *Horrors of the Half-Known Life* (New York, 1976), 175–88.

44. *Keeping Fit to Fight* (Washington, 1918), 6–7; "Lecture to Troops," 21.

45. "Lecture to Troops," 12; "Syllabus Accredited for Use in Official Supplementary Lectures on Sex Hygiene and Venereal Diseases," unpublished typescript, (February 1918), NA RG 165, Box 433.

46. "Lecture to Troops," 23–24.

47. Walter Clarke, "Social Hygiene and the War," *SocHy* 4 (April 1918): 266–73; Hilton Railey to Raymond B. Fosdick, September 17, 1917, NA RG 165, Box 426; H. E. Kleinschmidt, "Educational Prophylaxis of Venereal Diseases," *SocHy* 5 (January 1919): 29.

48. "Syllabus Accredited for Use in Official Supplementary Lectures on Sex Hygiene and Venereal Diseases," unpublished typescript, (February 1918), NA RG 165, Box 433; "Lecture to Troops," 9–10.

49. "Lecture to Troops," 9; "Syllabus Accredited for Use in Official Supplementary Lectures on Sex Hygiene and Venereal Diseases."

50. United States War Department, *Annual Report 1918* (Washington, 1918), 652–53; Walter Clarke, "Social Hygiene and the War," *SocHy* 4 (April 1918), 292; F. G. Barr, "Talk to Soldiers," unpublished typescript, March 1918, NA RG, Box 246; Edward J. Williams to Chief Surgeon, February 20, 1919, NA RG 120, Box 5170.

51. "Lecture to Troops," 20; *Keeping Fit to Fight* (Washington, 1918), 4.

52. "Lecture to Troops," 17. For a typical account of German atrocities in Belgium see Jennie H. Harris, "The Prostitute in Relation to Military Camps," *WMJ* 28 (June 1918): 127; also Newell Dwight Hillis, *The Blot on the Kaiser's Scutcheon* (New York, 1918).

53. "Lecture to Troops," 20.

54. See Peter T. Cominos, "Innocent Femina Sensualis in Unconscious Conflict," in Martha Vicinus, ed., *Suffer and Be Still: Women in the Victorian Age* (Bloomington, 1972), 155–72; "Lecture to Troops," 15, 18.

55. *Keeping Fit to Fight* (Washington, 1918), 4, 8.

56. Martin, ed., *Digest of the Proceedings of the Council of National Defense*, 150–51; M. J. Exner to Raymond B. Fosdick, December 17, 1917, NA RG 165, Box 420; Norman F. Coleman to Thomas D. Eliot, November 30, 1917, and January 23, 1918, NA RG 165, Box 431; Raymond B. Fosdick to Josephus Daniels, October 10, 1917, Daniels MSS, Box 458; T. A. Berryhill to Daniels, December 3, 1917, NA RG 165, Box 419; Fosdick to Daniels, December 28, 1917, Daniels MSS, Box 458.

57. H. E. Kleinschmidt, "Is Education a Worthwhile Factor in the Control of Venereal Diseases?" *SocHy* 5 (April 1919): 230. See also Martin S. Pernick, "Progressives, Propaganda, and Public Health: Army Medicine and Venereal Disease Education Films," unpublished paper, 1974; K. S. Lashly and J. B. Watson, "Psychological Study of Motion Pictures in Relation to Venereal Disease Campaigns," *SocHy* 7 (April 1921): 181–219.

58. E. H. Griffith quoted in Walter Clarke, "Social Hygiene and the War," *SocHy* 4 (April 1918): 294–97, 281–82; 295–96.

Some objections were raised concerning the film's advocacy of chemical prophylaxis. See, for example, Katharine C. Bushnell, "A Shameful Imposture," privately published pamphlet in Records of the Public Health Service, Division of Venereal Diseases, WNRC NA RG 90, Box 329.

59. Clarke, "Social Hygiene and the War," 297.

60. *Don't Take a Chance* (New York, 1918). On Progressive ideals of manhood see Peter Gabriel Filene, *Him/Her/Self: Sex Roles in Modern America* (New York, 1974), esp. pp. 68–115; also, James R. McGovern, "David Graham Phillips and the Virility Impulse of Progressives," *New England Quarterly* 39 (September 1966): 344–55.

61. Martin, ed., *Digest of Proceedings of the Council of National Defense*, 406; Walter Clarke, "The Promotion of Social Hygiene in War Time," *Annals* 79 (September 1918): 188.

62. On Victorian sexual attitudes and the "conspiracy of silence" see, for example, Nathan Hale, Jr., *Freud and the Americans: The Beginnings of Psychoanalysis in America* (New York, 1971), 24–46; Michel Foucault, *The History of Sexuality*, vol. 1, (New York, 1978), esp. pp. 3–35; and Peter Gay, "Victorian Sexuality," *American Scholar* (Summer 1980): 372–78.

63. Joseph Lee, "War Camp Community Service," *Annals* 79 (September 1918): 190.

64. Raymond B. Fosdick to Joseph Lee, May 20, 1917, NA RG 165, Box 570; Lee, "War Camp Community Service," 193.

65. Taft, ed., *Service With Fighting Men*, 1:104. Fosdick, *Chronicle of a Generation*, 144–45; Palmer, *Newton D. Baker: America at War*, 1:310; and John G. Buchanan, "War Legislation Against Alcoholic Liquor and Prostitution," *Journal of the American Institute of Criminal Law and Criminology* 9 (February 1919): 520–29.

66. All houses of prostitution and saloons within five miles of the military camps were declared illegal; the War Department later extended the ban to ten miles in some areas. "Zones of Safety," *Survey* 38 (June 21, 1917): 349–50; Bascom Johnson, "Eliminating Vice from Camp Cities," *Annals* 78 (July 1918): 60–64; Edward Frank Allen, *Keeping Our Fighters Fit* (New York 1918), 198.

Fosdick noted that sections 12 and 13 dramatically altered the original conception of the CTCA as a sponsor for voluntary agencies eager to do service in the camps. He later wrote: "I would have preferred to have the positive side of our work take precedence over the negative aspects, but there was no choice, and we were launched into a resounding battle." See Fosdick, *Chronicle of a Generation*, 144–45.

67. Newton D. Baker to Governors, May 26, 1917, NA RG 165, Box 417. Portions of this letter were widely reprinted. See, for example, *Survey* 38 (June 23, 1917): 273; Elwood Street, "When the Soldiers Come to Town," *Survey* 38 (August 18, 1917): 434; Gertrude Seymour, "The Health of Soldier and Civilian," *Survey* 40 (May 11, 1918): 156; and Fosdick, *Chronicle of a Generation*, 144–46;

68. Pusey, "Handling of the Venereal Disease Problem in the United States Army in the Present Crisis," *JAMA* 71 (September 28, 1918): 1017; Loyd Thompson and J. R. Bolsany, "Venereal Disease in the Thirty-Ninth Division," *JAMA* 71 (October 19, 1918):

1297; Frank Parker Stockbridge, "The Cleanest Army in the World," *Delineator* 93 (December 1918): 8; also Robert A. Woods, "Prohibition and Social Hygiene," *SocHy* 5 (April 1919): 137–45.

69. The discovery of the Wassermann reaction to detect syphilis and dark-field microscopic diagnosis of gonorrhea made it possible to determine infections clearly. Physicians suggested that these techniques had implicated the prostitute as the primary spreader of venereal disease. See, for example, Edward B. Vedder, *Syphilis and Public Health* (Philadelphia, 1918). On the relationship of alcohol and disease see Howard B. Woolston, *Prostitution in the United States* (New York, 1921), 179–180; "Venereal Disease Among Prostitutes," *SocHy* 5 (October 1919): 539–544; Victor Cox Pedersen, "Venereal Problems of the War," *Medical Record* 96 (July 19, 1919): 105. Raymond B. Fosdick to Livingston Farrand, August 2, 1919, in Records of the American National Red Cross, 1917–1934, Record Group 200, Box 558, National Archives.

70. John H. Stokes, *Today's World Problem in Disease Prevention* (Washington, 1919), 105; *Program of Protective Social Measures*, U.S. Interdepartmental Social Hygiene Board pamphlet (Washington, 1920), in Daniels MSS, Box 463.

71. J. Frank Chase to Raymond B. Fosdick, October 13, 1917, NA RG 165, Box 586; Gertrude Seymour, "The Health of Soldier and Civilian," *Survey* 40 (May 11, 1918): 158.

72. J. Frank Chase to Raymond B. Fosdick, October 13, 1917, NA RG 165, Box 586, George quoted in "How We Are Defending the Health of Our Soldiers and Sailors," circular of the California State Law Enforcement and Protection League, (March 1918) in Daniels MSS, Box 461; "Could the Kaiser Do Worse?" (1918) in Records of the Council of National Defense, WNRC RG NA 62, Box 437.

73. "Bascom Johnson, A.B., LL.B.," American Social Hygiene Association flyer, (1942), ASHA Papers, Box 7.

74. The CTCA enlisted investigators from the American Social Hygiene Association, the New England Watch and Ward Society, the Bureau of Social Hygiene, and the Committee of Fourteen. See "Minutes of the Commission on Training Camp Activities," unpublished notebooks, July 26, 1917, NA RG 165, Box 57; Bascom Johnson, "Eliminating Vice From Camp Cities," *Annals* 78 (July 1918): 62; George J. Anderson, "Making Camps Safe for the Army," *Annals* 79 (September 1918): 145.

75. Richard I. Manning to Josephus Daniels, July 30, 1917, Daniels MSS, Box 458; "Another Red Light District Gone," *Survey* 39 (October 27, 1917): 97; "Zones of Safety," *Survey* 38 (June 21, 1917): 349–50; Harrol B. Ayres, "Democracy at Work—San Antonio Being Reborn," *SocHy* 4 (April 1918): 211–17; Gertrude Seymour, "The Health of Soldier and Civilian," *Survey* 40 (May 11, 1918): p. 156; "How We Are Defending the Health of Our Soldiers and Sailors," circular of the California State Law Enforcement and Protection League, (March 1918) in Daniels MSS, Box 461. On efforts in Florida see James R. McGovern, "Sporting Life on the Line: Prostitution in Progressive Era Pensacola," *Florida Historical Quarterly* 54 (October 1975): 139–40; and Governor Sidney Catts to Josephus Daniels, September 14, 1917, NA RG 165, Box 586.

76. "Camp Sheridan Report on Control of Venereal Diseases," unpublished typescript, November 12, 1917, NA RG 165, Box 434; Jean M. Gordon to Newton D. Baker, September 14, 1917; also William M. Railey to Raymond B. Fosdick, September 6, 1917, NA RG 165, Box 582.

77. George J. Anderson, "Making the Camps Safe for the Army," *Annals* 79 (September 1918): 149; A. C. McKinney to Margaret Elias, July 16, 1917, NA RG 165, Box 582; Raymond B. Fosdick to Josephus Daniels, September 11, 1917, Daniels MSS, Box 458; George J. Anderson, "Report on Storyville," unpublished typescript, September 25, 1917, NA RG 165, Box 582.

78. Josephus Daniels to Governor Pleasant, September 24, 1917; Newton D. Baker to Raymond B. Fosdick, September 2, 1917; Fosdick to Bascom Johnson, September 10, 1917, NA RG 165, Box 582; Jean M. Gordon to Newton D. Baker, September 14, 1917, NA RG 165, Box 582; and Al Rose, *Storyville, New Orleans* (University, Alabama, 1974), 167, 170–77.

79. Raymond B. Fosdick to Josephus Daniels, March 26, 1918; Fosdick to Daniels, July 10, 1917, Daniels MSS, Box 458; and Fosdick, *Chronicle of a Generation*, 145.

80. Edward Frank Allen, *Keeping Our Fighters Fit*, 200; "Making Cities Safe for Soldiers," *Survey* 38 (July 17, 1917): 376–77; "Zones of Safety," *Survey* 38 (June 21, 1917: 349; Timothy Newell Pfeiffer, "Social Hygiene and the War," *SocHy* 4 (July 1918): 424; also Frank J. Osborne, "The Law Enforcement Program Applied," *SocHy* 5 (April 1919): 83–96.

81. Bascom Johnson, "Next Steps," *SocHy* 4 (January 1919): 10; J. Frank Chase to Raymond B. Fosdick, August 20, 1917, NA RG 165, Box 584.

82. "Suggestions for State Boards of Health Regulations," unpublished typescript, NA RG 165, Box 434; "Legal Measures for the Control of Venereal Disease," unpublished typescript, WNRC RG 90, Box 223; John G. Buchanan, "War Legislation Against Alcoholic Liquor and Prostitution," *Journal of the American Institute of Criminal Law and Criminology* 9 (February 1919): 525; Charles L. Miller to C. C. Pierce, October 15, 1919; and T. N. Pfeiffer to David Robinson, October 16, 1919, WNRC 90, Box 329.

83. Raymond B. Fosdick, "The Program of the Commission on Training Camp Activities With Relation to the Problem of Venereal Disease," *SocHy* 4 (January 1918): 76.

84. *Report of the Chairman of the Commission on Training Camp Activities* (Washington, 1918); "Report from Troy, New York," unpublished typescript, March 1, 1918, NA RG 165, Box 434; George J. Anderson, "Making the Camps Safe for the Army," *Annals* 79 (September 1918): 148; Buchanan, "War Legislation Against Alcoholic Liquor and Prostitution," 525.

85. United States War Department, *Annual Report 1918* (Washington, 1918), 21; United States War Department, *Annual Report 1917* (Washington, 1918), 343. U.S. Congress. Senate. Committee on Military Affairs. *Hearings on Army Appropriation Bill, 1919*. 65th Congress, 2nd session, June 10, 15, 17, 18, 1918, pp. 60–83.
    Granville MacGowan, "Discussion," *JAMA* 71 (October 19, 1918): 1296.

86. See, for example, William F. Snow and Wilbur A. Sawyer, "Venereal Disease Control in the Army," *JAMA* 71 (August 10, 1918): 457; United States War Department, *Annual Report 1918* (Washington, 1918), 509–13; Edmond R. Beckwith, "Venereal Diseases," *American Journal of Nursing* 18 (September 1918): 1137; "How the First Million Draft Recruits Measured Up Physically," *Current Opinion* 67 (September 1919): 195; Albert G. Love and C. B. Davenport, *Defects Found in Drafted Men* (Washington, 1920), 34; and F. F. Russell, "The Venereal Diseases in Civil and Military Life," *SocHy* 4 (January 1918): 43–46. William F. Snow testified that the annual rate of men infected with gonorrhea entering the army was 231.3 per 1000; with syphilis 53.5 per 1000. "For all venereal diseases we have 320 per 1000 as brought into the Army, contracted before entrance, compared to 16.8 per 1000 contracted after enlistment." See *Hearings on Army Appropriation Bill, 1919*, pp. 62–63; also, "Venereal Disease Statistics," unpublished typescript, 1919?, Records of the U.S. Interdepartmental Social Hygiene Board, NA RG 90. Snow and Sawyer, "Venereal Disease Control in the Army," 462.

87. United States War Department, *Annual Report 1918* (Washington, 1918), 343; Isaac W. Brewer, "The Incidence of Venereal Diseases Among 6,086 Men Drafted Into

Service," *BMSJ* 153 (January 10, 1919): 122; Victor C. Vaughan, "Discussion," *JAMA* 71 (August 10, 1918): 467.

88. Though established by the Council, the Civilian Committee to Combat Venereal Disease actually worked under the direction of the CTCA. "Minutes of the Council of National Defense," unpublished notebooks, 2 (December 9, 1917): 286–87, Records of the Council of National Defense, WNRC NA RG 62, Box 429; "Damaged Goods," flyer, 1918, in WNRC RG 62, Box 439; "Suggestions for a Citizens' Program for Combatting Prostitution and Venereal Diseases," Civilian Committee for Combatting Venereal Disease, 1918, WNRC RG 62, Box 443.

89. Franklin Martin, "Campaign Against Venereal Disease," mimeographed circular letter, April 5, 1918, WNRC RG 62, Box 437; *Smash the Line*, Commission on Training Camp Activities pamphlet (Washington, 1918); "Barring Sex Disease from the American Army," *New York Times Magazine*, (October 28, 1917), 11–12.

90. William F. Snow, "The Control of Venereal Diseases," unpublished typescript, n.d., WNRC RG 62, Box 437.

91. T. Clark to Henry P. Davidson, August 30, 1918, NA RG 200, Box 558; "The Venereal Peril to Our Army," *JAMA* 69 (September 1, 1917): 734; also Ann Doyle, "Venereal Diseases and Clinics for Civilians Near Military Camps," *Proceedings of the National Conference of Social Work 1918* (Chicago, 1919), 192–94.

The CCCVD also worked to ban quackery and the sale of venereal nostrums. See Franklin Martin, "Venereal Disease Remedies," circular letter, February 26, 1918, WNRC RG 62, Box 437; and John G. Buchanan to Franklin Martin, July 5, 1918, WNRC RG 62, Box 439.

92. Gertrude Seymour, "A Year's Progress in Venereal Disease Control," *SocHy* 5 (January 1919): 61. William H. Zinsser, "Social Hygiene and the War," *SocHy* 4 (October 1918): 497–524; *Your Side of the Fight: Keeping Them Fit to Work*, Commission on Training Camp Activities pamphlet (Washington, 1918); also, Victor Cox Pedersen, "Venereal Problems of the War," *MedRec* 96 (July 19, 1919): 104.

93. Zinsser, "Working With Men Outside the Camps," 197; Elwood Street, "When the Soldiers Come to Town" *Survey* 38 (August 18, 1917): 433; on the incidence of sex crimes see Joseph Mayer, *The Regulation of Commercialized Vice: An Analysis of the Transition From Segregation to Repression in the United States* (New York, 1922), 12; and Bascom Johnson, "Eliminating Vice From Camp Cities," *Annals* 78 (July 1918): 61.

94. Hilton Railey's series of articles in the *New York Evening Post* were widely cited. See *New York Evening Post*, July 14, 21, 28, August 4, 11, 18, 1917; also "The Prudery of the Press," *JAMA* 72 (May 29, 1919): 1547; and Paul S. Boyer, *Purity in Print* (New York, 1968), esp. pp. 53–98. Martin, ed., *Digest of Proceedings of the Council of National Defense*, 406.

95. Joseph Lee, "War Camp Community Service," *Annals* 79 (September, 1918): 190; Winthrop D. Lane, "Girls and Khaki," *Survey* 39 (December 1, 1917): 236

96. Henrietta S. Additon, "Work Among Delinquent Women and Girls," *Annals* 79 (September 1918): 154; Jennie H. Harris, "The Prostitute in Relation to the Military Camps," *WMJ* 28 (June 1918): 125.

97. U.S. Congress. House. Committee on Military Affairs. *Hearings on Training Camp Activities*. 65th Congress, 2nd session, March 14, 1918, p. 5; also Warren Olney, Jr., to Raymond B. Fosdick, August 4, 1917, NA RG 165, Box 585. Maude E. Miner to Raymond B. Fosdick, August 6, 1917, NA RG 165, Box 585; also Miner to Fosdick, March 9, 1918, NA RG 165, Box 431. Fosdick appointed Mrs. John D. Rockefeller, Jr., Mrs. James Cushman, and Mrs. William Dummer to the Committee on Protective

Work for Girls. Additon, "Work Among Delinquent Women and Girls," 152.

98. "Lecture for Women," unpublished typescript, n.d. (1918?), WNRC RG 62, Box 437; see also, Rachelle S. Yarros, "Experiences of a Lecturer," *SocHy* 5 (April 1919): 205–22.

99. "The rumor of numerous girls being pregnant appalls us." Amelia Dranga to Newton D. Baker, September 12, 1917, NA RG 165, Box 504; "Lecture for Women," 3; Katherine Bement Davis, "Social Hygiene and the War," *SocHy* 4 (October 1918): 532; Raymond B. Fosdick to Maude E. Miner, August 24, 1917, NA RG 165, Box 585.

100. Mrs. Woodallen Chapman, *A Nation's Call to Young Women*, Commission on Training Camp Activities pamphlet (Washington, 1918); "Lecture to Women," 2.

101. A copy of *End of the Road* is held at the Motion Picture Division, National Archives, RG 200.

102. The department store was frequently cited as an environment which could lead to chance encounters between men and women, resulting in moral degeneration. See, for example, David J. Rothman and Sheila M. Rothman, eds., *Sources of the American Social Tradition* (New York, 1975), 245–57.

103. "Protective Officers for Girls Wanted," *Survey* 39 (January 26, 1918); 465–66. Maude E. Miner quoted in Lane, "Girls and Khaki," *Survey* 39 (December 1, 1917): 236; and Miner, "Protective Work for Girls in War," *Proceedings of the National Conference of Social Work 1918* (Chicago, 1919), 657.

104. Arthur B. Towne, "Informal Discussion," *Proceedings of the National Conference of Social Work 1918* (Chicago, 1919), 131–32; Rachelle S. Yarros, "The Prostitute as a Health and Social Problem," *Proceedings of the National Conference of Social Work 1919* (Chicago, 1920), 223.

105. Jane Deeter Rippin, "Social Hygiene and the War," *SocHy* 5 (January 1919): 125–26. On the new mores see, for example, Kenneth A. Yellis, "Prosperity's Child: Some Thoughts on the Flapper," *AmQ* 21 (Spring 1969): 44–64; James R. McGovern, "The American Woman's Pre-World War I Freedom in Manners and Morals," *JAH* 55 (September 1968): 315–33; and Paula Fass, *The Damned and the Beautiful* (New York, 1977), esp. pp. 260–90.

106. Additon, "Work Among Delinquent Women and Girls," 153–54; Frank M. Warren to Raymond B. Fosdick, December 14, 1917, NA RG 165, Box 418; Mrs. Charles H. King to Woodrow Wilson, December 4, 1917, NA RG 165, Box 421.

107. Roy K. Flannagan to Ennion G. Williams, October 17, 1918, WNRC RG 90, Box 223; Facsimile (n.d.) in WNRC RG 90, Box 329; *Hearings on Training Camp Activities*, March 14, 1918; also Raymond B. Fosdick to Lord A'bernon, n.d.?, Fosdick MSS, Box 1; Gertrude Seymour, "A Summary of New Public Health Measures for Combatting Venereal Disease," *SocHy* 4 (July 1918): 391; and Joseph Mayer, "Social Hygiene Legislation in 1917," *SocHy* 5 (January 1919): 67–71.

108. T. W. Gregory, "Memorandum on Legal Aspects of the Proposed System of Medical Examination of Women Convicted Under Section 13, Selective Service Act," unpublished typescript, April 3, 1918, WNRC RG 90, Box 223; T. W. Gregory, "Circular No. 855," July 20, 1918; "Circular No. 812 and 813," April 3, 1918, WNRC RG 90, Box 223.

109. Katharine C. Bushnell, "What's Going On," privately published pamphlet, 1918, in WNRC RG 90, Box 329; Bushnell to David Robinson, February 14, 1920; Bushnell, "Plain Words to Plain People," privately published flyer, n.d., WNRC RG 90, Box 329; Ethel S. Dummer to Jessie Binford, December 24, 1918, Dummer Papers; J. S. Law-

rence to C. C. Pierce, November 24, 1919, WNRC RG 90, Box 329; Maude Miner to Ethel S. Dummer, April 17, 1918, Dummer Papers; Bushnell, "What's Going On," 4–10; Bushnell to Robinson, May 20, 1919, WNRC RG 90, Box 329; and Dummer to Alice Hamilton, April 8, 1920, Dummer Papers. See also B. S. Steadwell, "Wartime Measures Against Venereal Diseases," *Light*, (September-October, 1919): 5–7; and David J. Pivar, "Cleansing the Nation: The War on Prostitution, 1917–21," *Prologue* 12 (Spring 1980): 34–36.

110. Roy K. Flannagan to Ennion G. Williams, October 17, 1918; W. A. Brumfield to Surgeon General, November 18, 1918; ——— to C. C. Pierce, January 23, 1919; H. C. Hall to Division of Venereal Diseases, January 23, 1919; ——— to C. C. Pierce, February 8, 1919, WNRC RG 90, Box 223; Flannagan to Williams, October 17, 1918, WNRC RG 90, Box 223; "Valid Provisions for the Quarantining of Persons with Venereal Disease," *JAMA* 74 (May 8, 1920): 1348; "Detention of Persons Infected with Venereal Virus," *JAMA* 73 (December 6, 1919): 1791; and "Decisions of the State Supreme Courts on the Subject of Venereal Disease Laws," unpublished typescript, n.d., WNRC RG 90, Box 223.

111. C. C. Pierce, "The Value of Detention as a Reconstruction Measure," *AJObst* 80 (December 1919): 629.

112. Timothy Newell Pfeiffer, "Social Hygiene and the War," *SocHy* 4 (July 1918): 427.

113. Martha P. Falconer, "The Part of the Reformatory Institution in the Elimination of Prostitution," *SocHy* 5 (January 1919): 4, 5; and *Hearings on Army Appropriation Bill, 1919*, 80. Mary Macey Dietzler, *Detention Houses and Reformatories as Protective Social Agencies in the Campaign of the United States Government Against Venereal Diseases*, U.S. Interdepartmental Social Hygiene Board (Washington, 1922), 24, 25; T. A. Storey in Dietzler, *Detention Houses*, 2.

115. Dietzler, *Detention Houses*, 24–25.

116. Dietzler, *Detention Houses*, 41; see also *Hearings on Training Camp Activities*, 5; *Hearings on Army Appropriation Bill, 1919*, p. 80; United States War Department, *Annual Report 1918* (Washington, 1918), 27.

117. *Report of the United States Interdepartmental Social Hygiene Board* (Washington, 1920), 21–23; Dietzler, *Detention Houses*, 16–21, 23, 36–40; H. H. Moore, "Four Million Dollars for the Fight Against Venereal Diseases," *SocHy* 5 (January 1919): 15–26.

118. Estimates of the number of prostitutes apprehended during the war vary. Most sources suggest that the government, through the CTCA and ISHB, detained some 30,000 women. See C. C. Pierce, "The Value of Detention as a Reconstruction Measure," *AJObst* 80 (December 1919): 630; and Dietzler, *Detention Houses*, 16, 69; Timothy Newell Pfeiffer, "Social Hygiene and the War," *SocHy* 4 (July 1918): 426–27.

119. Dietzler, *Detention Houses*, 66; Bushnell, "What's Going On," 12–14.

120. Dietzler, *Detention Houses*, 74, 76; W. F. Draper, "The Detention and Treatment of Women as a Measure of Control of Venereal Diseases in Extra-Cantonment Zones," *AJObst* 80 (December 1919): 643.

121. Dietzler, *Detention Houses*, 8, 36; also, Jane Deeter Rippin, "Municipal Detention for Women," *Proceedings of the National Conference of Social Work 1918* (Chicago, 1919), 132–39; and Martha P. Falconer, "The Segregation of Delinquent Women and Girls as a War Problem," *Annals* 79 (September 1918): 160–66; Pierce, "The Value of Detention as a Reconstruction Measure," 629; Falconer, "The Part of the Reformatory Institution in the Elimination of Prostitution," 8.

122. *Manual for the Various Agents of the United States Interdepartmental Social*

Hygiene Board (Washington, 1920), 20, 22; Pierce, "The Value of Detention as a Reconstruction Measure," 629; Dietzler, *Detention Houses*, 33.

123. For examples of these sociological surveys see, "Study of 6,000 Case Records of Delinquent Women and Girls," in *Manual for the Various Agents*, 75–85; and *Report of the United States Interdepartmental Social Hygiene Board, 1921* (Washington, 1922), 163–176.

124. *Manual for the Various Agents*, 22, 81; for a description of the development of this individualistic orientation in case work see David J. Rothman, *Conscience and Convenience: The Asylum and Its Alternatives in Progressive America* (Boston, 1980), 53–55; also Roy Lubove, *The Professional Altruist: The Emergence of Social Work as a Career* (Cambridge, 1965), 43–49.

125. Pierce, "The Value of Detention as a Reconstruction Measure," 633; A. J. McLaughlin, "Pioneering in Venereal Disease Control," *AJObst* 80 (December 1919): 634, 642; W. F. Draper, "The Detention and Treatment of Infected Women as a Measure of Control of Venereal Disease in Extra-Cantonment Zones," 643–45; Dietzler, *Detention Houses*, 47. "Much of our best effort has been put into trying to make mental defectives act like normal human beings, and when this miracle could not be wrought, we grew discouraged with the whole project." Additon, "Work Among Delinquent Women and Girls," 156.

126. T. A. Storey in Dietzler, *Detention Houses*, 7, 8.

127. McLaughlin, "Pioneering in Venereal Disease Control," 639; "The Campaign Against Prostitution and Venereal Diseases," *JAMA* 74 (June 19, 1920): 1728.

128. *The Enemy at Home*, American Social Hygiene Association pamphlet (New York, 1918).

129. Raymond B. Fosdick, "The Commissions on Training Camp Activities," *Annals* 79 (September 1918): 142; Walter Clarke, "The Promotion of Social Hygiene in War Time," *Annals* 79 (September 1918): 188.

130. "Making the Cities Safe for Soldiers," *Survey* 38 (July 28, 1917): 377; Fosdick, "The Commissions on Training Camp Activities," 131; William H. Zinsser, "Social Hygiene and the War," *SocHy* 4 (October 1918): 520; also M. J. Exner, "Social Hygiene and the War," *SocHy* 5 (April 1919): 296–97.

131. Bascom Johnson, "Eliminating Vice from Camp Cities," *Annals* 78 (July 1918): 64.

132. Quoted in C.-E.A. Winslow, *The Life of Hermann M. Biggs* (Philadelphia, 1929), 158.

133. See, for example, George Rosen, *Preventive Medicine in the United States, 1900–1975* (New York, 1975), esp. pp. 14–19; also Christopher Lasch, *Haven in a Heartless World* (New York, 1977), 98–103. Martin, ed., *Digest of the Proceedings of the Council of National Defense*, 294.

134. The fullest description of "civilized morality" appears in Nathan Hale, *Freud and the Americans: The Beginnings of Psychoanalysis in America* (New York, 1971), 24–46.

135. Zinsser, "Social Hygiene and the War," 498–501.

Chapter III

1. On the relationship of the Progressive movement to the war see Allen F. Davis, "Welfare, Reform and World War I," *AmQ* 29 (Fall 1967): 516–533; also, William E. Leuchtenburg, "The New Deal and the Analogue of War," in *Change and Continuity in Twentieth-Century America*, ed. John Braeman *et al.* (Columbus, 1964), 84–94.

2. Secondary accounts of the efforts directed against venereal disease in the AEF are Fred D. Baldwin, "The Invisible Army," *AmQ* 16 (Fall 1964): 432–44; and Donald Smythe, "Venereal Disease: The AEF's Experience," *Prologue* (Summer 1977): 65–74.

3. Quoted in Edwin Frank Allen, *Keeping Our Fighters Fit* (New York, 1918), 1.

4. The threat of soldiers returning from the war with venereal infections is a recurring theme in the massive social hygiene literature generated by the war. See, for example, M. J. Exner, "Prostitution in its Relation to the Army on the Mexican Border," *SocHy* 3 (April 1917): 205–20; Franklin Martin, "Social Hygiene and the War," *SocHy* 3 (October 1917): 605–11; and Raymond B. Fosdick, "The War and Navy Departments Commissions on Training Camp Activities," *Annals* 79 (September 1918): 130–42; "Statement of One of the Y.M.C.A. Divisional Secretaries," unpublished typescript, n.d., in Records of the Surgeon General, NA RG 112, Box 5179; Mrs. J. W. Broughton to Raymond B. Fosdick, September 7, 1917, in Records of the War Department General and Special Staffs, NA RG 165, Box 585.

5. A general account of the introduction of germ theory into American medicine is contained in William G. Rothstein, *American Physicians in the Nineteenth Century* (Baltimore, 1972), esp. pp. 261–78. See also, Donald Fleming, *William H. Welch and the Rise of Modern Medicine* (Boston, 1954); P. M. Ashburn, *A History of the Medical Department of the United States Army* (Boston, 1929), esp. pp. 261–81; Walter Clarke, "The Promotion of Social Hygiene in War Time," *Annals* 79 (September 1918): 178–89.

The discoveries that American industry had made concerning labor productivity, efficiency, and organization were applied with vigor in the military. For an analysis of the new consciousness of efficiency during the Progressive period see, Samuel Haber, *Efficiency and Uplift* (Chicago, 1964); also, Samuel P. Hays, *Conservation and the Gospel of Efficiency* (Cambridge, 1959).

6. "Incidence of Gonorrhea and Syphilis, Total Army, 1819–1950," mimeograph in ASHA Papers, poster series; L. M. Maus, "A Brief History of Venereal Diseases in the United States Army and Measures Employed for Their Suppression," unpublished typescript, June 14, 1917, p. 1, ASHA Papers, Folder 131:2; William Lyster, "Venereal Disease and the New Army," *JAMA* 69 (October 13, 1917) 1258. See also, United States War Department, *Annual Report 1917* (Washington, 1917), 396.

7. Lyster, "Venereal Disease and the New Army," 1258; also, Valery Harvard, "Venereal Diseases in the Army and Their Prophylaxis," *TASSMP* 1 (1906): 123–30; United States War Department, *Annual Report 1918* (Washington, 1918), 652. The institution of the Wassermann reaction in the Army in the years between 1906 and 1911 brought many new cases of syphilis to the attention of Army medical personnel. See Maus, "A Brief History of Venereal Diseases," 5; Lyster, "Venereal Disease in the New Army," 1258.

8. *Annual Report 1918*, 652–54. Prophylactic packages refer to a chemical treatment to be applied by the soldier after sexual intercourse to prevent the development of an infection. For a discussion of its early development and use in the military see, L. Mervin Maus, "Further Observations on the Prophylaxis of Venereal Diseases in the United States Army," *MilSurg* 27 (December 1910): 636–44; Victor Cox Pedersen, "Venereal Problems of the War," *Medical Record* 96 (July 12, 1919): 60–61.

9. M. J. Exner to Raymond B. Fosdick, June 23, 1917, NA RG 165, Box 575. Exner was forced to admit that "to get England and France to join us in a moral sanitation program similar to ours . . . is probably too ideal and does not off hand look very encouraging." Exner to Fosdick, May 29, 1917, NA RG 165, Box 575; see also "Cleaning Up Behind French Lines," *Survey* 38 (September 29, 1917): 577; and William F. Snow, "Social Hygiene and the War," *SocHy* 3 (July 1917): 417–26; also, "The War and the Venereal Problem," *AJPH* 7 (July 1917): 612–13.

10. Frank E. Vandiver, *Black Jack: The Life and Times of John J. Pershing* (College Station, Texas, 1977), 2:662, 773; Hugh Hampton Young, *A Surgeon's Autobiography* (New York, 1940), 301; Exner to Fosdick, May 26, 1917, NA RG 165, Box 575.

11. Young, *A Surgeon's Autobiography*, 270. James G. Harbord, Pershing's Chief of Staff, later commented on the "terrifying" nature of these lectures. See Harbord, *The American Army in France, 1917–1919* (Boston, 1936), 73; Felix Frankfurter to Newton Baker, August 15, 1917, Baker MSS. The best discussions of Pershing's interest in the venereal disease problem are contained in Smythe, "Venereal Disease: The AEF's Experience," 70–71; and Frank E. Vandiver, *Black Jack*, 2:773–77.

12. Hugh Hampton Young, "Preventive Medicine as Applied to the Venereal and Skin Diseases," *JAMA* 73 (November 29, 1919): 1669–70; also, Young, *A Surgeon's Autobiography*, 277, 283–84.

13. H. H. Young, "Report on Conference with Colonel Parks of the New Zealand Contingent," June 9, 1917, unpublished typescript, Records of the American Expeditionary Forces, 1917–1923, NA RG 120; Young, *A Surgeon's Autobiography*, 273–74.

14. Hugh H. Young, "Research Society Reports," *Medical Bulletin* (Paris), 1 (May, 1918), 505–16; "Venereal Disease and its Prevention in the Army," unpublished typescript, n.d., NA RG 120.

15. See the classic Progressive study of prostitution, Abraham Flexner, *Prostitution in Europe* (New York, 1917), esp. pp. 130–36, 157–58, 216–18; Joseph Earle Moore, "Venereal Campaign in Paris District of the American Expeditionary Forces," *JAMA* 74 (April 24, 1920): 1159.

16. George Walker, *Venereal Disease in the American Expeditionary Forces* (Baltimore, 1922), 85, 84–89. Walker's book is the only full-scale account of the Medical Department's campaign against venereal disease. See also, P. M. Ashburn, "Factors Making for a Low Venereal Record in the American Expeditionary Forces," *JAMA* 73 (December 13, 1919): 1827; Wood quoted in Hermann Hagedorn, *Leonard Wood: A Biography* (New York, 1931), 2:255.

17. Charles Eliot, "Vice Behind the French Lines," *Survey* 38 (September 8, 1917): 509.

18. "Advice to Soldiers in Paris," *SocHy* 5 (January 1919): 111–12; "Colonel Care Series," posters in ASHA Papers, Folder 131:6.

19. For British and French venereal statistics see Young, *A Surgeon's Autobiography*, 279; Young, "Preventive Medicine," 1669; Thomas Parran and R. A. Vonderlehr, *Plain Words About Venereal Disease* (New York, 1941), 75; and Walker, *Venereal Disease in the AEF*, 134–36. On British attempts to control the venereal diseases during the war see, "London Letter," *JAMA* 71 (November 9, 1918): 1595; and Edward H. Beardsley, "Allied Against Sin: American and British Responses to Venereal Disease in World War I," *Medical History* 20 (April 1976): 189–203.

20. The General Orders regarding venereal disease are reproduced in Frank W. Weed, *Sanitation in the American Expeditionary Forces*, vol. 6 of *The Medical Department of the United States Army in the World War* (Washington, 1926), 936–37, 955–64. (Hereafter cited as Weed, *Sanitation in the AEF*). Though the order made explicit the command's position on venereal disease, some officers argued that the provision requiring court-martial encouraged soldiers to conceal infections. It also proved difficult to enforce. Weed, the official Army historian of the anti-venereal campaign, has compiled many important documents and statistics in this indispensable volume.

21. The institution of prophylaxis made it possible for the military to consider venereal diseases as purely discretionary, thus it was the only illness which was punished. Many medical officers felt that the provisions for court-martial did not have a great impact on reducing infections. See, Ashburn, "Factors Making for a Low Venereal Record

in the AEF," 1828. See also E. L. Keyes to Surgeon General, March 29, 1918, NA RG 120. Keyes believed the punishment might be unjust if the prophylactic treatment was not effective.

22. This order was based on Young's observation of the treatment of British venereal patients. See, Weed, *Sanitation in the AEF*, 956–57; Edward Hartman to Joseph Lee, September 14, 1917, NA RG 165, Box 365.

23. Young, "Preventive Medicine," 1670.

24. Young, *A Surgeon's Autobiography*, 308; see also, "Report to the Executive Committee—National War Work Council Y.M.C.A.," (New York, 1917), 49 in National Young Men's Christian Association Papers, Box E 174.

25. Young, *A Surgeon's Autobiography*, 309; Young, "Preventive Medicine," 1677.

26. Pershing quoted in Young, *A Surgeon's Autobiography*, 309; Young's report to the Chief Surgeon on conditions in St. Nazaire is reprinted in Weed, *Sanitation in the AEF*, 902–3; see also Young, "Success of the Campaign for Combatting Venereal Diseases in the A.E.F.," unpublished typescript, n.d., NA RG 120.

27. Weed, *Sanitation in the AEF*, 960–62; Young to A. E. Bradley, November 11, 1917, NA RG 120, Box 5167.

28. It should be noted that all officers in the Medical Corps did not agree with Young's prescription for the problems of St. Nazaire. Lieutenant Howard Cecil recommended that the Army "employ a number of prostitutes . . . who will be carefully inspected under military control." See, Howard L. Cecil to Commanding Officer, Base Section No. 1, October 4, 1917; and Clyde S. Ford to Surgeon, Base Section No. 1, October 10, 1917, NA RG 120. In fact, surveying conditions in St. Nazaire six months after Pershing's visit, George Walker found that the houses of prostitution had been reopened for U.S. troops, in violation of G.O. No. 77. See Walker, "Summary of Facts Relating to the Restricted District, St. Nazaire," unpublished typescript, April 1918, NA RG 120. American-run houses of prostitution were also established in other French towns. See, J. E. Moore to H. H. Young, April 26, 1918, NA RG 120.

29. Weed, *Sanitation in the AEF*, 961; Young, *A Surgeon's Autobiography*, 310.

30. Weed, *Sanitation in the AEF*, 906; and Walker, *Venereal Disease in the AEF*, 51.

31. Although portions of Simonin's memo are published in Weed, *Sanitation in the AEF* 907–10, the entire document is available in typescript in "Papers Relating to the Attitude of the A.E.F. in Relation to the Problem of Prostitution," August 20, 1918, Parran MSS.

32. "Simonin Memo," 17, 20, Parran MSS.

33. "Simonin Memo," 20, Parran MSS.

34. "Simonin Memo," 21, Parran MSS.

35. G. Clemenceau to Chief of the French Mission, AEF, February 17, 1918, in Weed, *Sanitation in the AEF*, 910; Raymond B. Fosdick, "The Fight Against Venereal Disease," *TNR* 17 (November 30, 1918): 132; Fosdick, *Chronicle of a Generation* (New York, 1958), 171.

36. H. H. Young and E. L. Keyes, "Reply to Simonin," unpublished typescript, n.d., p. 28, Parran MSS.

37. M. W. Ireland to J. Pershing, May 20, 1918, NA RG 120; E. L. Keyes, "Plan for Response to the Communication of the Minister of War," unpublished typescript, February 22, 1918, NA RG 120.

38. Young and Keyes, "Reply to Simonin," 27, Parran MSS; Ogier quoted in Walker, *Venereal Disease in the AEF*, 52; William Howard Taft, ed., *Service With Fighting Men* (New York, 1922), 1:116.

39. H. E. Kleinschmidt, "Is Education a Worthwhile Factor in the Control of Venereal Diseases?" *SocHy* 5 (April 1919): 229.

40. Isaac Brewer, "The Venereal Peril," *SocHy* 3 (January 1917): 104; Gertrude Seymour, "Health of Soldier and Civilian: II. Venereal Disease Abroad," *Survey* 39 (December 29, 1917): 367; Luther H. Gulick, *Morals and Morale* (New York, 1919), 48.

41. *Literary Digest* 57 (June 22, 1918): 19; Taft, ed., *Service With Fighting Men*, 1:109, 118; *Outlook* 117 (December 5, 1917): 552.

42. Gulick, *Morals and Morale*, 14; also, Elmer T. Clark, *Social Studies of the War* (New York, 1919), 17–45; "Exaggerated Reports of the Depravity of Our Soldiers in France," *Current Opinion* 64 (March 1918): 197; Mrs. M. B. Munson to R. B. Fosdick, September 27, 1917, NA RG 165, Box 585.

43. R. W. Bainbridge to William Redfield, January 8, 1918, NA RG 165, Box 447.

44. William F. Milburn and Charles H. Myers, August 2, 1917, NA RG 165, Box 585; and Newton Baker to Fosdick, July 13, 1917, NA RG 165, Box 570; also, Glen E. Holt, ed., *An American in the Army and YMCA, 1917–1920: The Diary of David Lee Shillingslaw* (Chicago, 1971), 42–47.

45. Gulick, *Morals and Morale*, 50–51; for a description of the work of YMCA women volunteers in France see, "Letters of Mary Lee," *Atlantic Monthly* 124 (October 1919): 520–31. See also, Marian Baldwin, *Canteening Overseas* (New York, 1920). One woman working for the YMCA in Paris walked the streets late at night, searching for soldiers with pick-ups. "After talking for a little while, the man as a rule became ashamed and was ready to take the warning." She reportedly "rescued" some 1,100 men from "dangerous companions." See, Walker, *Venereal Disease in the AEF*, 154.

46. Taft, ed., *Service With Fighting Men*, 1:143–51. In August 1918, company commanders in Base Section No. 1 were ordered to classify their men according to character. Those who rated highest could obtain all-day passes with a 9:30 curfew; men in class two received four hour passes; those assessed as having "poor character" received no privileges. Weed, *Sanitation in the AEF*, 915–917.

47. H. H. Young to A. E. Bradley, November 11, 1917, RG 120.

48. Taft, ed., *Service With Fighting Men*, 2:142–162; "Interview With Dr. J. H. McCurdy, Y.M.C.A.," unpublished typescript, January 16, 1920, p. 41, YMCA Papers, Box E 143.

49. Taft, ed., *Service With Fighting Men*, 2:142–43; Walker, *Venereal Disease in the AEF*, 178–91.

50. "Something to Think About for Men Going on Leave," unpublished mimeograph, April 12, 1919, NA RG 120, Box 5259.

51. Walker, *Venereal Disease in the AEF*, 20, 183; Weed, *Sanitation in the AEF*, 927–34.

52. Weed, *Sanitation in the AEF*, 932; also, William D. Jack and Herbert Foster to Chief Surgeon, February 16, 1919, NA RG 120, Box 5170. Jack and Foster estimated that 40 percent of the men had intercourse while on leave. Ashburn, "Factors Making for a Low Venereal Record in the AEF," 1827. The notion that American troops attracted more prostitutes because they received higher pay appears frequently in discussions of the venereal problem. See, Virgil V. Johnson, "Venereal Disease in France," *Survey* 39 (December 8, 1917): 300.

53. Walker, *Venereal Disease in the AEF*, 8; J. Pershing to Surgeon General, January 18, 1919, NA RG 120.

54. Weed, *Sanitation in the AEF*, 939–46.

55. Weed, *Sanitation in the AEF*, 939–46; Walker, *Venereal Disease in the AEF*, 10–19.

56. "Venereal Prophylaxis," *War Medicine* (Paris), 2 (September 1918), 283–84.

57. Weed, *Sanitation in the AEF*, 949–59; Walker, V*enereal Disease in the AEF*, 16–17; Joseph Earle Moore, "The Value of Prophylaxis Against Venereal Diseases," *JAMA* 75 (October 2, 1920): 911–15.

58. Weed, *Sanitation in the AEF*, 949; Walker, V*enereal Disease in the AEF*, 14–16. The ability of the AEF to get its members to accept prophylactic treatments was in itself a remarkable accomplishment in military discipline. Certainly the provision of a court-martial charge of neglect of duty for failure to obtain the treatment must have had a potent effect on attracting soldiers to the stations. "Both the medical and line officers of the French Army marvelled at our ability to force our men to take the prophylaxis," noted George Walker. "They claimed that they would not dare to do such a thing in their army" (p. 135).

59. Pershing to Chief Surgeon, April 8, 1919, in Weed, *Sanitation in the AEF*, 945–46; E. L. Keyes to Alfred Bradley, March 29, 1918, NA RG 120; also, Weed, *Sanitation in the AEF*, 952.

60. Edith Houghton Hooker, "A Criticism of Venereal Prophylaxis," *SocHy* 4 (April 1918): 189, 192; also, "Social Hygiene for Soldiers," *Survey* 39 (October 27, 1917): 99; and B. S. Steadwell, "The Modern Campaign Against Venereal Disease," *The Light*, January-February 1920, 6–8.

61. Edith Houghton Hooker, "The Case Against Prophylaxis," *SocHy* 5 (April 1919): 176; Hooker, "The Case Against Prophylaxis," 179.

62. Walker, V*enereal Disease in the AEF*, 31, 37–8; see also, Charles E. Riggs, "A Study of Venereal Prophylaxis in the Navy," *SocHy* 3 (July 1917): 299–312; and Moore, "The Value of Prophylaxis Against Venereal Diseases," 911.

63. R. C. Holcomb, "Have We Devised an Effective Propaganda of Venereal Prophylaxis," *SocHy* 4 (January 1918): 64. Journalist H. L. Mencken attacked reformers such as Hooker for attempting to deny soldiers the advances of science. He expressed the fear that prophylaxis would be repressed along with prostitution, projecting: "The disease rate, with an ineffective suppression in place of scientific watchfulness, will go up by at least 500 percent, and thousands of boys will be ruined for life." New York *Evening Mail*, September 18, 1917. Bailey K. Ashford, "Informal Talk Given to the Individual Companies of Command," unpublished typescript, n.d., NA RG 120.

64. Franklin Martin, "Social Hygiene and War," *SocHy* 3 (October 1917): 608; Hooker, "The Case Against Prophylaxis," 173.

65. Lyster, "Venereal Disease and the New Army," 1359.

66. L. Mervin Maus, "Further Observations on the Prophylaxis of Venereal Diseases in the United States Army," *MilSurg* 27 (December 1910): 639–40; also, Maus, "Prophylaxis of the Venereal Diseases in the Army and Navy," *Transactions of the International Congress of Hygiene and Demography* 5 (1913): 325–35; Weed, *Sanitation in the AEF*, 955; also, A. E. Bradley to General W. C. MacPherson, March 2, 1918, NA RG 120. Bradley explained that pro-kits were available only to officers and men on leave where no prophylactic station was accessible.

67. Weed, *Sanitation in the AEF*, 955; Walker, V*enereal Disease in the AEF*, 27. The provision of pro-kits has often been mistaken for the distribution of condoms. Although many officers urged the Medical Department to distribute condoms, they were never officially provided. See, T. C. Rhoads to Commanding General, March 13, 1919, NA RG 120, Box 5717.

68. Daniels to Commanding Officers, U.S. Navy, February 27, 1915, in *SocHy* 1 (June 1915): 483; Fosdick, *Chronicle of a Generation*, 162.

69. Walker, V*enereal Disease in the AEF*, 101; Ashburn, "Factors Making for a Low Venereal Record in the AEF," 1825–28. In Paris alone, where most members of the

AEF were not permitted to go, almost 100,000 official prophylactic treatments were administered. See Moore, "The Value of Prophylaxis Against Venereal Diseases," 912. Walker's estimate of 242,000 prophylactic treatments during the course of the war is far too low. Walker, *Venereal Disease in the AEF*, 32. See also H. H. Young, "Venereal Disease and its Prevention in the Army," unpublished typescript, n.d., p. 3; and Young, "Success of the Campaign for Combatting Venereal Diseases," unpublished typescript, n.d., NA RG 120.

70. Official Army venereal statistics are contained in Joseph Siler, *Communicable and Other Diseases*, vol. 9 of *The Medical Department of the United States Army in the World War* (Washington, 1928), esp. pp. 263–69; Alfred S. Crosby, *Epidemic and Peace* (Westport, Connecticut, 1976); "The Economic Loss from Venereal Diseases in the Army," *JAMA* 75 (November 13, 1920): 1353.

71. Siler, *Communicable and Other Diseases*, 263–64, 269; Albert S. Bowen, *Activities Concerning Mobilization Camps and Ports of Embarkation*, vol. 4 of *The Medical Department of the United States Army in the World War* (Washington, 1928), 332; W. C. Gorgas to Commanding Generals, Ports of Embarkation, November 8, 1917, NA RG 120; William F. Snow and Wilbur A. Sawyer, "Venereal Disease Control in the Army," *JAMA* 71 (August 10, 1918): 457.

72. Siler, *Communicable and Other Diseases*, 269; Ashburn, "Factors Making for a Low Venereal Record in the AEF," 1826–27; Moore, "The Value of Prophylaxis Against Venereal Disease," 911–15.

73. Siler, *Communicable and Other Diseases*, 264; Mimeographed flyer in NA RG 120, Box 5170; quoted in Weed, *Sanitation in the AEF*, 969; see also 978–81; the fullest description of the venereal camps is contained in Walker, *Venereal Disease in the AEF*, 197–213; "Interview with D.R. J. H. McCurdy, Y.M.C.A.," unpublished typescript, January 16, 1920, p. 50, YMCA Papers, Box E143.

74. Siler, *Communicable and Other Diseases*, 264; U.S. War Department *Annual Report 1918* (Washington, 1918), 507–8, 513; Albert G. Love and C. B. Davenport, *Defects Found in Drafted Men* (Washington, 1920), 34; on venereal disease among blacks; see, for example, H. H. Hazen, "Syphilis in the American Negro," *JAMA* 63 (August 8, 1914): 463–66; and Thomas Murrell, "Syphilis and the American Negro," *JAMA* 54 (March 12, 1910): 846–49; Arthur B. Spingarn, "The War and Venereal Disease Among Negroes," *SocHy* 4 (July 1918): 333–46; Spingarn, "The Health and Morals of Colored Troops," *Crisis* 16 (August 1918): 66–68; also, Arthur E. Barbeau and Florette Henri, *The Unknown Soldiers: Black Troops in World War I* (Philadelphia 1974), 52–55.

75. Weed, *Sanitation in the AEF*, 953–54; Walker, *Venereal Disease in the AEF*, 122–23; and Young, *A Surgeon's Autobiography*, 320–21; United States War Department, *Annual Report 1918*, 508–9.

76. "It is a difficult thing to demobilize any active organization," wrote Charles E. Barr, "but in the case of our army, in unaccustomed surroundings, amid a people whose habits of life and thought differed so radically from our own, and in associations that loosened all the usual conventions of their lives, the dangers of demoralization were intensified." "Public Health Education and the American Army in France," *SocHy* 5 (October 1919): 545; John J. Pershing to Chief Surgeon, January 18, 1919, NA RG 120; "Weekly Medical Circular No. 3," October 10, 1919, unpublished mimeograph, NA RG 120, Box 5167. These rates were computed by multiplying the monthly rate by twelve.

77. "Demobilization and Venereal Diseases," *JAMA* 71 (December 7, 1918): 1915; Walter Clarke, "The Promotion of Social Hygiene in War Time," *Annals* 79 (September 1918): 189.

78. "Proposed Bulletin," January 27, 1919, unpublished typescript, NA RG 120;

"Venereal Diseases and Birth Rates," *War Medicine* (Paris), 2 (January 1919), 1184; Walker, *Venereal Diseases in the AEF*, 74, 124–26. Almost 6,000 cases of venereal disease were discovered through embarkation exams. "Outline of Talk on Venereal Disease to be Given to Soldiers by Line Officers," Headquarters 2nd Army, January 25, 1919, unpublished typescript, NA RG 120, Box 3294. H. H. Young argued for frequent inspections of returning troops. See, Young to Chief Surgeon, November 16, 1918, NA RG 120, Box 5169; Young, *A Surgeon's Autobiography*, 341.

79. "Back in the Good Old U.S.A.," pamphlet, n.d., ASHA Papers, Folder 131:6; Edward J. Williams to Chief Surgeon, February 20, 1919, NA RG 120, Box 5170.

80. Quoted in Dixon Wecter, *When Johnny Comes Marching Home* (Boston, 1944), 330–31.

81. Frank Parker Stockbridge, "The Cleanest Army in the World," *Delineator* 93 (December 1918): 8; Raymond B. Fosdick, "The Fight Against Venereal Disease," *TNR* 17 (November 30, 1918): 134.

82. Gulick, *Morals and Morale*, 34; Newton Baker to State Governors, November 14, 1918, Josephus Daniels Papers, Library of Congress, Washington, D.C.; see also Daniel A. Poling, "Physically Competent and Morally Fit," *Outlook* 119 (July 10, 1918): 415–17.

83. Walker, *Venereal Disease in the AEF*, 223–25; see also, Magnus Hirschfeld, *The Sexual History of the World War* (New York, 1941).

84. Quoted in Peter Gabriel Filene, *Him/Her/Self: Sex Roles in Modern America* (New York, 1974), 105.

85. George Rosen, *Preventive Medicine in the United States, 1900–1975* (New York, 1975), esp. pp. 3–19.

Chapter IV

1. See New York State Department of Health, "Press Release," November 20, 1934, unp. typescript, TP MSS.

Many in the social hygiene movement protested CBS's censorship. See William F. Snow to William S. Paley, November 20, 1934; Snow, "Press Release," December 29, 1934; Albert Pfeiffer to Snow, January 4, 1934; Walter Brunet to Snow, January 8, 1935, in ASHA Papers, Folders 70:4–6.

A number of newspapers and magazines reported the incident. See, for example, New York *Post*, November 20, 1934; New York *Herald Tribune*, November 21, 1934; *Time*, December 3, 1934; and "Honi Soit Qui Mal y Pense," *NEJM* 211 (November 29, 1934): 1031.

2. Among the works which consider the "sexual revolution" of the 1920s see Paula S. Fass, *The Damned and the Beautiful* (New York, 1977), 260–90; Peter Gabriel Filene, *Him/Her/Self* (New York, 1975), 118–52; David M. Kennedy, *Birth Control in America* (New Haven, 1970), 136–75; and William E. Leuchtenburg, *Perils of Prosperity* (Chicago, 1958), 158–77.

3. "Great Pox," *Time*: 28 (October 26, 1936): 31.

4. Rachelle Yarros, "Shall We Finish the Fight?" *Life and Labor* 9 (January 1919): 19; Neva R. Deardorff, "Throttling Social Hygiene," *Survey* 45 (March 19, 1921): 884; M. W. Ireland to Attorney General, June 7, 1922, USISHB Papers, NA RG 90.

5. "Record of a Conference, March 25, 1921," unp. typescript; also, T. A. Storey to C. C. Pierce, June 27, 1921; T. A. Storey, "Facts Justifying the Investment of Congress in the Interdepartmental Social Hygiene Board," unp. typescript, NA RG 90.

See also, "Some Facts Bearing on the Campaign Against Venereal Disease in America," unp. typescript' in Josephus Daniels Papers, Library of Congress, Box 463.

"The Passing of the Interdepartmental Social Hygiene Board," *JAMA* 76 (January 8, 1921): 117.

For the official response of the ISHB see "Concerning Inaccuracies Carried in a Recent Issue of the *Journal of the American Medical Association*," unp. typescript, n.d., NA RG 90.

See Ronald L. Numbers, *Almost Persuaded: American Physicians and Compulsory Health Insurance* (Baltimore, 1978), for an extended discussion of the response to proposals for programs during the 1920s.

6. Gilchrist quoted in Martin Pernick, "Progressives, Propaganda, and Public Health," unp. mss., November 1974, p. 11; J. E. Rush, "Critical Comment on Current Methods of Public Education in Venereal Disease," *American Journal of Sociology* 27 (November 1921): 329.

7. The Public Health Service conducted an extensive poll of state boards of health to determine their policies concerning prophylaxis. See, for example, C. A. Harper (Wisconsin State Board of Health) to Taliaferro Clark, December 23, 1930, WNRC RG 90, Box 232. American Social Hygiene Association, "The Case Against the Prophylactic Packet," unp. circular, n.d. (1920?), WNRC RG 90, Box 231.

8. Roy K. Flannagan to Mark J. White, April 14, 1923, WNRC RG 90, Box 232. O. C. Wenger of the PHS wrote: "The whole subject of prophylaxis is T.N.T. at this stage of the game as far as the Service is concerned because we might innocently start some unwelcome comment." Wenger to Thomas Parran, October 23, 1926, TP MSS. S. Leon Gans to C. C. Pierce, April 30, 1920; also, Paul Popenoe to H. H. Moore, June 29, 1920, WNRC RG 90, Box 232. A similar experiment was attempted in Kentucky. See William Riley to Thomas Parran, November 1, 1927, WNRC RG 90, Box 232.

9. George H. Bigelow, "Letter to the Editor," *The Independent* (Boston), 118 (June 25, 1927): 667; H. S. Cumming to Stewart Beach, July 11, 1927, WNRC RG 90, Box 232.

10. Thomas Parran to William Pentz, December 31, 1927; Parran, "Atlanta Speech," unp. typescript, November 1926, WNRC RG 90, Box 232.

11. There is, unfortunately, inadequate biographical material on Parran. See, however, his obituary by Alden Whitman, *New York Times*, February 17, 1968; also, *Current Biography*, (August 1940), 629–31. A *curriculum vitae* is in the TP MSS.

12. "The Reminiscences of Thomas Parran," Columbia Oral History Collection, (1965), 64; O. C. Wenger to Walter Brunet, April 3, 1926, WNRC RG 90, Box 231.

13. Thomas Parran to Taliaferro Clark, March 15, 1933, TP MSS.

14. See, for example, Maurice A. Bigelow, "Youth and Morals," *JSocHy* 14 (January 1928): 1–5.

15. Paul E. Bowers, "Some Sociological and Psychiatrical Aspects of the Venereal Disease Problem," unp. typescript, n.d., 79, WNRC RG 90, Box 231. On the response to Freud see John Chynoweth Burnham, *Psychoanalysis and American Medicine, 1894–1918* (New York, 1967), 180–216; also Nathan Hale, *Freud and the Americans* (New York, 1971), esp. pp. 397–433. All-American Conference on Venereal Disease, *Preliminary Report of Proceedings* (Washington, 1921), 51.

16. Bowers, "Some Sociological and Psychiatrical Aspects of the Venereal Problem," 77; Ford quoted in Roderick Nash, *The Nervous Generation: American Thought, 1917–1930* (Chicago, 1970), 167; American National Association of Masters of Dancing, "Rules, Regulations, and Suggestions Governing Social Dancing," pamphlet, 1919, ASHA Papers, Folder L2:3.

17. O. C. Wenger, "The Prevention of the Venereal Diseases," unp. typescript, n.d. (1924?), 2, WNRC RG 90, Box 231; James R. McGovern, "Sporting Life on the Line: Prostitution in Progressive Era Pensacola," *Florida Historical Quarterly* 54 (October 1975): 139–40. Also, Charles Winick and Paul M. Kinsie, *The Lively Commerce: Prostitution in the United States* (Chicago, 1971).

18. "To Dance Hall Managers and Proprietors of the U.S.," circular letter, September 1919, WNRC RG 90, Box 328.

19. Charlotte Perkins Gilman, "Parasitism and Civilized Vice," in V. F. Calverton and S. D. Schmalhausen, eds., *Woman's Coming of Age* (New York, 1931), 125; also, Gilman, "The New Generation of Women," *Current History* 18 (August 1923): 735–36. See Edwin O. Smigel and Rita Seiden, "The Decline and Fall of the Double Standard," *Annals* 376 (March 1968): 7–17.

20. Questionaires for these studies are contained in the files of the Venereal Disease Division of the PHS, WNRC RG 90, Boxes 253–59; "How Prevalent is Syphilis?" *AJPH* 22 (September 1932): 987–88; Thomas Parran, "Public Health Control of Syphilis," *Annals of Internal Medicine* 10 (July 1936): 65; on incidence among blacks see Taliaferro Clark, *The Control of Syphilis in Southern Rural Areas* (Chicago, 1932).

21. Thomas Parran, "The Eradication of Syphilis as a Practical Public Health Objective," *JAMA* 97 (July 11, 1931): 73–76; also, Matthias Nicoll, Jr. and Marjorie T. Bellows, "Effects of a Confidential Inquiry on the Recorded Mortality from Syphilis and Alcoholism." *AJPH* 24 (August 1934): 813–20; Ira S. Wile, "Sex Education in Relation to Mental and Social Hygiene," *Mental Hygiene* 18 (January 1934): 40–50; Thomas Parran and Lida J. Usilton, "The Extent of the Problem of Syphilis and Gonorrhea in the United States," *American Journal of Syphilis* 14 (April 1930): 145–55; Louis Dublin to Ruth Topping, April 7, 1932, BSH Papers, Box 10.

22. See John H. Stokes, *Modern Clinical Syphilology* (Philadelphia, 1926), 113–35; Joseph Earle Moore, *The Modern Treatment of Syphilis* (Baltimore, 1933), 32–109.

23. Thomas Parran, "Syphilis: A Public Health Problem," *Science* 87 (February 18, 1938): 148. An exception to this pattern was research done at "Department L," the syphilis clinic at Johns Hopkins. For a comprehensive survey see A. McGehee Harvey, "Clinical Investigation of Chronic Diseases: Its successful Pursuit in an Outpatient Setting." *Journal of Chronic Diseases* 33 (1980): 529–66. In addition to the wide range of arsenical regimens, some physicians treating tertiary syphilis in mental institutions during the 1920s and 1930s employed "fever therapy." Patients were deliberately infected with malaria, which, it was hoped would kill off the infecting spirochete. The efficacy of this treatment was never conclusively verified. See, for example, Max A. Bahr and W. L. Bruetsch, "Two Years' Experience with the Malarial Treatment of General Paralysis in a State Institution," *American Journal of Psychiatry* 84 (March 1928): 715–27; and Nolan D. C. Lewis, Lois Hubbard and Edna G. Dyar, "The Malarial Treatment of Paretic Neurosyphilis," *American Journal of Psychiatry* 81 (October 1924): 175–89.

24. Thomas Parran, *Shadow on the Land: Syphilis* (New York, 1937), 284; Thomas Parran, "Memorandum Relative to Syphilis Research," March 6, 1929, WNRC RG 90, Box 325. Also, Committee on Research in Syphilis, "Report of the Chairman of the Scientific Committee," January 1, 1930, WNRC RG 90, Box 327; and "The Reminiscences of Thomas Parran," COHC, 72.

25. Parran, *Shadow on the Land,* 285. Also, Harry F. Dowling, *Fighting Infection* (Cambridge, 1977), 94–95; Dowling, "The Emergence of the Cooperative Clinicial Trial," *Transactions and Studies of the College of Physicians and Surgeons of Philadelphia,* 4th Series, 43 (July 1975): 22–29; Surgeon General, *Annual Report of the U.S. Public Health Service,* 1939 (Washington, 1939), 129; O. C. Wenger, R. A. Vonderlehr, and T. Clark, "The Past, Present, and Future of the Syphilis Problem," unp. typescript, n.d. (1933?),

WNRC RG 90, Box 225. Members of the Cooperative Clinicial Group included Harold N. Cole of Western Reserve, J. E. Moore of Johns Hopkins, Paul A. O'Leary of the Mayo Clinic, John H. Stokes of the University of Michigan, and Thomas Parran.

26. "Social Hygiene and Unemployment," unp. typescript, n.d. (1932?), ASHA Papers, Folder 18:6.

27. "The City's Care of Syphilis," *Survey* 69 (June 1933): 228; "What St. Louis Pays for Venereal Disease," *Survey* 69 (May 1933): 196; Costs of Venereal Disease to St. Louis," unp. typescript, January 1, 1933, p. 40, ASHA Papers, Folder 100:3.

28. Joseph Earle Moore, *The Modern Treatment of Syphilis* (Baltimore, 1933), 39–42; Albert Keidel, "Economic Aspects of the Management of Syphilis," *Archives of Dermatology and Syphilology* 25 (March 1932): 479, 477; J. Frank Schamburg, "Discussion," *Archives of Dermatology and Syphilis* 25 (March 1932): 480.

29. Ruth Topping, "Visits to Venereal Disease Clinics at Vanderbilt and Harlem Hospitals," April 14, 1932, BSH Papers, Box 10. Also, Mary S. Edwards, "Venereal Disease Clinics," November 11, 1932, p. 2, BSH Papers, Box 10. On hospital admission of venereal patients see H. S. Cumming to Albert S. Hyman, February 23, 1923, WNRC RG 90, Box 223; Keidel, "Economic Aspects of the Management of Syphilis," 478.

30. See, for example, John H. Stokes to A. Warren Stearns, February 6, 1929, BSH Papers, Box 7; John H. Stokes, "Education of the Physician and the Movement for Venereal Disease Control," *JAMA* 107 (September 12, 1936): 866–71; see also "A Report on Instruction Regarding Syphilis in American Medical Schools," unp. typescript (1933), ASHA Papers, Folder 165:8; and A. W. Stearns to Lawrence B. Dunham, January 2, 1929, BSH Papers, Box 7. N. A. Nelson in U.S. Congress. Senate. Committee on Commerce. *Hearings on Investigation and Control of Venereal Diseases.* 75th Congress, 3rd Session, February 14–15, 1938, p. 13. (Hereafter, Senate *Hearings*); Joseph Earle Moore, "The Public Health Officer and the Control of Syphilis," *AJPH* 25 (January 1935): 37;

John H. Stokes, "Clinical Problems in Syphilis Control Today," *JAMA* 108 (March 6, 1937): 780–85.

31. "Report of a Survey of Medical Aspects of Social Hygiene in San Francisco, California, 1931," unp. typescript, ASHA Papers, Folders 98:4–5. "Drug Stores in Relation to Venereal Diseases in Chicago," (March 18, 1931), unp. typescript, ASHA Papers, Folder 9; see also, "Advertising Men's Specialists in Newark, N.J.," (June-July, 1933), ASHA Papers, Folder 100:5. Walter M. Brunet and Samuel M. Auerbach, "Present Day Charlatanism in the Venereal Disease Field," *JSocHy* 14 (1928): 342–47; "The Essence of Quackery," *JSocHy* 16 (1930): 497–98.

32. N. A. Nelson and Gladys L. Crain, *Syphilis, Gonorrhea and the Public Health* (New York, 1938), 2.

33. Thomas Parran and Lida J. Usilton, "The Extent of the Problem of Syphilis and Gonorrhea in the United States," *American Journal of Syphilis* 14 (April 1930): 152; "For War on Social Diseases," *Business Week* (October 10, 1937), 34.

34. Morris Fishbein, "Social Diseases," *Hygeia* 16 (January 1938): 10; Parran and Usilton, "The Extent of the Problem," 152; Charles H. Babcock to Edwards Stettinius, Jr., September 4, 1937, ASHA Papers, Folder 22:5.

35. Thomas Parran, "Speech to Conference on Life and Property Conservation," unp. typescript, May 1, 1929, WNRC RG 90, Box 226. On welfare capitalism see James R. Green, *The World of the Worker* (New York, 1980), 100–32.

36. American Social Hygiene Association, "Hidden Costs in Industry," publication number 751, 1931; O. C. Wenger, "Syphilis Among Railroad Employees," unp. typescript, November 1, 1927, WNRC RG 90, Box 233; James R. Garner, "Syphilis vs.

Railroad Manpower," *International Journal of Medicine and Surgery*, 43 (October 1930): 551–53; E. V. Milholland, "Safeguarding the Physical Welfare of Employees, the Travelling Public and the Property of Railroads," *International Journal of Medicine and Surgery*, 45 (January 1932): 36–38. Baseball players, on the road for half the season, were reportedly subject to frequent infection. See Harold Seymour, *Baseball: The Golden Age* (New York, 1971), 106.

37. "Consultant Service," unp. typescript, n.d. (1937?), ASHA Papers, Folder 22:5; also, William F. Snow, "Syphilis in Industry," November 1, 1937, ASHA Papers, Folder 167:5; "For War on Social Diseases," *Business Week* (October 30, 1937), 34–35; G. H. Gehrman, "Syphilis in Large Industrial Organizations," *VDI* (1936); James W. Long, "Industrial Aspects of Venereal Disease Control," *JSocHy* 24 (January 1938): 1–10; Albert E. Russell, "The Control of Syphilis in Industry," *JSocHy* 24 (January 1938): 11–14. Organized labor often supported physical exams. See Samuel Gompers to Rupert Blue, June 30, 1919; and William Green to Mark J. White, February 24, 1925, WNRC RG 90, Box 232. See also Thomas Parran, *Shadow on the Land*, 192; "Fighting Venereal Disease," *Business Week* (March 12, 1938), 38–39; R. R. Sayers, "Syphilis Control in Industry and Society," *AJPH* 28 (February 1938): 157.

38. Ray S. Dixon, "Economic Losses to Industry and Society," unp. typescript, January 1933, ASHA Papers, Folder 100:3.

39. Senate *Hearings*, 159.

40. During the 1920s, the ASHA had continued its emphasis on anti-vice activities, sex education, and added a new "Family Life Division" devoted essentially to child-rearing guidance. See, for example, Alphonse M. Schwitalla, "The Aims and Achievements of Social Hygiene," *JSocHy* 15 (January 1929): 1–7; also, Harry Emerson Fosdick, "What is Happening to the American Family," *JSocHy* 15 (March 1929): 139–51. "Fruits of a Great Crusade," *American Mercury* 28 (July 1931): 288. H. L. Mencken, the editor of the *American Mercury*, seems to have had a particular animus against the social hygienists and their propensity for euphemism. See *The American Language* (New York, 1937), 300–306. Michael M. Davis to Thomas Parran, June 29, 1936, TP MSS.

41. Anthony M. Turano, "Mrs. Grundy's Disease," *American Mercury* 40 (April 1937): 401; Parran, *Shadow on the Land*, 225; Haven Emerson, "Public Health Awaits Social Courage," *AJPH* 24 (October 1934): 1012.

42. Thomas Parran, "The Eradication of Syphilis as a Practical Public Health Objective," *JAMA* 97 (July 11, 1931): 73.

43. Bundesen in Senate *Hearings*, 35; "Control of Syphilis as the Next Public Health Objective," *JAMA* 106 (April 18, 1936): 1390; N. A. Nelson, "The Civilian Education Program in the Control of Syphilis," *JAMA* 107 (September 17, 1936): 872; Walter Clarke, "Should We Say 'Venereal' Disease?" unp. typescript, October 22, 1930, ASHA Papers, Folder 162:4.

44. Several studies on the history of birth control in America have addressed the growing authority of the medical profession in the realm of sexuality. See Linda Gordon, *Woman's Body, Woman's Right* (New York, 1976); David Kennedy, *Birth Control in America* (New Haven, 1970); and James Reed, *From Private Vice to Public Virtue* (New York, 1978).

45. Thomas Parran, "The Next Great Plague to Go," *Survey Graphic* 25 (July 1936): 405–11; and "Why Don't We Stamp Out Syphilis," *Reader's Digest* (July 1936): 65–73.

46. Parran, "The Next Great Plague to Go," 411.

47. Parran, "The Next Great Plague to Go," 411.

48. Parran, "The Next Great Plague to Go," 411; Parran, *Shadow on the Land*, 111–

16; Thomas Parran, "The Public Health Control of Syphilis," *Annals of Internal Medicine* 10 (July 1936): 66–67; also, "Venereal Disease Control in Scandinavian Countries and the Netherlands," *JAMA* 111 (July 30, 1938): 430–31; and "Syphilis and Gonorrhea in Sweden," *JAMA* 110 (February 26, 1938): 655–56. On the impact of Scandinavian programs on New Deal social welfare policy see William E. Leuchtenburg, "Great Depression," in C. Vann Woodward, ed., *The Comparative Approach to American History* (New York, 1968), 301.

49. Parran, "Next Great Plague to Go," 409–10; Parran to Fred W. Taylor, July 7, 1936, TP MSS; Parran to Mary Ross, May 20, 1936, TP MSS.

50. "Great Pox," *Time* 28 (October 26, 1936). On the media response see "Education of the Public on Syphilis—A Warning," *JAMA* 108 (February 6, 1937): 478–79; "Syphilis in the News in New York State," *AJPH* 25 (May 1935): 643; "Bringing Syphilis Into the Light," *JAMA* 107 (September 5, 1936): 792; and David Resnick, "Social Hygiene and the Public Mind," *JSocHy* 23 (October 1937): 334–37; "Newspapers and Venereal Disease Control," *AJPH* 27 (September 1937): 959.

51. Paul De Kruif to Thomas Parran, October 7, 1936, TP MSS; Thomas Parran and Paul De Kruif, "We Can End This Sorrow," *LHJ* 54 (August 1937): 23, 88–90; also Bruce Gold and Beatrice Blackmar Gold, "By Reading This You Might Save a Child's Life," *LHJ* 55 (April 1938): 24. The *Journal* was also the first popular magazine to discuss cancer openly. New York *Hearld Tribune*, June 6, 1938.

52. Thomas Parran to Thomas F. Laurie, October 26, 1936, TP MSS; John Stokes to Parran, February 27, 1937, TP MSS; Clipping in TP MSS, n.d. (October 1936?).

53. Sinclair Lewis, *Arrowsmith* (New York, 1925). Lewis received the Pulitzer Prize for *Arrowsmith*. See also, Paul De Kruif, *Microbe Hunters* (New York, 1926). De Kruif advised Lewis on the scientific aspects of *Arrowsmith*. Charles E. Rosenberg, "Martin Arrowsmith: The Scientist as Hero," *AmQ* 15 (1963): 447–58; and John C. Burnham, "American Medicine's Golden Age: What Happened to It?" *Science* 215 (March 19, 1982): 1474–79.

54. Thomas Parran, *Shadow on the Land: Syphilis* (New York, 1937). The book received universally positive notices. See, for example, *Nation* 145 (September 25, 1937): 325; *New Republic* 92 (October 6, 1937): 249; *Yale Review* 27 (Autumn 1937): 196; *New York Times Book Review*, (August 1, 1937), 4. Paul Kellogg to Parran, December 17, 1937, TP MSS; Parran to Franklin D. Roosevelt, December 21, 1936, TP MSS.

55. George Gallup, "Youth Declares War," *Literary Digest* 125 (January 1, 1938): 13–15.

56. Parran, *Shadow on the Land*, 261; "The Veneral Disease Conference," *AJPH* 27 (February 1937): 178–79. Roosevelt letter in "Proceedings of the Conference on Venereal Disease Control Work," December 28–30, 1936, VDI Supplement 3 (Washington, 1937); *Time* (January 11, 1937), 38.

57. Surgeon General, *Annual Report of the U.S. Public Health Service, 1936* (Washington, 1936).

58. "Proceedings of the Conference on Venereal Disease Control Work," 8.

59. See William E. Leuchtenburg, "The New Deal and the Analogue of War," in John Braeman, Robert H. Bremner, and Everett Walters, eds., *Change and Continuity in the Twentieth Century* (Columbus, 1964), 88–144.

60. U.S. Congress. House. Committee on Interstate and Foreign Commerce. *Hearings on Investigation and Control of Venereal Diseases.* 75th Congress, 3rd Session, April 12–14, 1938, 3, 55. (Hereafter, House *Hearings*).

61. William F. Snow, "Syphilis and Federal Assistance to the States," *JSocHy* 24 (1938): 417–21.

62. Senate *Hearings*, 10, 145; Paul De Kruif to Parran, March 9, 1938, TP MSS.

63. Senate *Hearings*, 145; House *Hearings*, 23. Congressmen and Senators frequently noted this shift in public opinion in their speeches. See, for example, John F. Dockweiler, *Congressional Record* 83 (March 29, 1938): 1226–27; John M. Houston, *Congressional Record* 83 (April 14, 1938): 1538–39; and Alfred N. Phillips, *Congressional Record* 83 (March 17, 1938): 1092–93.

64. On the battle against national health legislation and the AMA's role see Daniel S. Hirshfield, *The Lost Reform: The Campaign for Compulsory Health Insurance in the United States from 1932 to 1943* (Cambridge, 1970); Young in House *Hearings*, 86.

65. John H. Stokes, *Modern Clinical Syphilology* (Philadelphia, 1926), 1081–82; Joseph Earle Moore, *The Modern Treatment of Syphilis* (Baltimore, 1933), 40.

66. House *Hearings*, 120–121; "Report of the General Director, American Social Hygiene Association," unp. typescript, December 18, 1936, TP MSS.

67. "Millions vs. Germs," *Time* (May 30, 1938), 31; also *New York Times*, May 26, 1938; Surgeon General, *Annual Report of the U.S. Public Health Service, 1938*, (Washington, 1938), 127.

68. Surgeon General, *Annual Report of the U.S. Public Health Service, 1940*, (Washington, 1940), 6–7, 132–35.

69. T. Clark to Fowler, December 13, 1932, WNRC RG 90, Box 225. See also, Fred S. Hall, *Medical Certification for Marriage* (New York, 1925); Bernard C. Roloff, "The 'Eugenic' Marriage Laws of Wisconsin, Michigan, and Indiana," *JSocHy* 6 (April 1920): 227–54.

70. Edward A. Macy, "Marriages Insured Against Syphilis," *Survey* 74 (August 1938): 262–63; also Bascom Johnson, "New Laws to Protect Marriage and Babies," *JSocHy* 25 (June 1939): 285–87. On medical aspects of marriage and non-infectiousness see Moore, *The Modern Treatment of Syphilis*, 469–74. "Premarital Tests," *Literary Digest* 123 (July 3, 1937): 22; also Mary S. Edwards, "Facts Behind the Laws," *JSocHy* 24 (November 1938): 469–76; Paul Cornell, "Shall We Break With Tradition in Marriage Laws," *JSocHy* 24 (November 1938): 463–68.

71. "Syphilis Tests," *Time*, October 31, 1938, p. 37; Senate *Hearings*, 6–7.

72. Macy, "Marriages Insured Against Syphilis," 263; "Venereal Diseases," *Survey* 74 (October 1938): 326; John Hall, "How the New Jersey Premarital Medical Examination Law Passed," *JSocHy* 24 (November 1938): 497; also, Francis P. Cavanaugh, "Catholic Attitude Toward Some Social Hygienic Legislation," *JSocHy* 24 (November 1938): 513.

73. J. Whitridge Williams, "The Significance of Syphilis in Prenatal Care and in the Causation of Fœtal Death," *Bulletin of the Johns Hopkins Hospital* 31 (1920): 141–45; Williams, "The Influence of the Treatment of Syphilitic Pregnant Women Upon the Incidence of Congenital Syphilis," *Bulletin of the Johns Hopkins Hospital* 33 (1922): 383–86; Walter Clarke to Taliaferro Clark, November 8, 1930, WNRC RG 90, Box 246; also, "Prenatal Health Laws," *VDI* 19 (May 1938): 128–31; and Sylvester W. Trythall, "The Premarital Law," *JAMA* 187 (March 21, 1964): 900–903.

74. Edward C. Kienle, "Public Opinion and New York's 'Baby Health Bill'," *JSocHy* 24 (November 1938): 487–92. The *New York Post* vigorously backed the campaign for the bill. See the editorial "13,000 Babies," January 5, 1938.

75. A. Frank Brewer and Florence E. Olson, "Evaluation of California's Prenatal Law Requiring a Serologic Test for Syphilis," *American Journal of Syphilis* 31 (1947): 633–39.

76. "Outlawing Syphilis, *JSocHy* 24 (November 1938): 521.

77. Thomas Parran, "Discussion," *JAMA* 101 (December 16, 1933), 1957. See also,

Joseph Earle Moore, "Development of Adequate Treatment Facilities for Control of Syphilis," *JAMA* 107 (September 5, 1936): 787–90; Dudley C. Smith, "Practical Epidemiology of Syphilis," *JAMA* 107 (September 5, 1936): 784–86; Dudley C. Smith and William Brumfield, "Tracing the Transmission of Syphilis," *JAMA* 101, (December 16, 1933): 1955.

78. "Persuasive Methods in the Control of Syphilis," *Science*, Supplement 84, (December 18, 1936): 6–7. Also, William L. Munson, "Epidemiology of Syphilis and Gonorrhea," *AJPH* 23 (August 1933): 797–808; and Charles W. Arthur, "Function of the Laboratory in the Epidemiological Control of Syphilis," *AJPH* 25 (July 1935): 846; Senate *Hearings*, 102–3, 23–30; and R. C. Kimbrough, D. M. Cowgill, and E. P. Bowerman, "Rural Syphilis—A Localized Outbreak," *AJPH* 28 (June 1938): 756–58.

79. Arthur Harris Rosenberg, "Compulsory Disclosure Statutes," *NEJM* 280 (June 5, 1969): 1287–88.

80. The Chicago Syphilis Project is described in Paul De Kruif, "Can We Now Fight Syphilis?" *LHJ* 54 (November 1937): 29, 96–100; De Kruif, *The Fight for Life* (New York, 1938), 284–311; and De Kruif "Chicago Against Syphilis," *Reader's Digest* 38 (March 1941): 23–33.

81. Arnold Sundgaard, *Spirochete*, in Hallie Flanagan, ed., *Federal Theatre Plays* (New York, 1938); also, John S. O'Connor, "*Spirochete* and the War on Syphilis," *Drama Review* 21 (March 1977): 91–98. A collection of the highly favorable notices which *Spirochete* received is in the Library of Congress Federal Theatre Project Archives, George Mason University, Fairfax, Virginia.
De Kruif to Parran, June 14, 1937; also May 1, 1938, TP MSS; also, De Kruif to Arnold Sundgaard, March 10, 1938, Federal Theatre Project Archives; and Florence S. Kerr to Hallie Flanagan, March 12, 1938, NA RG 69 and FTP Archives.

82. See O. C. Wenger, "Annual Report, Chicago Syphilis Control Program," July 1, 1940—June 30, 1941, NA RG 69; Senate *Hearings*, 8.

83. Bill Pitchford, "Combatting Syphilis Among University Students," *Hygeia* 17 (March 1939): 261; in 1927, Parran conducted a speaking tour for college fraternities. See Parran to Tau Delta Phi, May 6, 1927, WNRC RG 90, Box 216. "Venereal Disease," *Survey* 74 (October 1938): 326; Senate *Hearings*, 27; John A. Kolmer, "The Wassermann Test," *Hygeia* 12 (December 1934): 1106–1109; H. H. Hazen "The Serodiagnosis of Syphilis," *JAMA* 108 (March 6, 1937): 785–88; Walsh McDermott, "Evaluating the Physician and His Technology," *Dædalus* 106 (Winter 1977): 144.

84. William F. Snow, "Syphilis and Social Security," *JSocHy* 22 (1936): 343; see also, Dowling, *Fighting Infection*, 104. N. A. Nelson to Parran, July 1, 1936, TP MSS; also, P.S. Pelouze, "Modern Clinical Management of Gonorrhea," *JAMA* 108 (March 6, 1937): 788–90. "Venereal Diseases," *AJPH* 26 (August 1936): 824.

85. Parran, "The Next Great Plague to Go," 410; "Syphilis;" *Hygiea*; 16 (May 1937): 392.

86. Ruth Ellen Lindenberg, "Are You Afraid of Syphilis," *Survey* 74 (February 1938): 44; Thurman B. Rice to Parran, August 7, 1936, TP MSS; Ben Reitman, "Syphilophobia," VDC #94, n.d. (1937?), unp. typescript, Reitman MSS, University of Illinois at Chicago.

87. "Fact vs. Propaganda," *NYStJM* 40 (May 15, 1940): 764; "Inflated Statistics," *NYStJM* 40 (May 1, 1940): 693–94.
For a response to these critiques see Walter Clarke to Thomas Parran, May 10, 1940, ASHA Papers, Folder 115:1.

88. Walter Clarke to C. Wright MacMillan, February 7, 1940, ASHA Papers, Folder L2:8; also, "Domestic Servants and Syphilis," *AJPH* 27 (August 1937): 802. Senate

Hearings, 132. Even Parran, well aware of the scientific aspects of venereal transmission, frequently cited an epidemic which apparently originated from a "kissing game" played at a teenage party. Though this mode of transmission is not absolutely impossible, the emphasis on such a story would, it seems, support the injunctions against liberalizing sexual mores. See Parran, "The Next Great Plague to Go," 409.

89. Morris Fishbein, "Social Diseases," *Hygeia* 16 (January 1938): 10; Senate *Hearings*, 43.

90. See James Jones, *Bad Blood* (New York, 1981), 16–29.

91. Allan M. Brandt, "Racism and Research: The Case of the Tuskegee Syphilis Study," *Hastings Center Report* 8 (December 1978): 21–28; also Jones, *Bad Blood*.

92. R. W. Williams to Alexander Fitz-Hugh, October 14, 1943, ASHA Papers, Folder 118:8. For similar traditional views see also: G. Frank Lydston, "The Race Problem in America in its Relation to Criminal Sociology," *AJClinMed* 17 (February 1910): 170–175; Thomas W. Murrell, "Syphilis and the American Negro," *JAMA* 54 (March 12, 1910): 846–849; Daniel David Quillian, "Racial Peculiarities: A Cause of the Prevalence of Syphilis in Negroes," *AJDerm* 10 (July 1906): 277–79. H. L. McNeil "Syphilis in the Southern Negro" *JAMA* 67 (September 30, 1916): 1001–1004; H. H. Hazen, "Syphilis in the American Negro," *JAMA* 63 (August 8, 1914): 463–68; as well as George M. Frederickson, *The Black Image in the White Mind* (New York, 1971), 228–55; and John H. Haller, *Outcasts From Evolution* (Urbana, Illinois, 1971), 40–68.

93. Lester B. Granger to Walter Clarke, January 15, 1943, ASHA Papers, Folder 117:6; see also, "Statement Regarding Interracial Program of the American Social Hygiene Association," February 21, 1933, ASHA Papers, Folder 166:6.

94. Ben Reitman to Public Affairs Committee, November 25, 1938, Reitman MSS.

95. Ruth Topping "File Memorandum," February 15, 1932, BSH Papers, Box 7; Topping, "File Memorandum," March 3, 1932, BSH Papers, Box 10. On the extensive use of condoms see "The Business of Birth Control," *JAMA* 110 (February 12, 1938): 513.

96. Woodbridge Morris to Ray Lyman Wilbur, August 15, 1940, ASHA Papers: Walter Clarke to Ray Lyman Wilbur, August 16, 1940, ASHA Papers; also Robert L. Dickinson to William F. Snow, January 31, 1934, ASHA Papers, Folder 9:3.

97. Parran, *Shadow on the Land*, 209.

Chapter V

1. For a fuller discussion of the biomedical model see René Dubos, *The Mirage of Health* (New York, 1959); and Bernard Dixon, *Beyond the Magic Bullet*, (New York, 1978). On Ehrlich's discovery, see Paul De Kruif, *Microbe Hunters* (New York, 1926), 314–377; and Robert Reid, *Microbes and Men*, (London, 1974), 125–33. On contemporary incidence of disease see John Powles, "On the Limitations of Modern Medicine," *Science, Medicine, and Man* 1 (1973): 1–30; and Thomas McKeown, "A Historical Appraisal of the Medical Task," in McKeown and Gordon McLachlan, eds., *Medical History and Medical Care* (London, 1971), 29–50.

2. Medical Department, U.S. Army, *Preventive Medicine in World War II, Communicable Diseases*, (Washington, 1960), 5:140–41 (hereafter, *Preventive Medicine in World War II*); also "The American Social Hygiene Association and World War II," unpublished typescript, n.d., ASHA Papers, Folder 130:4.

3. Thomas Parran and Raymond Vonderlehr, *Plain Words About Venereal Disease* (New York, 1941), 87.

4. *Preventive Medicine in World War II*, pp. 142–43; also, A. J. Aselmeyer, "Civil-

ian Measures for the Control of Venereal Diseases in World War II," *JAMA* 120 (November 21, 1942): 880–83.

5. Parran and Vonderlehr, *Plain Words:* 90,1.

6. William F. Snow to A. J. Chesley, November 17, 1941; see also, Chesley to Snow, November 23, 1941, ASHA Papers, Folder 141:8; on press reports see Alfred Deutsch to Raymond Vonderlehr, November 19, 1941, ASHA Papers, Folder 141:8. See also, Eliot Ness to Charles P. Taft, November 24, 1941, TP MSS; Franklin D. Roosevelt to Paul McNutt, November 18, 1941, TP MSS; Roosevelt to McNutt, December 5, 1941, TP MSS; McNutt to Parran, November 27, 1941, TP MSS.

7. Parran to McNutt, November 23, 1941, TP MSS; Jean Pinney to William F. Snow, November 26, 1941, ASHA Papers, Folder 141:8; "Prostitution is an Axis Partner," *AJPH* 32 (January 1942): 85–86. See also "The New York Academy of Medicine on 'Plain Words About Venereal Disease,' " *AJPH* 32 (January 1942): 113.

8. William Bisher, "Venereal Disease Control as Applied to the Army," *NYStJM* 43 (October 1, 1943): 1833; Granville W. Larimore and Thomas H. Sternberg, "Does Health Education Prevent Venereal Disease?" *AJPH* 35 (August 1945): 801.

9. James P. Pappas, "The Venereal Disease Problem in the U.S. Army," *MilSurg* 93 (August 1943): 182; Larrimore and Sternberg, "Does Health Education Prevent Venereal Disease?" 801–802; Leo Shifrin, "Venereal Disease: A Navy Problem" *NYStJM* 43 (1943): 1829; Herman Goodman, "Venereal Disease Education Program and the Public Health Agencies," *MedRec* 157 (February 1944): 70–76, (March 1944): 138–42; and "The Public Knowledge of Venereal Disease," *AJPH* 30 (May 1940): 548–49.

10. Joel T. Boone, "The Sexual Aspects of Military Personnel," *JSocHy* 27 (March 1941): 123; Bisher, "Venereal Disease Control as Applied to the Army," 1833; Michael Wishengrad, "Discussion," *NYStJM* 43 (October 1, 1943): 1831.

11. Morris Leider, "Theoretical Considerations in Venereal Disease Control Planning," *AmJSyph* 31 (May 1947): 330–33.

12. "Catholics and Venereal Disease," *TNR* 111 (October 9, 1944): 446; see also "Catholics vs. V. D. Frankness," *Newsweek* 24 (September 18, 1944): 84–86. Theodore Schroeder, "The Spiritual Value of Syphilis," *Arch Derm Syph* 40 (September 1942): 470–74.

13. George Lieby and Granville Larimore, "A Study of Factors Allied with Venereal Disease," unpublished typescript (August 1945), ASHA Papers, Folder 145:10; See also the classic study by Samuel A. Stouffer *et al.*, *The American Soldier: Adjustment During Army Life* (Princeton, 1949), 1:176–78, 545–49. *Preventive Medicine in World War II*, p. 253. Following the cessation of hostilities, supplies dropped from an average of 8 condoms per man each month, to 4 per man per month.

14. Walter Clarke, "Syphilis, Gonorrhea and the National Defense Program," *JSocHy* 26 (November 1940): 341; "The American Social Hygiene Association and World War II," unpublished typescript, n.d., ASHA Papers, Folder 130:4; Henry L. Stimson to Governors, March 20, 1942, ASHA Papers, Folder 130:4.

15. *Preventive Medicine in World War II*, pp. 164–65.

16. Paul McNutt, "The Federal Fight Against Venereal Disease," *JSocHy* (March 1942): 122; *Preventive Medicine in World War II*, p. 174; also, Eliot Ness, "Repression of Prostitution in War Time," unpublished typescript, November 20, 1942, ASHA Papers, Folder 68:4.

17. Harry Benjamin, "Sex in the Army," *American Mercury* 54 (March 1942): 580; see also Raymond Vonderlehr, "The Impact of the War on the Venereal Disease Problem," *NEJM* 227 (August 6, 1942): 203–4; and Irwin Ross, "Sex in the Army," *American Mercury* 53 (December, 1941): 661–69. "Proceedings of the National Police Ad-

visory Committee," unpublished typescript, August 7, 1942, NA RG 215, Box 119; *Preventive Medicine in World War II*, p. 141; see also "The Certification of Prostitutes," unpublished typescript, August 27, 1942, ASHA Papers, Folder 59:2.

18. Eliot Ness, "The New Offensive Along the Police Front," *JSocHy* 28 (October 1942): 371; see also Thomas B. Turner, "Immediate Wartime Outlook and Indicated Postwar Conditions with Respect to the Control of Venereal Disease." *AJPH* 33 (November 1943): 1311; and Ness, "Venereal Disease Control in Defense," *Annals of the American Academy* (March 1942): 89–93. James D. Lade, "The Legal Basis for Venereal Disease Control," *AJPH* 35 (October 1945): 1043; "Proceedings of the National Police Advisory Committee for Social Protection," unpublished typescript, August 7, 1942, NA RG 215, Box 119; Helen V. Tooker, "Venereal Disease—Far From Beaten," *Harper's Magazine* 189 (November 1944): 551; see also Charles R. Reynolds, "Prostitution as a Source of Infection with the Venereal Diseases in the Armed Forces," *AJPH* 30 (November 1940): 1276–81; and A. B. Price and F. J. Weber, "Control of the Venereal Diseases in Civilian Areas Adjacent to Concentrations of Armed Forces," *AJPH* 31 (September 1941): 912.

19. E. W. Norris, A. F. Doyle, A. D. Iskrant, "VD Epidemiology, Third Service Command," *SMJ* 37 (1943): 244; Albert Deutsch, "Danger! Venereal Disease," *Nation* 161 (September 22, 1945): 285.

20. John Stokes, "Discussion" *JAMA* 120 (November 21, 1942): 882; also, James P. Pappas, "The Venereal Disease Problem in the U.S. Army," *MilSurg* 93 (August 1943): 172–73. "She Looked Clean, But . . ." Washington, D.C., (1944); see also "Differences in Places of Procurement and Places of Exposure used by Three Types of Contact," unpublished mimeograph, (August 1944), NA RG 215, Box 1. "Techniques for Repressing of Unorganized Prostitution," (1943), ASHA Papers, Folder 128:8.

21. Turner, "Immediate Wartime Outlook and Indicated Post-War Conditions with Respect to the Control of Venereal Diseases," *AJPH* 33 (November 1943): 1311; Stokes quoted in R. R. Willcox, "Some American Ideas on Venereal Disease Control," *BrMedJ* (November 30, 1946): 827; see also Thomas Devine to Barbara Dudd, January 11, 1946, NA RG 215, Box 2. Bascom Johnson to Arthur Fink, May 14, 1945, ASHA Papers, Folder 128:9.

22. *Preventive Medicine in World War II*, p. 143.

23. *Preventive Medicine in World War II*, p. 146; Turner, "Immediate Wartime Outlook," 1330.

24. *Preventive Medicine in World War II*, p. 83; R. A. Vonderlehr and Lida J. Usilton, "The Extent of the Syphilis Problem at the Beinning of World War II," *NYStJM* 42 (October 1, 1943): 1823–33.

25. *Preventive Medicine in World War II*, p. 266; Turner, "Immediate Wartime Outlook," 1309.

26. J. F. Mahoney, R. C. Arnold, and A. Harris, "Pencillin Treatment of Early Syphilis: A Preliminary Report," *AJPH* 33 (December 1943): 1387–91; J. E. Moore, J. F. Mahoney, U. Schwartz, T. Sternberg, and U. B. Wood, Jr. "The Treatment of Early Syphilis with Penicillin: A Preliminary Report of 1,418 Cases," *JAMA* 126 (September 9, 1944): 67–73; J. D. Ratcliff, *Yellow Magic* (New York, 1945), 118–33; David Wilson, *In Search of Penicillin* (New York, 1976); also John Parascandola, *The History of Antibiotics* (Madison, Wisc., 1980) and John C. Sheehan, *The Enchanted Ring: The Untold Story of Penicillin* (Cambridge, 1982). Harry F. Dowling, "Comparisons and Contrasts Between the Early Arsphenamine and Early Antibiotic Periods," *BHM* 47 (May–June 1973): 248–9; *Preventive Medicine in World War II*, p. 331.

27. Harry F. Dowling, *Fighting Infection: Conquests of the Twentieth Century*

(Cambridge, 1977), 146–47; C. C. Dauer, "A Demographic Analysis of Recent Changes in Mortality, Morbidity, in Age Group Distribution of Our Population," in Iago Galdston, ed., *The Impact of the Antibiotics on Medicine and Society* (New York, 1958), 98–120.

28. Quoted in Louis Lasagna, *The VD Epidemic* (Philadelphia, 1975), 1; W. H. Aufranc, "Are Venereal Diseases Disappearing? Over-All Picture Throughout the Country," *AJSyph* 35 (March 1951): 135–37; William J. Brown, J. F. Donohue, N. W. Axnick, J. H. Blount, O. G. Jones, N. H. Ewen, *Syphilis and Other Venereal Disease* (Cambridge, 1970), 44; *STD Fact Sheet* (Washington: DHHS, 1981), 16, (See Appendix); John F. Mahoney, "The Effect of the Antibiotics on the Concepts and Practices of Public Health," in Galdston, ed., *The Impact of the Antibiotics*, 213.

29. "CG For GI's" *Newsweek* 39 (January 21, 1952): 85; also Joseph Hirsh, "The Army's 'New Approach' to Venereal Disease Control," unpublished typescript, (May 13, 1948?), ASHA Papers, Folder 145:11; "Resurgent Venereal Disease," *Newsweek* 30 (August 18, 1947): 48–51; "Changing Attitude of the Army with Regard to Venereal Diseases," *AJPH* 38 (August 1948): 150–52.

30. John Stokes in "Proceedings of the National Conference on Postwar Venereal Disease Control," *VDI*, Supplement 20 (Washington, 1944), 153, 155; Stokes, "The Practitioner and the Antibiotic Age of Venereal Disease Control," *VDI* 31 (January 1950), 1–13; William Styron, *In the Clap Shack* (New York, 1973), 10–11. Styron's play is the story of a young Marine private, diagnosed as syphilitic and subjected to a sadistic, moralistic physician.

31. John H. Stokes, "The Status of Venereal Disease Control," *AJPH* 40 (July 1950): 864–66; "Proceedings of the National Police Advisory Committee for Social Protection and Venereal Disease," unpublished typescript, August 7, 1942, NA RG 215, Box 119. (Italics mine). William F. Snow in "Proceedings of the National Conference on Postwar Venereal Disease Control," *VDI*, Supplement 20 (Washington, 1944), 202; "Casefinding in the Control of Syphilis," *AJPH* 36 (May 1946): 527–29.

32. Stokes, "The Practitioner and the Antibiotic Age of Venereal Disease Control," *VDI* 31 (January 1950): 13; William F. Draper, unpublished typescript, February 6, 1946, NA RG 215, Box 150; see also Thomas B. Turner, "Venereal Disease in the Postwar Period." unpublished typescript, (February 7, 1945), NA RG 215, Box 150.

33. *New York Times*, November 18, 1979; *New York Times* April 26, 1978; also *STD Fact Sheet* (Washington, DHHS, 1981); *STD Fact Sheet* (Washington, DHHS, 1981). (See appendix).

34. Alfred E. Kinsey, Wardell B. Pomeroy, Clyde E. Martin, *Sexual Behavior in the Human Male* (Philadelphia, 1948). On Kinsey's research see Regina Markell Morantz, "The Scientist as Sex Crusader: Alfred C. Kinsey and American Culture," *AmQ* 29 (Winter 1977): 563–589.; and Paul Robinson, *The Modernization of Sex* (New York, 1976), 42–119. The problem with these data are legion, nevertheless, they do serve as a rough indication of changing behavior. See James Moneymaker and Fred Montanino, "The New Sexual Morality: A Society Comes of Age," in James M. Henslin and Edward Sagarin, eds., *The Sociology of Sex* (New York, 1978), 27–40; also Mervin B. Freedman, "The Sexual Behavior of American College Women: An Empirical Study and an Historical Study," in Ailon Shiloh, ed., *Studies in Human Sexual Behavior: The American Scene* (Springfield, Illinois, 1970), 135–50; and Morton Hunt, *Sexual Behavior in the 1970s* (Chicago, 1974). See also Jeffrey Weeks, *Sex, Politics and Society: The Regulation of Sex Since 1800* (London, 1981), 249–72. Although Weeks is writing about England many of his points are clearly applicable to the United States.

35. William Darrow, "Changes in Sexual Behavior and Venereal Disease," *Clinical*

Obstetrics and Gynecology 18 (March 1975): 255–67; William M. McCormack, "Sexually Transmitted Diseases: Women as Victims," *JAMA* 248 (July 9, 1982): 177–78; Joseph Kelaghan, George L. Rubin, Howard Ory, and Peter Layde, "Barrier-Method Contraception and Pelvic Inflammatory Disease," *JAMA* 248 (July 9, 1982), 184–87; G. S. Berger, L. Keith, and W. Moss, "Prevalence of Gonorrhea Among Women Using Various Methods of Contraception," *British Journal of Venereal Diseases* 51 (1975), 307–309; John C. Cutler, et. al., "Vaginal Contraceptives as Prophylaxis Against Gonorrhea and other Sexually Transmissible Diseases," *Advances in Planned Parenthood* 12 (1977), 45–56; also Darrow, "Social and Behavioral Aspects of the Sexually Transmitted Diseases," *Sexuality Today—And Tomorrow* (1976), 134–151.

36. Simon Podair, "Shall Our Schools Teach About Venereal Disease?" *Saturday Review* 49 (March 19, 1966): 72–73, 88; also *New York Times*, February 27, 1977; Jessica Mitford, *Poison Penmanship* (New York, 1979), 108–27, "NBC Turns Down a Gold Chance," *Saturday Review* 47 (December 12, 1964): 61. "The Price of Prudery," *Nation* 200 (April 19, 1965): 406; also David Sanford, "The AMA and that Disease," *TNR* 153 (September 18, 1965): 10. *New York Times*, October 31, 1982. The Texas State Commissioner later rescinded his decision.

37. The best discussion of public health funding for venereal disease is Odin W. Anderson, "Syphilis and Society: Problems of Control in the United States, 1912–1964," Health Information Foundation, *Research Series* 22 (1965); Thomas H. Sternberg, "Adjusting Venereal Disease Control to the Antibiotic Era," *AJSyph* 36 (September 1952): 446.

38. James K. Shafer, "Applied Epidemiology in Venereal Disease Control," *AJPH* 44 (March 1954): 355–59; *Today's V.D. Control Problem* (Washington, 1957), 2; also "The Tainted Young," *Newsweek* 46 (December 5, 1955): 68; and "Too Soon Forgotten," *Newsweek* 47 (July 11, 1956): 68.

39. Yehudi Felman, "Should Premarital Syphilis Serologies Continue to be Mandated by Law?" *JAMA* 240 (August 4, 1978): 459–60; also *JAMA* 241 (May 11, 1979): 2007–8. Yehudi Felman, "A Plea for the Condom, Especially for Teenagers," *JAMA* 241 (June 8, 1979): 2517–18; William W. Darrow, "Innovative Health Behavior," Ph.D. dissertation, Emory University, 1973; Phyllis Franck and Diana S. Hart, "VD: The Neglected Epidemic," Washington *Post*, April 17, 1978.

40. "Case-finding in the Control of Syphilis," *AJPH* 36 (May 1946): 527–29; Howard Ennes, Jr., and T. G. Bennett, "The Contact Education Interview," *AJSyph* 29 (November 1945): 647; "VD Quiz Man," *Newsweek* 37 (July 11, 1954): 86–87.

41. Franck and Hart, "VD: The Neglected Epidemic," Washington *Post*, April 17, 1977.

42. "More Kinds and Cases of VD" *Medical World News* 16 (July 28, 1975): 37–54; Melvin S. Rosenthal, "Genital Herpes Simplex Virus Infections," *Primary Care* 6 (September 1979): 517–520; and Daniel Laskin, "The Herpes Syndrome," *New York Times Magazine*, February 21, 1982, pp. 94–98, 108. There are no requirements for reporting herpes infections to public health officials and thus statistics remain sketchy.

43. Lawrence Corey, "The Diagnosis and Treatment of Genital Herpes," *JAMA* 248 (September 3, 1982): 1041–1044. The drug acyclovir, recently approved by the Food and Drug Administration, apparently helps to improve external lesions and relieve discomfort, but is not a cure. Stephen E. Straus, et al., "Suppression of Frequently Recurring Genital Herpes," *NEJM* 310 (June 14, 1983): 1545–50; see also Washington *Star*, July 9, 1981; *Wall Street Journal*, September 3, 1982; *New York Times*, July 10, 1984.

44. "Herpes: The New Sexual Leprosy," *Time* 116 (July 28, 1980): 76; "The New

Scarlet Letter," *Time* 120 (August 2, 1982): 62–66; "The Misery of Herpes II," *Newsweek* 96 (November 10, 1980): 105; Lois Draegin, "Sex Makes You Sick," *Soho Weekly News* 9 (November 24, 1981): 12–14.

45. Draegin, "Sex Makes You Sick," 14.

46. *The Daily Tar Heel* (University of North Carolina, Chapel Hill), October 1, 1982.

47. "The New Scarlet Letter," *Time* 120 (August 2, 1982): 63, 66; Jack McClintock, "Love Labor's Lost," *Esquire* 48 (November 1982): 145–55.

48. Washington *Post*, October 11, 1982; Nora Gallagher, "Fever All Through the Night," *Mother Jones* 7 (November 1982): 36–43. "Sexually Transmitted Diseases," *The Harvard Medical School Health Letter* 6 (April 1981); Corey, "The Diagnosis and Treatment of Genital Herpes," 1041–49; also, *New York Times*, November 26, 1980; Washington *Post*, August 17, 1980; Washington *Star*, May 9, 1981; quotation in Ezekiel Emanuel, "Harping on Herpes," *TNR* (September 13, 1982): 15.

49. "The New Scarlet Letter," 64.

50. "The New Scarlet Letter," 65; Draegin, "Sex Makes You Sick," 12.

51. Although the organization is still called HELP, the ASHA has removed the explanation of the acronym from its most recent literature. The word "herpetic" is still commonly used.

52. "The New Scarlet Letter," 62, 66.

Chapter VI

The title for this chapter comes from William H. McNeill, *Plagues and Peoples* (New York, 1976).

1. A number of books on the AIDS epidemic offer valuable overviews. See especially, National Academy of Sciences, *Mobilizing Against AIDS: The Unfinished Story of a Virus* (Cambridge, 1986); Dennis Altman, *AIDS in the Mind of America* (New York, 1986); Jacques Leibowitch, *A Strange Virus of Unknown Origin*, trans. Robert Howard (New York, 1985); Ann Giudici Fettner and William Check, *The Truth About AIDS* (New York, 1984). See also, Ruth Kulstad, ed., *AIDS: Papers from Science, 1982–1983* (Washington, 1986).

2. U.S. Department of Health and Human Services, *Morbidity and Mortality Weekly Report*, June 5, 1981; see also, Jean L. Marx, "New Disease Baffles Medical Community," *Science* (August 13, 1982), in Kulstad, ed.: 11–16.

3. For an excellent summary of the early medical history of the epidemic see June E. Osborn, "The AIDS Epidemic: An Overview of the Science," *Issues in Science and Technology* 2 (Winter 1986): 40–55.

4. See National Academy of Sciences, *Mobilizing Against AIDS*; also, Sheldon H. Landesman, et al., "The AIDS Epidemic," *NEJM* 312 (February 21, 1985): 521–25; and Anthony S. Fauci, "The Acquired Immunodeficiency Syndrome: An Update," *Annals of Internal Medicine* 102 (1985): 800–813.

5. See Colin Norman, "AIDS Virology: A Battle on Many Fronts," *Science* 230 (November 1, 1985): 518–21; and Jean L. Marx, "Human T-Cell Leukemia Virus Linked to AIDS," *Science* (May 20, 1983), in Kulstad, ed.: 24–32; and Jean L. Marx, "Strong New Candidate for AIDS Agent," *Science* 224 (May 4, 1984): 475–77.

6. See "Status Report on the Acquired Immunodeficiency Syndrome: HTLV-III Testing," *JAMA* 254 (September 13, 1985): 1342–45; Stanley H. Weiss, et al., "Screening Test for HTLV-III Antibodies: Specificity, Sensitivity, and Applications," *JAMA* 253 (1985): 221–25.

7. Colin Norman, "Patent Dispute Divides AIDS Researchers," *Science* 230 (No-

vember 8, 1985): 640–43; Norman, "AIDS Priority Fight Goes to Court," *Science* 231 (January 1, 1986): 11–12; *Wall Street Journal*, May 1, 1986; see also *New York Times*, July 1, 1986; July 10, 1986.

8. *Time*, 126 (August 12, 1985): 47. On the scientific aspects of vaccine development see also *Wall Street Journal*, June 23, 1986; June 26, 1986; *New York Times*, November 27, 1985; May 27, 1986; *Washington Post*, May 7, 1986. On the complexity of the virus see *Science* 233 (July 18, 1986): 282.

9. On the problem of vaccine liability see Edmund W. Kitch, "The Vaccine Dilemma," *Issues in Science and Technology* 2 (Winter 1986): 108–21; and Peter Huber, "AIDS and Lawyers," *TNR* 194 (May 5, 1986): 14–15.

10. On AIDS drug testing see *New York Times*, July 1, 1986 and June 26, 30, 1985; also Deborah H. Barnes, "In Search of the Best Drugs Against AIDS," *Science* 233 (July 25, 1986): 419.

11. See June E. Osborn, "The AIDS Epidemic: Multidisciplinary Trouble," *NEJM* 314 (March 20, 1986): 779–82.

12. See National Institutes of Health, Consensus Development Conference Statement, "The Impact of Routine HTLV-III Antibody Testing of Blood and Plasma Donors on Public Health," July 7–9, 1986; also Deborah M. Barnes, "Keeping the AIDS Virus Out of the Blood Supply," *Science* 233 (August 1, 1986): 514–15; *New York Times*, July 18, 1986; and Michael T. Osterhom, et al., "Screening Donated Blood and Plasma for HTLV-III Antibody," *NEJM* 312 (May 2, 1985): 1185–88.

13. On heterosexual transmission see, for example, U.S. Department of Health and Human Services, *Morbidity and Mortality Weekly Report*, September 20, 1985; Robert R. Redfield, et al., "Heterosexually Acquired HTLV-III/LAV Disease (AIDS-Related Complex and AIDS)," *JAMA* 254 (October 18, 1985): 2094–96; also *Wall Street Journal*, March 7, 1986 and June 26, 1986; *New York Times*, July 28, and August 1, 1986.

14. Eugene McCray, "Occupational Risk of the Acquired Immunodeficiency Syndrome Among Health Care Workers," *NEJM* 314 (April 24, 1986): 1127–32; Stanley H. Weiss, et al., "HTLV-III Infection Among Health Care Workers," *JAMA* 254 (October 18, 1985): 2089–93; several health care workers have become HIV-positive after inadvertent needle sticks with contaminated specimens. According to the CDC, such risks are minimal, if proper procedures are followed. On casual transmission see Gerald H. Friedland, et al., "Lack of Transmission of HTLV-III/LAV Infection to Household Contacts of Patients with AIDS or AIDS-Related Complex with Oral Candidiasis," *NEJM* 314 (February 6, 1986): 344–49; also *New York Times*, February 6, 1986. Also, USHHS, *Morbidity and Mortality Weekly Report*, November 15, 1985.

15. On AIDS epidemiology see James W. Curran, et al., "The Epidemiology of AIDS: Current Status and Future Prospects," *Science* 229 (September 27, 1985): 1352–57; *Wall Street Journal*, May 30, 1986; *New York Times*, January 14, 1986, and June 13, 1986; *Washington Post*, June 5, 1986; and Deborah M. Barnes, "Grim Projections for AIDS Epidemic," *Science* 232 (June 27, 1986): 1589–90; and Victor De Gruttola et al., "AIDS: Has the Problem Been Adequately Assessed?" *Reviews of Infectious Disease* 8 (March-April 1986): 295–305.

16. See Jonathan Lieberson, "The Reality of AIDS," *New York Review of Books* (January 16, 1986): 43–48; also, *New York Times*, June 24, 1986.

17. *Washington Post*, June 5, 1986; *New York Times*, June 13, 1986.

18. Colin Norman, "Politics and Science Clash on African AIDS," *Science* 230 (December 6, 1985): 1140–42; also *Science* 233 (July 18, 1986); *New York Times*, November 21, 24, December 9, 15, 1985.

19. *New York Times*, June 13, 1986; *Washington Post*, June 5, 1986.

20. On the response to AIDS in the gay community see especially Altman, *AIDS in the Mind of America*, 82–109; Frances FitzGerald, "The Castro-II," *New Yorker* (July 28, 1986): 44–63; Seymour Kleinberg, "Life After Death," *TNR* 195 (August 11, 18, 1986): 28–33; *New York Times*, June 16, 17, 1983, and July 22, 1985.

21. *New York Times*, June 16, 1983.

22. On the debates about closing the bathhouses, see FitzGerald, "The Castro-II," *New Yorker* (July 28, 1986): 44–63; also, *New York Times*, October 24, November 1, 7, 8, 1985. Also, Ronald Bayer, "AIDS and the Gay Community: Between the Specter and Promise of Medicine," *Social Research* 52 (Autumn 1985): 581–606.

23. *New York Times*, November 8, 1985.

24. *New York Times*, July 22, 1985; Altman, *AIDS in the Mind of America*, 82–109.

25. Leon McKusick, et al., "AIDS and Sexual Behavior Reported by Gay Men in San Francisco," *AJPH* 75 (May 1985): 493–96; Leon McKusick, et al., "The AIDS Epidemic: A Model for Developing Intervention Strategies for Reducing High-Risk Behavior in Gay Men," *Sexually Transmitted Diseases* 12 (1985): 229–34; Donald E. Riesenberg, "AIDS-Prompted Behavior Changes Reported," *JAMA* 255 (January 10, 1986): 171, 176. See also *New York Times*, January 5, 1986; *Washington Post*, June 24, 1985.

26. *New York Times*, December 1, 1985, and April 18, 1984. In May 1986, James Curran of the CDC announced that he would support a test program to provide sterile needles to addicts. See *New York Times*, May 30, 1986. New Jersey has recently proposed such a program. *New York Times*, July 24, 1986.

27. *New York Times*, June 17, 1986.

28. *New York Times*, October 20, 1985.

29. "AFRAIDS," *TNR* (October 14, 1985): 7–9. See also Charles Krauthammer, "The Politics of a Plague," *TNR* (August 1, 1983): 18–21.

30. *New York Times*, June 26, 1985.

31. Jay A. Winsten, "Fighting Panic on AIDS," *New York Times*, July 26, 1983.

32. "The Fear of AIDS," *Newsweek* 106 (September 23, 1985): 18–25. On the school controversy see *New York Times*, October 13, 24, 1985, December 8, 1985. Also David J. Rothman, "Public Policy and Risk Assessment in the Case of AIDS," forthcoming United Hospital Fund (1986).

33. Leon Eisenberg, "Private Trust/Public Confidence in Science and Medicine: The Genesis of Fear," American Society for Law and Medicine, April 1986; Robert Balzell, "The History of an Epidemic," *TNR* 189 (August 1, 1983): 14–18; Richard Goldstein, "The Uses of AIDS," *Village Voice* (November 5, 1985): 25–27.

34. "Fear and AIDS in Hollywood," *People* (September 23, 1985): 28–33; *New York Times*, November 7, 1985; *Washington Post*, July 28, 1985.

35. *Life*, 8 (July 1985): 12–21.

36. See Ronald Bayer, *Homosexuality and American Psychiatry: The Politics of Diagnosis* (New York, 1981).

37. *The New York Post*, May 24, 1983.

38. Quoted in *New York Times*, March 18, 1986.

39. Erving Goffman, *Stigma: Notes on the Management of Spoiled Identity* (Englewood Cliffs, N.J., 1963).

40. On the Justice Department ruling see *New York Times*, June 23, 27, 1986; *Wall Street Journal*, June 27, 1986.

41. *New York Times*, June 26, 1986.

42. Charles Krauthammer, "Fear Him and Fire Him," *Washington Post*, June 27, 1986.

43. *New York Times*, July 1, 1986.

44. On military testing, see *New York Times*, October 13, 1985, January 31, February 2, 1986; *Science* 223 (July 18, 1986). The results of military screening have shown relatively high rates of infection. In Manhattan, 2 percent of individuals applying to enter the service has been found to be infected; these numbers are 15 to 20 times higher than the estimated national prevalence.

45. Among those who have recommended mandatory screening for those at high risk are Lewis Kuller, professor of epidemiology at University of Pittsburgh, and Paul Starr, professor of sociology at Princeton. See *Chronicle of Higher Education*, June 4, 1986.

46. William F. Buckley, Jr., "Identify All the Carriers," *New York Times*, March 18, 1986.

47. See for example, Mark Senak, "Ban AIDS Blood Tests," *New York Times*, May 27, 1986.

48. *New York Times*, June 11, 1986. See also the full-page advertisement of the American Council of Life Insurance and the Health Insurance Association of America, *Washington Post*, May 11, 1986.

49. Quoted in *Washington Post*, June 20, 1986; June 28, 1986.

50. *New York Times*, June 8, January 10, 1986, November 3, 1985; on the problem of financing AIDS see also George R. Seage, "The Medical Cost of Treatment of AIDS/ARC Patients," Boston Department of Health and Hospitals, May 12, 1985; Philip R. Lee, "AIDS Allocating Resources for Research and Patient Care," *Issues in Science and Technology* 2 (Winter 1986): 66–73; and especially Rashi Fein, "AIDS and Economics," AIDS Institute of the New York State Department of Health, May 29, 1986.

51. *Washington Post*, May 25, 1983, July 23, 1985; *New York Times*, June 15, 1983, July 29, October 24, 1985; and especially, Office of Technology Assessment (U.S. Congress), "Review of the Public Health Service's Response to AIDS: A Technical Memorandum," Washington, D.C., February 1985.

52. Harvey V. Fineberg, "A Way to Tackle AIDS Education," *New York Times*, July 13, 1986; also Paul Cleary et al., "Health Education about AIDS Risk," *Health Education Quarterly* (forthcoming).

53. *New York Times*, July 6, 1986.

54. For an analysis of the difficult social policy questions raised by AIDS, see Ronald Bayer, "AIDS, Power and Reason," *Milbank Quarterly* (forthcoming). On legal issues see William Curran and Larry Gostin, "First Line of Defense in Controlling AIDS," *American Journal of Law and Medicine* (forthcoming).

55. See Eisenberg, "Private Trust/Public Confidence in Science and Medicine: The Genesis of Fear," American Society of Law and Medicine, Boston, April 1986; also Peter Conrad, "The Social Meaning of AIDS," *Social Policy* (forthcoming).

56. Robin Marantz Henig, "AIDS: A New Disease's Deadly Odyssey," *New York Times Magazine* (February 6, 1983): 36.

57. See, for example, John H. Knowles, "The Responsibility of the Individual," *Daedalus* 106 (Winter 1977): 68; and Robert Carlen, "Against Free Clinics for Sexually Transmitted Diseases," *NEJM* 307 (November 18, 1982): 1350.

58. Dowling, *Fighting Infection*, 228–50; *New York Times*, January 23, 1977.

Index

Acquired Immune Deficiency Syndrome (AIDS), 3, 182, 183-204; in Africa, 186, 187, 189; and behavioral change, 191, 202; and blood transfusions, 185-86; casual transmission of, 186, 192; civil liberties and, 199-201; costs of, 197-98; discrimination and, 192, 194-95; epidemiology of, 187-88; funding for, 198-99; Haitians and, 184, 186, 187; homosexuality and, 183-90, 192-97, 199-202; intravenous drug use and, 184, 190-91; media coverage of, 192-93; prevention of, 188-90, 199; screening for, 195-98; treatments for, 185; vaccines for, 185
Addams, Jane, 32, 34
Additon, Henrietta, 81
AIDS. *See* Acquired Immune Deficiency Syndrome
AIDS-Related-Complex (ARC), 186-87
Alcohol, 59, 72, 96, 98, 102-3, 108, 109
American Expeditionary Forces (AEF), 96-121
American Federation for Sex Hygiene, 25, 38
American Medical Association, 123, 145, 176
American Red Cross, 79, 108
American Social Health Association, 181
American Social Hygiene Association, 38, 53, 92, 128; in 1920s, 124, 130, 131, 134, 135, 150, 159; during World War II, 162, 166
American Society for Sanitary and Moral Prophylaxis (ASSMP), 24-26, 29-31, 35, 37, 52-53
American Vigilance Association, 37-38
Anderson, George, 77
Antibiotics, 161, 171, 173. *See also* Penicillin
Army. *See* Military
Ashburn, Percy, 110, 115-16
Ashford, Bailey, 113
Automobile, 76, 128

Baker, Herman, 144
Baker, Newton D., 53, 55-59, 71, 77-78, 106
Behrman, Martin, 75
Benjamin, Harry, 166
Bernays, Edward L., 47
Berryhill, T. A., 68
Bigelow, George, 124-25
Bigelow, Maurice, 27, 28
Biggs, Hermann, 42, 43, 94
Birth control, 159-60, 175-76
Bisher, William, 163
Blacks, 104, 116, 129, 152, 157-58, 169-70
Bok, Edward, 24